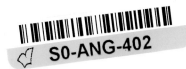

Infectious Disease Pathology: Clinical Cases

Gail L. Woods, M.D.
Professor of Pathology and Director of Clinical Microbiology,
The University of Texas Medical Branch at Galveston

Vicki J. Schnadig, M.D.
Associate Professor of Pathology and Associate Director
of Division of Cytopathology, The University of Texas
Medical Branch at Galveston

David H. Walker, M.D.
Professor and Chair of Pathology, The University of Texas
Medical Branch at Galveston

Washington C. Winn, Jr., M.D., MBA
Professor of Pathology, University of Vermont College
of Medicine, Burlington; Director, Clinical Microbiology
Laboratory, Fletcher Allen Health Care, Burlington

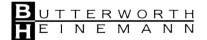

Boston • Oxford • Auckland • Johannesburg • Melbourne • New Delhi

Copyright © 2000 by Butterworth–Heinemann

A member of the Reed Elsevier group

All rights reserved.

No part of this publication may be reproduced, stored in a retrieval system, or transmitted in any form or by any means, electronic, mechanical, photocopying, recording, or otherwise, without the prior written permission of the publisher.

Every effort has been made to ensure that the drug dosage schedules within this text are accurate and conform to standards accepted at time of publication. However, as treatment recommendations vary in the light of continuing research and clinical experience, the reader is advised to verify drug dosage schedules herein with information found on product information sheets. This is especially true in cases of new or infrequently used drugs.

 Recognizing the importance of preserving what has been written, Butterworth–Heinemann prints its books on acid-free paper whenever possible.

 Butterworth–Heinemann supports the efforts of American Forests and the Global ReLeaf program in its campaign for the betterment of trees, forests, and our environment.

Library of Congress Cataloging-in-Publication Data
Infectious disease pathology / Gail L. Woods ... [et al.].
        p. cm.
    Includes index.
    ISBN 0-7506-9673-7
    1. Communicable diseases--Histopathology Case studies.
 2. Communicable diseases--Cytodiagnosis Case studies.
 3. Communicable diseases--Histopathology Atlases. 4. Communicable
 diseases--Cytodiagnosis Atlases. I. Woods, Gail L.
    [DNLM: 1. Communicable Diseases--pathology Case Report. WC 100
I40275 1999]
RC113.3.I55 1999
616.9'047--DC21
DNLM/DLC
for Library of Congress   99-27855
                                                                                      CIP

British Library Cataloguing-in-Publication Data
A catalogue record for this book is available from the British Library.

The publisher offers special discounts on bulk orders of this book.

For information, please contact:
Manager of Special Sales
Butterworth–Heinemann
225 Wildwood Avenue
Woburn, MA 01801-2041
Tel: 781-904-2500
Fax: 781-904-2620

For information on all B-H publications available, contact our World Wide Web home page at:
http://www.bh.com

10 9 8 7 6 5 4 3 2 1

Printed in China

Infectious Disease
Pathology:
Clinical Cases

To the memory of Dr. Gbo Yuoh

Contents

Preface

With this book, we bring to the practicing pathologist, pathology resident, infectious diseases physician, and medical student our collective experience in establishing the etiologic diagnosis of infectious diseases by interpretation of the histopathology of microscopic lesions in diseased tissue and cytopathology samples. Patients whose clinical diseases are most difficult to identify by clinical criteria and microbiological evaluation of readily available specimens often undergo a surgical biopsy, which yields a definitive diagnosis. Our emphasis on the morphologic diagnosis is a result of the relatively high level of success that this approach brings to these frequently difficult clinical cases.

This book may be used as an atlas for learning the morphology of a particular infection and for comparison with cases in the reader's own practice by virtue of its high-quality illustrations of infectious diseases encountered by the anatomic pathologist. However, the presentation is intended to provide a more useful function. Although most books about infectious diseases that include pathology texts are organized according to the taxonomy of infectious agents, clinical problems do not arrive with etiologic labels. They come through the pathologist's door as clinical problems with an associated histologic lesion or pattern of injury. Thus, this text is clinically based and diagnostic problem–oriented. The organization is according to the clinical syndrome and organ of principal involvement, and the most important

way station en route to the etiologic diagnosis is the histopathologic lesion. The clinical and histopathologic problem leads to the development of a differential diagnosis, a process that this book can guide.

Using the clinical presentation to introduce the differential diagnosis reflects the real-life situation that the pathologist and infectious disease physician face. We hope these case-based presentations reinforce the practical clinical use and didactic value of this book. The case-based discussions are designed to review the optimal tests for a definitive diagnosis, including microbiology, virology, parasitology, serology, and, when practical, molecular diagnostics. The most important aspects of the disease and pathogen are presented. We provide pearls rather than an exhaustive treatise.

The appendices provide additional sets of illustrations that allow side-by-side comparisons of the morphologic appearance of organisms within a category and of viral cytopathic effects. These may aid in selecting or rejecting entities within the differential diagnosis.

It is our sincere wish that the reader will find the concepts presented useful, the photographs esthetically enjoyable, and the mode of presentation painlessly informative.

Gail L. Woods
Vicki J. Schnadig
David H. Walker
Washington C. Winn, Jr.

Acknowledgments

The authors thank and acknowledge the late Gbo Yuoh, M.D., for his help in the tracking and compilation of several of the cases illustrated in this text.

The case histories, gross photographs, and histologic sections featured in this volume represent the efforts of numerous people. The authors gratefully acknowledge the many former and current members of the University of Texas Medical Branch and University of Vermont College of Medicine/Fletcher Allen Health Care Divisions of Autopsy and Surgical Pathology, whose postmortem protocols and gross organ photographs were incorporated in our book. We also thank our colleagues in the Clinical Microbiology Laboratory, who so greatly enhance the study of infectious diseases.

Dr. Schnadig thanks former fellow residents and faculty mentors from the Louisiana State University (New Orleans) Department of Pathology and former pathology residents from the Tulane University Department of Pathology who, approximately 20 years ago, nurtured her interest in infectious disease pathology by providing her with histologic sections and wet tissue from some extraordinary cases. This archived material was photographed and put to use in this volume.

Infectious Disease Pathology:
Clinical Cases

C H A P T E R

1

Approaches to the Detection of Infectious Agents in Tissue

Stains useful for the diagnosis of infectious diseases from tissue specimens vary depending on the type of organism responsible for infection (i.e., virus, bacterium, fungus, or parasite). In all cases, the first step in making a diagnosis is examination of sections stained with hematoxylin and eosin (H and E). An H and E stain allows detection of some pathogens or, in the case of viruses, the cytopathic changes they induce. It also enables recognition of the nature of the inflammation, on which the selection of special stains is partly based (Table 1-1). Different patterns of inflammation and examples of pathogens associated with each are illustrated in Appendices A–D. It is important to remember, however, that the inflammatory response varies depending on the immune status of the host.

VIRUSES

Individual viruses cannot be seen with a light microscope, but many induce cytopathic changes that are easily recognized in H and E–stained tissue sections or smears of cells stained by the Papanicolaou technique (see Appendix A). Occasionally, the changes visualized by the H and E or Papanicolaou stain are insufficient for diagnosis, and additional stains or tests are required. Few nonspecific "special stains" have been useful for diagnosis of viral infections. Lendrum's phloxine-tartrazine method enhances detection of some viral inclusion bodies; Parson's stain and Schleifstein's method have been used for detection of Negri bodies associated with rabies virus; and orcein, modified trichrome, and Victoria blue–nuclear fast red have been used for confirmation of chronic infection with hepatitis B virus. For the most part, however, immunohistochemical methods using commercial virus-specific antibodies are preferred. These antibodies are more expensive than the chemical reagents used in nonspecific special stains; therefore,

limiting their use to specific situations is reasonable. For example, immunohistochemical studies for herpes simplex virus and cytomegalovirus seldom are convincingly positive in the absence of viral inclusions; thus, they are most helpful when the cytopathic changes are not typical, such as when "smudge cells" caused by adenovirus infection cannot be distinguished by H and E morphology from dying cells infected with cytomegalovirus that are shrunken and smudged with poorly defined inclusions.

BACTERIA

Individual bacteria usually are difficult to detect in tissue sections stained with H and E, although exceptions exist. In cases of actinomycosis, granules are present, and clumps of amphophilic material, representing small colonies of bacteria, may be seen in cases of overwhelming infection with one of the pyogenic bacteria, particularly *Staphylococcus aureus*. The presence of bluish-purple, granular staining surrounding blood vessel walls suggests bacterial vasculitis, characteristic of infection with *Pseudomonas aeruginosa* or *Vibrio vulnificus*. Eosinophilic to amphophilic, granular microcolonies of *Bartonella henselae* or *Bartonella quintana* often are visible in lesions of bacillary angiomatosis or hepatic peliosis. Curved bacilli of *Helicobacter pylori* may be seen in the layer of mucus on the crypt epithelium of H and E–stained sections of gastric biopsy specimens that show acute gastritis.

The stain most commonly used for detection of bacteria in tissue sections is a modification of Gram stain. The Brown-Brenn tissue Gram stain and the Gram-Weigert stain are preferred for visualization of gram-positive bacteria, whereas the Brown-Hopps and Goodpasture methods are better for demonstrating gram-negative organisms. Silver impregnation methods using modifications of Warthin-

1

Starry, Dieterle's, or Steiner and Steiner stains are among the most sensitive stains for detecting bacteria in tissue sections, including those that stain weakly with a tissue Gram stain (e.g., legionellae and bartonellae) and spirochetes, which do not stain at all with Gram stain.

A variety of other special stains are useful for detection of specific bacteria or groups of bacteria in tissue sections. For example, the modified Giemsa stain, acridine orange, Wright-Giemsa, and toluidine blue show bacilli of *H. pylori*, although none is as sensitive as the Warthin-Starry stain. A combination stain consisting of Steiner and Steiner, H and E, and alcian blue (pH 2.5) allows simultaneous detection of *H. pylori* bacilli and histopathologic features of the gastric mucosa, including the precise location of the organisms. Actinomycetes frequently are visualized with Grocott-Gomori's methenamine silver stain, which generally is used for detection of fungal elements (discussed in the following section Fungi). A modified acid-fast stain (either Fite's method or Coates' modified Fite's method) usually distinguishes the stained bacilli of *Nocardia* species from the unstained *Actinomyces* species; however, *Nocardia* species do not invariably stain, and filaments of *Streptomyces* species occasionally are weakly acid-fast, making culture essential for accurate diagnosis. *Legionella micdadei* also can be seen in tissue with an acid-fast stain, a feature best recognized with Kinyoun

carbol fuchsin stain, Fite's method, and, less frequently, Ziehl-Neelsen stain. All *Legionella* species appear to stain with the Wolbach modification of the Giemsa stain, and specific antibodies for immunofluorescence staining are useful for tissue diagnosis of Legionella pneumonia caused by the most common serotypes of *Legionella pneumophila*.

Stains used for detection of mycobacteria (acid-fast bacilli) in tissue sections are Ziehl-Neelsen, Kinyoun carbol fuchsin, and fluorochrome (i.e., auramine O and auramine-rhodamine), the latter of which is the most sensitive, as is true for smears. For optimal visualization of bacilli of *Mycobacterium leprae*, Fite's method is preferred. Bacilli of *Mycobacterium avium* complex also stain positively with periodic acid-Schiff, which appears to be unique among the mycobacteria and is therefore a useful diagnostic feature. Commercial polyclonal antibodies against *Mycobacterium bovis* and *Mycobacterium duvalii* may be used for detection of human mycobacterial pathogens in tissue by immunohistochemical techniques. Immunohistochemistry appears to be more sensitive than Kinyoun carbol fuchsin stain and Fite's method; for detection of bacilli of *Mycobacterium tuberculosis*, it is comparable to that of Kinyoun carbol fuchsin and fluorochrome stains and Fite's method combined. These antibodies are more expensive than reagents used for the standard staining methods; there-

Table 1-1. Relationship of Host Inflammatory Response, Infectious Agent, and Staining Method for Its Detection

Inflammatory Response	Common Infectious Causes	Tissue Stains or Staining Methods
Acute inflammation (with or without abscesses)	Pyogenic bacteria	Brown-Brenn, Brown-Hopps, Gram Weigert
	Actinomycetes	H & E (granules), Brown-Brenn, Gram Weigert, GMS, Fite's or Coates' modified Fite's[a]
	Candida species, *Aspergillus* species[b]	H & E, PAS, GMS
	Zygomycetes	H & E, PAS
Nonorganizing mixed acute and chronic or chronic inflammation	*Legionella* species	Silver impregnation,[c] Wolbach modification of Giemsa, Brown-Hopps, Kinyoun carbol fuchsin or Fite's,[d] specific antibodies for immunofluorescence
	Helicobacter pylori	Silver impregnation,[c] "triple stain" (Steiner–H & E–alcian blue), H and E, Giemsa, toluidine O, acridine orange
	Cryptosporidium species	H & E, Fite's
	Microsporidia	H & E, Brown-Brenn, Brown-Hopps, Warthin-Starry, modified trichrome
	Treponema pallidum	Silver impregnation[c]
Mixed suppurative and granulomatous inflammation	Nontuberculous mycobacteria	Kinyoun carbol fuchsin, Ziehl-Neelsen, auramine-rhodamine[e]
	Blastomyces dermatitidis, Coccidioides immitis, Paracoccidioides brasiliensis	H & E, PAS, GMS
	Sporothrix schenckii[f]	PAS (particularly with diastase digestion), GMS
	Chromoblastomycosis, systemic phaeohyphomycosis[g]	H & E, Fontana-Masson
	Acanthamoeba species	H & E, PAS

Table 1-1. *(continued)*

Inflammatory Response	Common Infectious Causes	Tissue Stains or Staining Methods
Granulomatous inflammation		
Noncaseating "mature" granulomas	Mycobacteria	Kinyoun carbol fuchsin, Ziehl-Neelsen, auramine-rhodamine
	Histoplasma capsulatum	GMS, PAS, H & E
	Brucella species, *Coxiella burnettii*,[h] *Ehrlichia chaffeensis*, Cytomegalovirus	ND
	Toxoplasma gondii	H & E, PAS
	Schistosoma species	H & E; Kinyoun carbol fuchsin or Ziehl-Neelsen (for eggs)
	Dirofilaria immitis	H & E
Caseating granulomas	Mycobacteria	Kinyoun carbol fuchsin, Ziehl-Neelsen, auramine-rhodamine
	H. capsulatum	GMS, PAS
	Coccidioides immitis	H & E, PAS, GMS
	Cryptococcus neoformans[i]	H & E, GMS, PAS, mucicarmine, colloidal iron, Fontana-Masson
Necrotizing granulomas	*Yersinia enterocolitica*, *Yersinia pseudotuberculosis*	Brown-Hopps
	Bartonella henselae	Brown-Hopps, Warthin Starry, Dieterle
	Francisella tularensis, *Chlamydia trachomatis* (serotypes L₁–L₃)	ND
Histiocytic aggregates or diffuse infiltrates	*Mycobacterium avium* complex, *Mycobacterium genavense*	Kinyoun carbol fuchsin, Ziehl-Neelsen, auramine-rhodamine, PAS[j]
	H. capsulatum[k]	GMS, PAS, ±H & E
	Mycobacterium leprae	Fite's
	Leishmania species	H & E, Giemsa
	Listeria monocytogenes	Brown-Brenn, Brown-Hopps, Gram Weigert

H & E = hematoxylin and eosin; GMS = Grocott-Gomori's methenamine silver; PAS = periodic acid-Schiff; ND = organisms generally are not visualized in tissue.
[a]*Nocardia* species are positive; *Actinomyces* species are negative.
[b]Hyphae of other hyaline moulds, such as *Pseudallescheria boydii* and *Fusarium* species, have a similar appearance in tissue.
[c]Includes Warthin-Starry, Dieterle, and Steiner and Steiner stains.
[d]*Legionella micdadei* is positive.
[e]*M. fortuitum-chelonae* complex may not stain by fluorochrome techniques.
[f]Yeast cells of *S. schenckii* often are not detected in tissue (regardless of the staining method) because of their paucity.
[g]*Fonsecaea pedrosoi* and *Cladosporium carrionii* are the most frequent causes of chromoblastomycosis. Frequent causes of systemic phaeohyphomycosis are *Exophiala jeanselmei*, *Curvularia* species, *Bipolaris* species, *Xylohypha* species, *Phaeoannellomyces werneckii*, and *Wangiella dermatitidis*.
[h]Typically associated with, but not specific for, lipogranuloma (epithelioid granuloma with fibrinoid material and a clear central space).
[i]Reaction elicited by capsule-deficient strains in immune competent hosts; immune compromised hosts infected with an encapsulated strain typically show minimal or no inflammatory response.
[j]*M. avium* complex is positive.
[k]Reaction in immune compromised hosts, especially patients infected with human immunodeficiency virus.

fore, limited use of immunohistochemistry (e.g., only for situations in which the clinical history is suggestive of mycobacterial disease, but the standard stains for detection of mycobacteria are negative) is reasonable.

FUNGI

Several stains are useful for detection of fungal elements in tissue sections. The H and E stain allows detection of many of the commonly encountered fungi, especially aspergilli, various yeasts, and zygomycetes. For optimal detection of fungal elements in H and E–stained tissue sections, the substage condenser should be lowered so that hyphal walls refract the unfocused light. Moreover, many fungi demonstrate autofluorescence when the H and E–stained tissue is examined under ultraviolet illumination. Autofluorescence appears to be most useful for detection of elements of *Coccidioides immitis*, *Candida* species, and *Aspergillus* species, whereas yeast cells of *Histoplasma capsulatum* and hyphae of zygomycetes do not demonstrate this feature.

Stains other than H and E often enhance visualization of fungal elements, and in some cases the fungus present may be identified based on a characteristic morphology (examples are summarized in Appendix C). Probably the most commonly used of these special stains are Grocott-Gomori's methenamine silver (GMS) and Hotchkiss-McManus periodic acid-Schiff (PAS) stains, which allow detection of virtually all fungi. Stains that may be substituted for the GMS and PAS include Gridley's stain and various fluorescent techniques, such as calcofluor white, Congo red, and Uvitex 2B.

Some special stains are useful for identification of particular fungi. Two approaches relatively specific for *Cryptococcus neoformans* are (1) Mayer's mucicarmine, alcian blue, and colloidal iron, which stain acid mucopolysaccharides in the yeast's capsule; and (2) the Fontana-Masson stain, which stains capsule-deficient cells of *C. neoformans* and thus differentiates them from cells of *H. capsulatum* and *Blastomyces dermatitidis*, which are Fontana-Masson–negative. When individual stains fail to provide a definitive diagnosis, combining the Fontana-Masson technique with a capsular stain gives cells of *C. neoformans* a distinctive appearance not seen with other fungi. Commercial antibodies specific for *Pneumocystis carinii* are available for use in immunohistochemical assays, but because of their cost, limiting the use of antibodies to difficult diagnostic situations, such as an atypical host immune response (discussed in Chapter 2) or suspected disseminated disease is wise.

PARASITES

Many protozoal and helminthic parasites are visualized in sections stained with H and E, but in certain situations, special stains enhance their detection. For example, extremely small organisms such as microsporidia and cryptosporidia are easily missed in H and E–stained sections. Tissue Gram stains (Brown-Brenn is preferred) probably are the most useful for diagnosis of microsporidiosis, although microsporidia also can be detected by silver impregnation techniques, the Chromotrope-2R modified trichrome stain, and the Giemsa stain. Fite's method can be used for detection of cryptosporidia, which lose their acid-fast quality in histologic preparations and appear bright blue in tissue sections stained by this method.

Special stains also help differentiate parasites from inflammatory cells and aid in identification. For example, the PAS stain helps to distinguish trophozoites of *Entamoeba histolytica* from host macrophages and ganglion cells and to differentiate positively staining intracellular yeasts of *H. capsulatum* from unstained *Leishmania* species. Cysts of *Acanthamoeba* stain with GMS, PAS, and calcofluor white, which helps distinguish them from macrophages. Commercial antibodies against *Toxoplasma gondii* are useful for diagnosis in necrotic brain lesions, because organisms often are difficult to recognize in H and E–stained sections. Hooklets of *Echinococcus granulosus* and schistosome eggs are demonstrated with acid-fast stains. Weigert's iron hematoxylin and Russell-Movat pentachrome stains enhance visualization of the exoskeleton of helminths, thus providing an aid to identification when features are not distinctive in H and E–stained sections.

RECOMMENDED READING

Brinn NT. Rapid metallic histological staining using the microwave oven. J Histotechnol 1983;6:125–129.

Debongnie JC, Beyaert C, Legros G. Touch cytology, a useful diagnostic method for diagnosis of upper gastrointestinal tract infections. Dig Dis Sci 1989;34:1025–1027.

Debongnie JC, Delmee M, Mainguet P, et al. Cytology: a simple, rapid, sensitive method in the diagnosis of *Helicobacter pylori*. Am J Gastroenterol 1992;87:20–23.

Deodhar KP, Tapp E, Scheuer PJ. Orcein staining of hepatitis B antigen in paraffin sections of liver biopsies. J Clin Pathol 1975;28:66–70.

Genta RM, Lew GM, Graham DY. Changes in the gastric mucosa following eradication of *Helicobacter pylori*. Mod Pathol 1993;6:281–289.

Genta RM, Robason GO, Graham DY. Simultaneous visualization of *Helicobacter pylori* and gastric morphology: a new stain. Hum Pathol 1994;25:221–226.

Graham AR. Fungal autofluorescence with ultraviolet illumination. Am J Clin Pathol 1983;79:231–234.

Green LK, Moore DG. Fluorescent compounds that nonspecifically stain fungi. Lab Med 1987;18:456–458.

Gridley MR. A stain for fungi in tissue sections. Am J Clin Pathol 1953;23:303–307.

Gubetta L, Rizzetto M, Crivelli O, et al. A trichrome stain for the intrahepatic localization of the hepatitis B surface antigen (HBsAg). Histopathology 1977;1:277–288.

Kommaredii S, Abramowsky CR, Swinehart GL, Hrabak L. Nontuberculous mycobacterial infections: comparison of the fluorescent auramine-O and Ziehl-Neelsen techniques in tissue diagnosis. Hum Pathol 1984;15:1085–1089.

Lazcano O, Speights VO Jr., Strickler JG, et al. Combined histochemical stains in the differential diagnosis of *Cryptococcus neoformans*. Mod Pathol 1993;6:80–84.

Loffeld RJLF, Stobberingh E, Flendrig JA, Arends JW. *Helicobacter pylori* in gastric biopsy specimens. Comparison of culture, modified Giemsa stain, and immunohistochemistry. A retrospective study. J Clin Pathol 1991;165:69–73.

Ro JA, Lee SS, Ayala AG. Advantage of Fontana-Masson stain in capsule-deficient cryptococcal infection. Arch Pathol Lab Med 1987;111:53–57.

Slifkin M, Cumbie R. Congo red as a fluorochrome for the rapid detection of fungi. J Clin Microbiol 1988;26:827–830.

Strickler JG, Manivel JC, Copenhaver CM, Kubic VL. Comparison of in situ hybridization and immuno-histochemistry for detection of cytomegalovirus and herpes simplex virus. Hum Pathol 1990;21:443–448.

Tanaka K, Mori W, Suwa K. Victoria blue-nuclear fast red stain for HBs antigen detection in paraffin section. Acta Pathol Jpn 1981;31:93–98.

Walker DH, Dumler JS. Issue of the day: will patholo-gists play as important a role in the future as they have in the past against the challenge of infectious diseases? Infect Agents Dis 1995;4:167–170.

Watts JC, Chandler FW. The surgical pathologist's role in the diagnosis of infectious diseases. J Histotech-nol 1995;18:191–193.

Weber R, Bryan RT, Schwartz DA, Owen RL. Human microsporidial infections. Clin Microbiol Rev 1994;7:426–461.

Wiley EL, Mulhollan TJ, Beck B, et al. Polyclonal anti-bodies raised against Bacillus Calmette-Guerin, *Mycobacterium duvalii,* and *Mycobacterium paratuberculosis* used to detect mycobacteria in tis-sue with the use of immunohistochemical tech-niques. Am J Clin Pathol 1990;94:307–312.

Winn WC, Myerowitz RL. The pathology of the Legionella pneumonias. A review of 74 cases and the literature. Hum Pathol 1981;12:401–422.

Woods GL, Walker DH. Detection of infection or infec-tious agents by use of cytologic and histologic stains. Clin Microbiol Rev 1996;9:382–404.

2

Infections of the Respiratory Tract

Infection of the lower respiratory tract is a frequent and serious medical problem. Pathologists, clinicians, microbiologists, and radiologists have different perspectives regarding the etiologic diagnosis of pneumonia. For every specialist, establishing an etiologic diagnosis is frequently difficult; successive elimination from a list of etiologic diagnoses is not a reasonable approach. Clinicians generally derive differential diagnoses by using epidemiologic approaches (e.g., considering community-acquired versus nosocomial infections and previously healthy versus immunocompromised patients) to focus on a limited array of potential causative agents. Radiologists are able to describe images that the gross pathology determines by plain films, computed tomography (CT), or magnetic resonance imaging (MRI), but they can only play the odds in determining a likely etiology. A pathologist who combines expertise in both diagnostic anatomic pathology and clinical laboratory medicine can ultimately afford the patient's salvation. Not only must the pathologist skillfully interpret respiratory tract biopsy, fine-needle aspiration, bronchoalveolar lavage and bronchial brush material, but he or she must also provide a proficient microbiology laboratory to cultivate microorganisms and perform serologic assays. These clinical laboratory studies definitively identify the presence of the infectious agents presumptively diagnosed by histology or cytology. Diagnostic tissue samples may be collected at substantial cost and finite risk to the patient. A meticulous pathologist should communicate with the surgeon or bronchoscopist before the diagnostic procedure to ensure that vital specimens are appropriately collected and submitted for laboratory evaluation. Mate-

rial is separated aseptically for culture and for storage at −70°C or 4°C for additional studies, including cultures that were not considered useful initially. Multiple imprint smears are gently prepared from tissue samples for immediate or future staining. Identifying Gram-stained and acid-fast bacteria (AFB) on smears is much easier than in paraffin sections. Direct immunofluorescence methods are available for specific identification of some etiologic agents and can be applied effectively to properly prepared smears.

Microbiological methods alone cannot establish the clinical significance of endogenous, colonizing, and ubiquitous flora that are recovered in culture of sputum (e.g., *Streptococcus pneumoniae*, *Haemophilus influenzae*, *Pseudomonas aeruginosa*, or *Klebsiella pneumoniae*). The specimen might have been contaminated heavily by oropharyngeal flora.

At autopsy, gross pathology offers pathologists additional clues regarding the likely etiology of the pneumonia. The cases in this chapter illustrate a practicing pathologist's approach to the diagnosis of respiratory infections. The case studies describe clinical settings, pathologic appearances, and diagnostic evaluations. In practice, however, a diagnosis cannot be established in all cases, sometimes because of omissions in the diagnostic workup by the pathologist, particularly in autopsy cases. Pathologists are the best potential sentinels for the recognition of new diseases, whether emerging infections or others. Pathologists should pursue problems until solutions are discovered and remember that noninfectious causes—such as exogenous toxins, drugs, or allergic exposure—can also be culprits.

SINUSITIS

Clinical History

A 33-year-old woman was evaluated as an outpatient for facial discomfort and nasal obstruction. Over the past several years, she had experienced multiple bouts of acute exacerbation of chronic sinusitis, which had been treated with several different antimicrobial agents and steroids without relief. On physical examination, the patient was afebrile, with a pulse rate of 92 beats per minute, respiratory rate of 20 breaths per minute, and blood pressure of 107/74 mm Hg. A diffuse, obstructing polyposis of the nasal cavity, more pronounced on the left side, and a thin, mucopurulent exudate were present. A computed tomographic scan of the sinuses showed bilateral diffuse obliteration of the ethmoid, sphenoid, and maxillary sinuses. Endoscopic sinus surgery with polypectomy was performed, and resected tissue was submitted for histologic studies and fungal culture.

Pathologic Findings

Histologic examination of the resected tissue fragments showed intact respiratory epithelium overlying an accumulation of mucus (Figure 2-1). Examination of the mucus under higher power magnification revealed degenerating eosinophils, Charcot-Leyden crystals (Figure 2-2), and a few dematiaceous fungal hyphae (Figure 2-3). To identify the inciting organism, fungal culture of the resected tissue is necessary.

Differential Diagnoses

Three types of fungal infections may involve the nasal sinuses: (1) allergic fungal sinusitis, (2) invasive fungal sinusitis or zygomycosis, and (3) fungus ball. The pathologic findings in this case are consistent with a diagnosis of allergic fungal sinusitis, which may be elicited by hyaline or dematiaceous moulds. Fungi that have been associated with allergic fungal sinusitis include *Aspergillus* species and several dematiaceous fungi: *Alternaria* species, *Bipolaris* species, *Curvularia* species, *Drechslera* species, *Exserohilum* species, and *Helminthosporium* species. In contrast to allergic fungal sinusitis, invasive fungal sinusitis is characterized by intrusion of the fungal hyphae into viable tissue. The pathology of a fungus ball involving the sinuses (Figures 2-4 and 2-5) is identical to that of a fungus ball in the lung (discussed under Recurrent Hemoptysis and Radiologic Pulmonary Lesion).

Microbiology

The fungal culture grew *Bipolaris* species.

Comment

In most cases of allergic fungal sinusitis, more than one sinus is involved, as occurred in this case. Pathologic features characteristic of allergic fungal sinusitis include sloughing of the respiratory mucosa and thick mucus

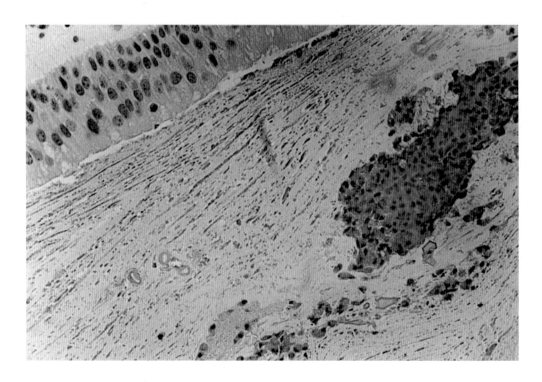

FIGURE 2-1. Section of tissue resected from the nasal sinuses shows a strip of respiratory epithelium and overlying mucus that contain degenerated eosinophils (hematoxylin and eosin stain; original magnification, ×100).

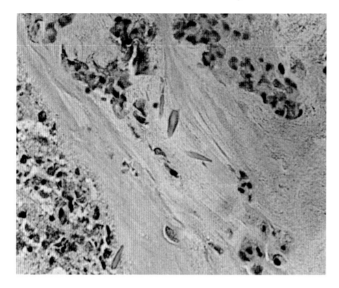

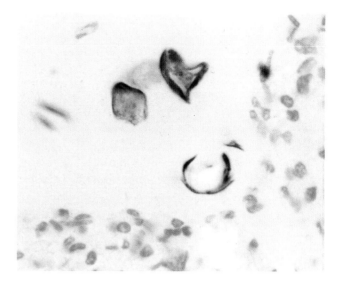

FIGURE 2-2. Higher-power magnification of the tissue illustrated in Figure 2-1 reveals many Charcot-Leyden crystals, one of the characteristic pathologic features of allergic fungal sinusitis (hematoxylin and eosin stain; original magnification, ×100).

FIGURE 2-3. Staining the tissue section illustrated in Figure 2-1 with a melanin stain demonstrates a few fragmented dematiaceous fungal hyphae (Fontana-Masson stain; original magnification, ×250). Fungal culture of tissue from this case grew *Bipolaris* species.

FIGURE 2-4. Section of tissue resected from the maxillary sinus shows focal ulceration of the respiratory mucosa, edema and a predominantly lymphoplasmacytic infiltrate in the submucosa, and a large mass of fungal hyphae in the lumen, with no evidence of tissue invasion by the fungus (hematoxylin and eosin stain; original magnification, ×25). These features are characteristic of a fungus ball.

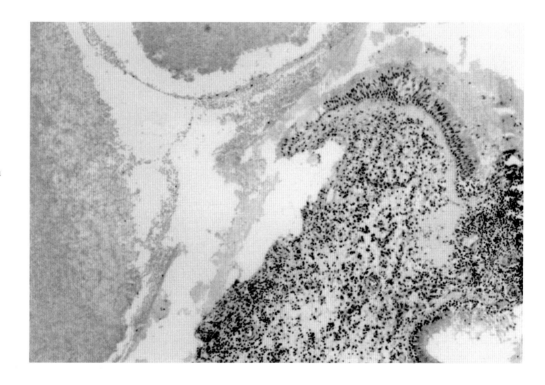

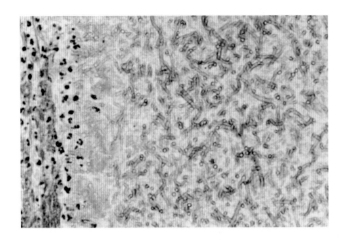

FIGURE 2-5. Higher magnification of the section illustrated in Figure 2-4 shows the mass of hyaline fungal hyphae that are septate and relatively uniform in diameter and that branch at acute angles (hematoxylin and eosin stain; original magnification, ×100). These features are consistent with *Aspergillus* species, but identification requires fungal culture.

containing degenerated eosinophils, many Charcot-Leyden crystals, and few fungal hyphae. No evidence of invasion of blood vessels by the fungus is found.

This case illustrates the features typical of allergic fungal sinusitis caused by a dematiaceous fungus. If *Aspergillus* species were the inciting mould, branching and septate hyaline hyphae would be present instead of brown-pigmented dematiaceous hyphae.

Diagnosis

Allergic fungal sinusitis.

LOWER RESPIRATORY TRACT INFECTION WITH WHEEZING IN AN INFANT

Clinical History

A 3-month-old male infant was brought to a pediatrician after 4 days of upper respiratory tract congestion and 1 day of cough. The baby was febrile, and physical examination revealed coarse rhonchi and otitis media. Despite antimicrobial therapy appropriate for otitis media, his condition worsened over the next 3 days with deeper cough and tachypnea (50 breaths per minute). Examination revealed expiratory wheezes, rales, prolonged expirations, and intercostal reactions. A chest radiograph demonstrated hyperaeration with flattened diaphragm, peribronchial thickening, and multifocal interstitial infiltrates. The patient's arterial Po_2 was 51 mm Hg. He was admitted to the hospital, where he developed an episode of apnea witnessed by the mother and could not be resuscitated.

The medical history included premature birth with pulmonary immaturity and infantile respiratory distress syndrome. Bronchopulmonary dysplasia was a sequela.

At the time of onset of illness (late winter), a high incidence of respiratory illness, with many cases of lower respiratory infection in infants and young children, was present in the community.

Pathologic Findings

At autopsy, the lungs within the opened chest cavity were overexpanded and did not collapse. On the cut surface, patchy alternating areas of atelectasis and overinflation with no regions of frank consolidation were present. Microscopic evaluation demonstrated severe bronchiolitis (Figure 2-6) and moderate interstitial pneumonia. The bronchiolar mucosa contained intraluminal projections of papilliform tufts of epithelial cells and occasional multinucleate syncytial giant cells (Figure 2-7 and Figure 2-8). A mucosal and submucosal infiltration of lymphocytes and macrophages extended into the adjacent alveolar septa. The alveoli were unevenly involved, with some showing interstitial and alveolar mononuclear cells, alveolar edema, and a few hyaline membranes.

Microbiology

Enzyme immunoassay detected antigens of respiratory syncytial virus (RSV) in respiratory secretions collected on a nasopharyngeal swab performed in the pediatrician's office on the day of hospital admission. The characteris-

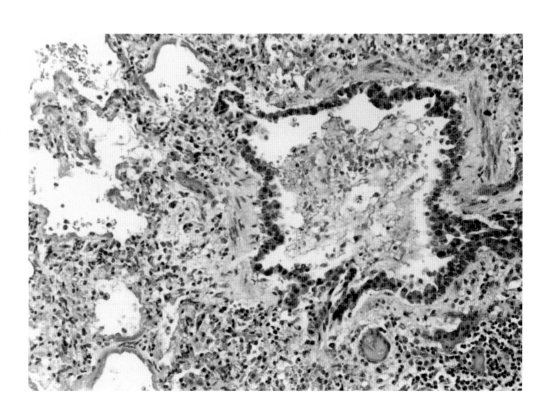

FIGURE 2-6. Section of lung shows respiratory syncytial virus bronchiolitis characterized by bronchiolar epithelial hyperplasia, intraluminal cellular debris and inflammatory cells, and interstitial and peribronchiolar infiltrate that is predominantly mononuclear (hematoxylin and eosin stain; original magnification, ×50).

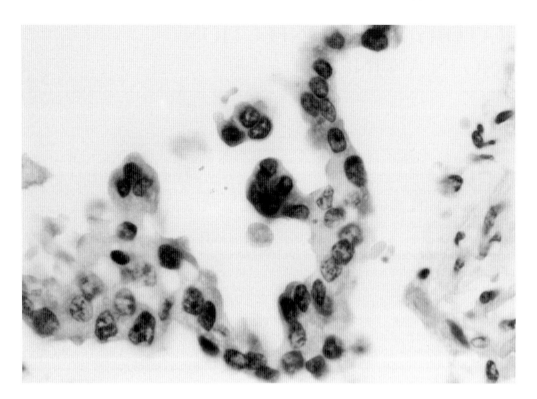

FIGURE 2-7. Section of lung from a patient with respiratory syncytial virus infection shows a papillalike projection of epithelial cells into the lumen and a syncytial giant cell (hematoxylin and eosin stain; original magnification, ×250).

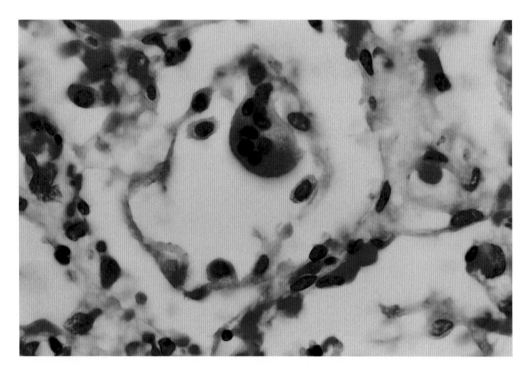

FIGURE 2-8. Section from the lung of a patient with respiratory syncytial virus infection shows a syncytial giant cell in an alveolar space (hematoxylin and eosin stain; original magnification, ×250).

tic cytopathic effect of RSV, syncytia formation, was observed in cell culture 5 days after inoculation with a nasal wash sample collected on admission and in lung tissue obtained at necropsy.

Comment

Viral infections are frequently the cause of lower respiratory infections in infants and young children. Wheezing

and air-trapping are characteristic clinical manifestations of bronchiolitis. The etiology is most often RSV, followed by parainfluenza virus type 3. Parainfluenza viruses types 1 and 2, adenoviruses, influenza viruses A and B, rhinoviruses, and *Mycoplasma pneumoniae* can occasionally cause bronchiolitis. RSV infects the airway epithelium and stimulates numerous host immune and inflammatory mechanisms leading to epithelial cytopathology, luminal exudate, and inflammation around the airways. The accumulation of RSV antigen in epithelial cytoplasm is easily detected by immunofluorescence, but only in a small minority of cells does it stain sufficiently differently from the cytoplasm to be detected as an inclusion body (Figure 2-9). Syncytial giant cells, although readily seen in this case, are not a constant feature of RSV infection in immunocompetent individuals. In severely immunocompromised patients with prolonged viral infections, syncytial giant cells and intracytoplasmic inclusions are usually prominent (Figure 2-10 and Figure 2-11). Patients at increased risk of severe or fatal infection include premature infants with bronchopulmonary dyplasia, infants with congenital heart disease (especially types associated with pulmonary hypertension), and children with cystic fibrosis or severe immunodeficiency diseases.

RSV infections occur as annual epidemics affecting all age groups. Reinfections occur throughout life, but the most severe cases occur as the primary infection in the youngest infants, even in the presence of maternal antibodies against RSV. An epidemiologic clue is the rise in incidence of bronchiolitis and pediatric pneumonia in

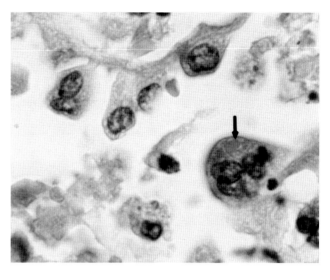

FIGURE 2-9. Section from a lung with respiratory syncytial virus infection shows a syncytial giant cell with a cytoplasmic inclusion (*arrow*; hematoxylin and eosin stain; original magnification, ×250).

FIGURE 2-10. Section of lung from an immunocompromised patient with a chronic persistent respiratory syncytial virus infection shows a multinucleate syncytial giant cell containing cytoplasmic inclusions of various sizes (hematoxylin and eosin stain; original magnification, ×250).

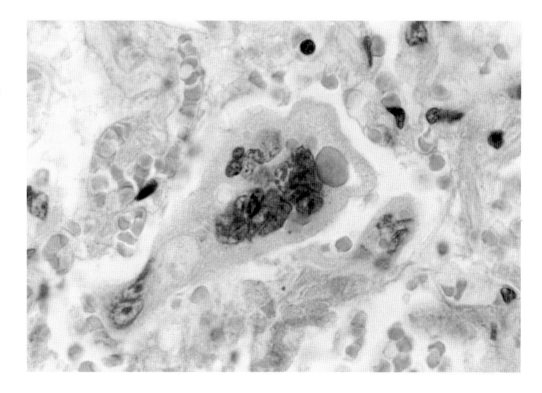

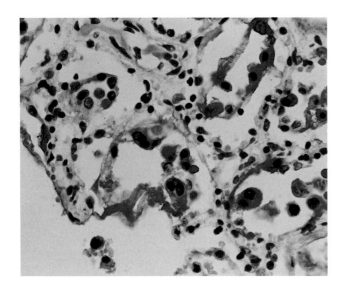

FIGURE 2-11. Section of lung from a patient with respiratory syncytial virus pneumonia shows viral antigen in the cytoplasm of alveolar lining cells, many of which have formed multinucleate syncytia. A striking interstitial mononuclear cell pneumonia is present (original magnification, ×100). (Respiratory syncytial virus immunostained section provided by Dr. Richard Cartun.)

the community. However, definitive diagnosis is readily achieved by rapid antigen detection in respiratory secretions collected by a nasal washing or swab or, if available, by viral isolation.

Diagnosis

Respiratory syncytial viral bronchiolitis.

DIFFUSE ALVEOLAR DAMAGE

Clinical History

A 68-year-old man, diagnosed with malignant lymphoma (diffuse lymphocytic type) 3 years earlier, was admitted to the hospital for evaluation of weakness, malaise, confusion, nausea and vomiting, and fever with shaking chills. Diffuse lower lobe infiltrates were present bilaterally. Empiric antimicrobial therapy was initiated for presumed viral and superimposed bacterial infection. On the third hospital day, the patient had not responded, and a lung aspirate was nondiagnostic. The patient was started on appropriate treatment for presumed *Pneumocystis carinii* infection and for possible anaerobic bacterial infection. By the seventh hospital day, all lung fields were opacified. He died the next day, 11 days after the illness began.

Pathologic Findings

The lung was diffusely consolidated and beefy red (Figure 2-12). Microscopically, the changes were relatively uniform throughout multiple sections. The interstitium was expanded by fluid and mononuclear cells. In the airspaces, a large amount of fibrin and a collection of macrophages and pneumocytes were present (Figure 2-13). Occasional hyaline membranes lined the alveolar walls. Focally, pneumocytes proliferated at the alveolar membrane, and the epithelium of the terminal and respiratory bronchioles showed reactive hyperplasia (Figure 2-14).

Microbiology

Influenza A virus was isolated from the lung. Aerobic cultures of sputum antemortem did not yield pathogens. Aerobic and anaerobic bacterial cultures of lung postmortem were negative.

Comment

Influenza viruses are enveloped RNA viruses that produce infection worldwide. The ribonucleoprotein antigen in the viral core defines the three types A, B, and C. Although this virus can produce severe, even fatal, disease in previously healthy young people, the elderly and debilitated are at greatest risk of mortality. The most serious complications of influenza are primary influenza virus pneumonia and secondary bacterial pneumonia, both of which occur in a small minority of cases. In fatal cases in epidemics, distinguishing pathologically between pure viral pneumonia and early bacterial superinfection has sometimes been difficult. A variety of respiratory bacteria may cause secondary infection. *H. influenzae* received its name because it was originally thought to have an etiologic relationship to influenza symptoms. In recent epidemics, *Staphylococcus aureus* and *S. pneumoniae* have figured most prominently. Secondary infections may also be produced by fungi and even other viruses, such as HSV.

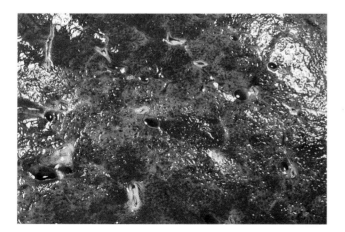

FIGURE 2-12. Photomicrograph of unfixed lung from a patient who died from influenza pneumonia shows solid, firm, and beefy red parenchyma. The distal airways can be discerned because they are held open by the thickened interstitium.

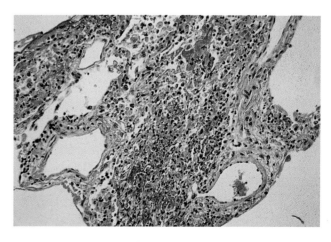

FIGURE 2-13. Section of the lung illustrated in Figure 2-12 shows thickening of the interstitium due to a mononuclear cell infiltrate and intensely eosinophilic hyaline material, cells, and cellular fragments within the alveoli (hematoxylin and eosin stain; medium-power magnification).

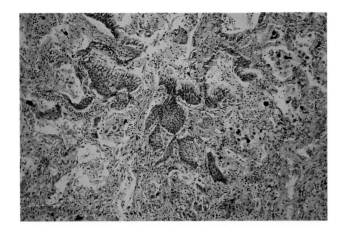

FIGURE 2-14. The interstitium is thickened, and the airspaces are filled with macrophages and pneumocytes. Abundant squamous metaplasia of the epithelium in the distal airways is present (hematoxylin and eosin stain; low-power magnification).

The histologic response to pure viral infection has been remarkably similar among multiple influenza virus epidemics. The response in aggregate represents the picture of diffuse alveolar damage. This histologic response to pneumocyte injury can be elicited by many insults, including high concentrations of oxygen under pressure, radiation, and some chemotherapeutic agents. It is similar to the histologic reaction in "shock lung," which is mediated by polymorphonuclear neutrophils. The histologic response in this case is typical of the response to many viral infections. No viral inclusions are available to aid in the morphologic identification of the etiology. The diagnosis may be made presumptively by occurrence of the histologic response in the setting of an influenza epidemic, but definitive diagnosis must be made by culture of the virus or demonstration of viral antigen in respiratory secretions. Residual changes after influenza infection of the lower respiratory tract include interstitial fibrosis and bronchiolitis obliterans with organizing pneumonia.

Diagnosis

Influenza pneumonia.

ACUTE VIRAL PNEUMONIA WITH AN INTENSE NEUTROPHILIC RESPONSE

Clinical History

A 48-year-old woman with myasthenia gravis, treated chronically with steroids, developed the acute onset of fever, malaise, dyspnea, and a nonproductive cough. She was admitted to the hospital with increasing respiratory distress. Her myasthenia gravis was maintained under control, but empiric antimicrobial therapy for suspected bacterial pneumonia failed to halt the progression of her pulmonary disease. A chest radiograph demonstrated patchy pulmonary infiltrates, which progressed to bilateral disease (Figure 2-15). She died 5 days after admission to the hospital.

Pathologic Findings

The lungs were diffusely consolidated without hemorrhage or abscess formation. Two patterns of histologic response were present. The first was diffuse alveolar damage, characterized by interstitial thickening and mononuclear cell inflammation, accumulation of fibrin and alveolar macrophages in the airspaces, and hyaline membranes lining the alveoli (Figure 2-16). The second pattern consisted of an intense neutrophilic exudate, rich in fibrin, in the small bronchioles and airspaces. Many of the neutrophils and macrophages in the exudate were disintegrating with fragmentation of the nuclei (karyorrhexis), a process some-

times called *leukocytoclasis* (Figure 2-17). Under close inspection, intranuclear inclusions could be found in the airspace exudate, the alveolar membrane, and the bronchiolar epithelium (Figure 2-18). The intranuclear inclusions were eosinophilic, with peripheralization of the nuclear chromatin. Some inclusions were separated from the chromatin by an artefactual clearing (halo). Occasional multinucleated cells with intranuclear inclusions were evident.

Differential Diagnoses

Differential diagnoses include causes of diffuse alveolar damage and necrotizing inflammatory infiltrates in the airspaces. Varicella-zoster virus may produce similar lesions, and the intranuclear inclusions are identical. Historical information is usually sufficient to implicate chickenpox, which typically has the viremic pattern demonstrated by type 2 herpes simplex virus (HSV) in the neonate. Cytomegalovirus (CMV) infections usually occur in somewhat different clinical situations, and the inflammatory process rarely displays a necrotizing component. The viruses can be distinguished by the morphology of the viral inclusions, although analysis of individual cells may be problematic. Adenovirus infection of the lung provides the greatest diagnostic challenge, because it also has a mixture of diffuse

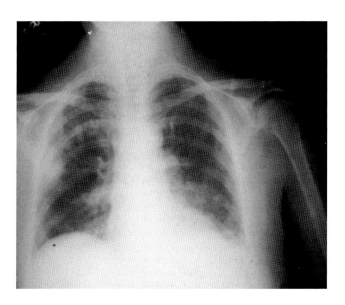

FIGURE 2-15. Chest radiograph shows bilateral patchy infiltrates, which suggest bronchopneumonia, most commonly caused by a variety of bacteria.

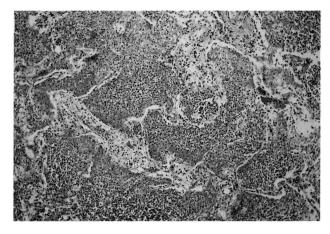

FIGURE 2-16. Section of lung from a patient with herpes simplex virus pneumonia shows an intense inflammatory infiltrate and abundant eosinophilic fibrin in the terminal airways and airspaces (hematoxylin and eosin stain; low-power magnification).

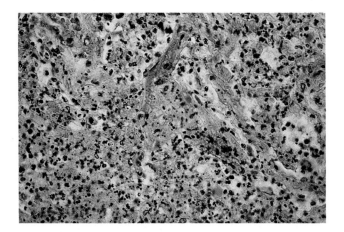

FIGURE 2-17. Higher-power magnification of the section illustrated in Figure 2-16 shows a predominance of polymorphonuclear neutrophils, many of which are undergoing karyorrhexis and karyolysis (hematoxylin and eosin stain; medium-power magnification).

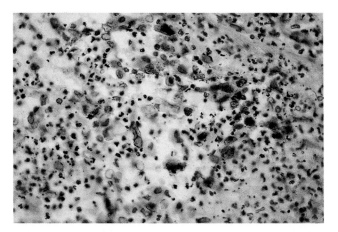

FIGURE 2-18. Focal areas of the section illustrated in Figure 2-16 demonstrate numerous intranuclear viral inclusions with peripheralization of the nuclear chromatin, consistent with herpes simplex virus. Many of the inclusions lack the artifactual halo, and thus resemble degenerating nuclei (hematoxylin and eosin stain; high-power magnification).

alveolar damage and necrotizing inflammation. The early inclusions of adenovirus resemble those of herpes simplex, but the adenoviral inclusions mature to an amorphous basophilic mass that fills the nucleus and spills beyond it (smudge cells). Adenoviral pneumonia is rare and usually occurs in the setting of severe immunosuppression, whereas herpes simplex pneumonia is more common, and the patient may be minimally immunocompromised in the classic sense.

Microbiology

Postmortem cultures of lung tissue yielded HSV. No bacteria were isolated or seen on Gram stain.

Comment

HSV produces pneumonia in two clinical situations. Neonatal pneumonia, usually caused by type 2 virus, occurs as a part of disseminated infection after acquisition from the maternal genital tract during delivery. Multifocal disease reflects the vascular dissemination of virus in this clinical situation, although primary herpes pneumonia with clinical manifestations limited to the pulmonary system has been described in neonates. The second and more common situation is found in adult patients who are debilitated, although not necessarily immunosuppressed. HSV type 1 is commonly present in the oral cavity of older children and adults as a latent infection. Five to 10 percent of individuals excrete the virus asymptomatically. The pathogenesis of the infection is probably aspiration of virus-infected secretions from the upper respiratory tract into the lung, resulting in multifocal airspace infiltrates. This process is quite analogous to most bacterial pneumonias. The risk factors for development of herpes pneumonia in

adults are, accordingly, conditions that predispose to aspiration, including chronic respiratory disease, mechanical ventilation, and diseases that reduce the level of consciousness or interfere with glottic integrity.

The histologic response to HSV infection of the lower respiratory tract takes two forms, which may coexist. The first is the pattern of diffuse alveolar damage that is associated with other viral respiratory infections. Proliferation of alveolar lining cells and an interstitial mononuclear infiltrate occur. In the airspaces, an intense accumulation of fibrin is present, which may form hyaline membranes along the alveolar walls. Alveolar macrophages and sloughed alveolar lining cells are prominent in the exudate. The second pattern is a more intensely inflammatory, even necrotizing exudate in the airspaces. Polymorphonuclear neutrophils are a prominent part of the exudate, and extensive karyorrhexis and karyolysis of the exudate are present, producing an appearance that has been described as leukocytoclastic. The epithelium of the alveolar wall, bronchioles, and bronchi often contain intranuclear inclusions in necrotic epithelial cells. At low power, the overall appearance is that of an intensely inflammatory purulent pneumonia. If the pathologist does not inspect the tissue carefully, the process may be assumed to be bacterial and the true nature of the process entirely misinterpreted. When a bacterial etiology is suspected, tissue Gram stain should be performed, and the pathologist should examine the section under high magnification, after which the viral inclusions should be appreciated.

Diagnosis

HSV pneumonia.

RAPIDLY PROGRESSIVE ADULT RESPIRATORY DISTRESS SYNDROME IN A PREVIOUSLY HEALTHY WOMAN

Clinical History

A 27-year-old woman had been ill at home for 4 days with fever, myalgia, headache, cough, and nausea that she attributed to a flulike illness. When she suffered an episode of vomiting, she sought medical attention. On physical examination, she had a temperature of 39°C, a pulse rate of 115 beats per minute, a respiratory rate of 24 breaths per minute, and a blood pressure of 90/70 mm Hg. Physical examination and radiograph of the chest were within normal limits. Abnormal laboratory studies included hematocrit of 49%, leukocytosis (21,450 per μl) with 12% bands and 3% metamyelocytes, and thrombocytopenia (85,000 per μl).

She was admitted for further evaluation and rapidly developed respiratory failure with rales (owing to pulmonary edema) and hypoxemia. She was intubated, ventilated mechanically, and developed intractable hypotension. Chest radiograph revealed extensive bibasilar airspace-filling opacification. Laboratory data included hemoconcentration (hematocrit, 50%) despite intravenous fluid therapy, marked leukocytosis (65,600 per μl) with left shift and circulating immunoblasts, thrombocytopenia (45,000 per μl), metabolic acidosis with decreased serum bicarbonate concentration (15 mmol/liter), increased serum aspartate aminotransferase (98 IU/liter), and hypoalbuminemia (2.6 g/liter). Thirty hours after admission, the patient developed cardiomechanical dissociation and could not be resuscitated.

Pathologic Findings

At autopsy, the lungs were heavy, weighing 1,070 g combined (normal, 780–920 g), and abundant fluid flowed from the cut surfaces, which were consolidated with a rubbery consistency. The pleural surfaces contained numerous petechiae, and massive bilateral serosanguinous pleural effusions (right, 1,675 ml; left, 1,350 ml) were present. Microscopic examination of sections of lung revealed interstitial pneumonia with pulmonary edema containing identifiable fibrin in some alveoli and focal hyaline membranes (Figures 2-19 and 2-20). The interstitial infiltration was mild to moderate and consisted of lymphocytes, immunoblasts, and macrophages. The red pulp and periarteriolar lymphoid sheaths of the spleen also contained abundant prominent immunoblasts (Figure 2-21).

Microbiology

Routine bacterial and viral cultures of the lung did not yield any isolate. Samples of lung were sent to the Centers for Disease Control and Prevention (CDC), where immunohistochemical evaluation with a monoclonal antibody to a Hantavirus antigen demonstrated extensive specific staining, most prominently in the pulmonary endothelium. RNA extracted from fresh-frozen lung was processed by reverse transcriptase and polymerase chain reaction with oligonucleotide primers specific for Hantavirus, and a

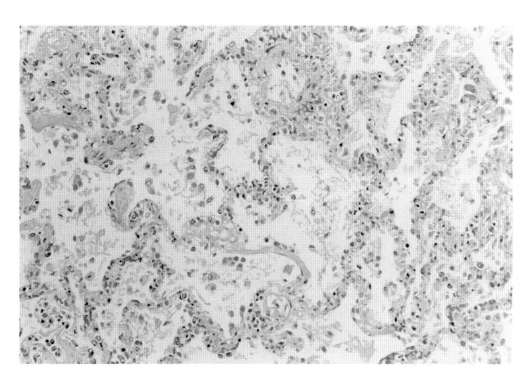

FIGURE 2-19. Section of lung from a patient who died from hantavirus pulmonary syndrome shows pulmonary edema and thickening of the alveolar walls due to a mononuclear cell infiltrate (hematoxylin and eosin stain; original magnification, ×50).

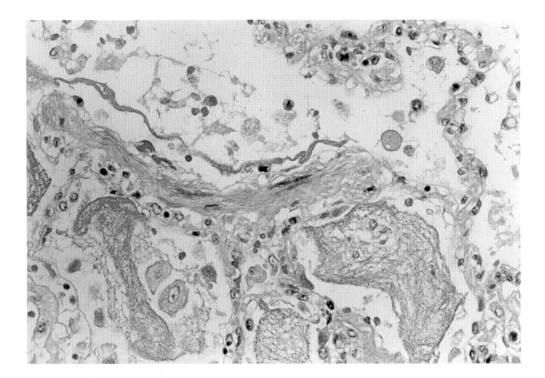

FIGURE 2-20. Higher-power magnification of the section illustrated in Figure 2-19 demonstrates intra-alveolar fibrin and an interstitial mononuclear cell infiltrate (hematoxylin and eosin stain; original magnification, ×100).

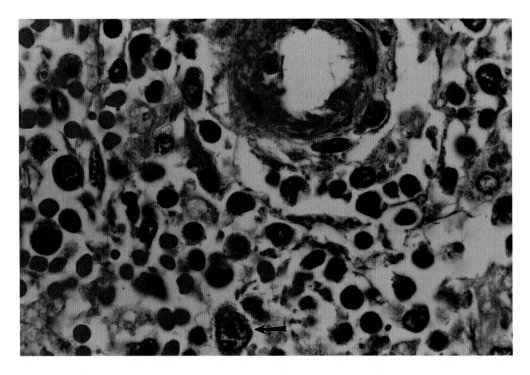

FIGURE 2-21. Section of spleen from a patient who died from hantavirus pulmonary syndrome shows a periarteriolar mononuclear infiltrate, including occasional immunoblasts (*arrow*; hematoxylin and eosin stain; original magnification, ×250).

DNA band of the appropriate size was detected. Sequencing of the DNA product confirmed that the patient was infected with Sin Nombre virus.

Comment

This case of hantavirus pulmonary syndrome is typical of this recently recognized, relatively uncommon infection.

The biphasic illness is characterized by a mild, nonspecific early stage and a severe, rapidly progressive phase of noncardiogenic pulmonary edema and massive pleural effusions with approximately 50% mortality. Like other emerging infectious diseases, hantavirus pulmonary syndrome has occurred since the distant past but was only relatively recently elucidated. An outbreak in the southwestern states in 1993 prompted laboratory evaluation at CDC that unexpectedly revealed antibodies reacting with several hantaviruses. The infectious disease pathologist, Sherif Zaki, immediately developed and applied an immunohistochemical method for conserved Hantavirus antigen and demonstrated that the endothelium of the pulmonary microcirculation was the major target. Simultaneously, Stuart Nichol, using primers based on conserved Hantavirus sequences, performed reverse transcriptase-polymerase chain reaction, and DNA sequencing identified the novel etiologic agent. Hantaviruses are members of the *Bunyaviridae* family—enveloped, trisegmented, negative-sense, single-stranded RNA viruses including Hantaan virus (Korean hemorrhagic fever or hemorrhagic fever with renal syndrome in eastern Eurasia), Puumala virus (nephropathia epidemica in Scandinavia), and Prospect Hill virus, which is nonpathogenic and is the only Hantavirus previously known to be native to North America. The discovery of Sin Nombre virus has led to the recognition of hantavirus pulmonary syndrome throughout the Americas and to recovery of novel hantaviruses from rodents in many locations.

Like other hantaviruses, Sin Nombre virus is maintained in nature in its own rodent host, *Peromyscus maniculatus*, which is widely distributed in the United States and serves as the source of infecting virus for humans. The differential diagnosis of this disease includes pneumonic plague, psittacosis, influenza, tularemic pneumonia, legionellosis, meningococcemia, leptospirosis, and rickettsial infections (e.g., Rocky Mountain spotted fever and murine typhus). That pathologists missed the diagnosis for so many years bespeaks the lack of knowledge, effective diagnostic tools, and effort devoted to determination of the etiology of pneumonia and adult respiratory distress syndrome even when an autopsy is performed.

Diagnosis

Hantavirus pulmonary syndrome.

VIRAL PNEUMONIA
IN THE IMMUNOCOMPROMISED HOST

Clinical History

A 34-year-old man presented to the emergency department with complaints of abdominal pain, blood in his stools, and edema of both legs for several days. History included alcohol and cocaine abuse and asthma. On physical examination, scleral icterus, diffuse abdominal tenderness, pitting edema to the knees bilaterally, and heme-positive stool were found. He was afebrile, his pulse rate was 97 beats per minute, and his respiratory rate was 18 breaths per minute. Chest radiograph showed subsegmental atelectasis in the lower lobes bilaterally. Pertinent abnormal laboratory test results included a total bilirubin of 13.1 mg/dl, elevation of all liver enzymes, and minimally prolonged prothrombin and partial thromboplastin times. He was admitted for evaluation and treatment of his liver disease.

During the first 2 days of hospitalization, the patient became febrile (temperature, 38.7°C), lethargic, and unable to follow commands. Abdominal examination showed increased distension, with the development of shifting dullness. Blood cultures grew gram-negative bacilli (later identified as *Providencia rettgeri*), for which he received appropriate antimicrobial therapy. On day 5, he became dyspneic; chest radiograph showed extensive bilateral lung opacities, reported as consistent with edema, pneumonia, or adult respiratory distress syndrome. He was unable to

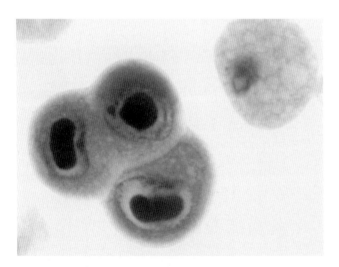

FIGURE 2-22. Cytologic preparation of bronchoalveolar lavage fluid shows a cluster of alveolar pneumocytes with typical cytopathic changes induced by infection with cytomegalovirus: enlarged cells with a large, oval intranuclear inclusion surrounded by a clear area (or "halo"; Papanicolaou stain; original magnification, ×250).

produce an expectorated sputum specimen; bronchoscopy with BAL was performed. A portion of the fluid was submitted to the clinical microbiology laboratory for bacterial, viral, fungal, and mycobacterial studies. No organisms were detected in cytospin preparations of the BAL fluid stained with Gram stain or auramine O. BAL fluid also was submitted to the cytopathology laboratory, and smears stained with the Papanicolaou and Giemsa stains showed enlarged cells with intranuclear and intracytoplasmic inclusions, typical of CMV (Figure 2-22). Based on these reports, appropriate antiviral therapy was added to the therapeutic regimen, but his condition deteriorated, and he died 2 days later.

Pathologic Findings

At autopsy, the lungs weighed 2,790 g combined, and the parenchyma was firm and rubbery throughout. Sections of formalin-fixed tissue stained with hematoxylin and eosin (H and E) showed enlarged alveolar pneumocytes with large, round amphophilic intranuclear inclusions, some of which appeared to be surrounded by an indistinct halo; numerous granular, often basophilic intracytoplasmic inclusions; or a combination of both (Figure 2-23). These morphologic features are characteristic of the cytologic changes induced by CMV infection.

Differential Diagnoses

Based on the cytopathologic and histopathologic findings in this case, the most likely etiologic agent is CMV. However, other viruses that induce cytopathic changes that occasionally may appear similar to those caused by CMV are adenovirus and HSV.

Microbiology

Centrifugation cell culture of the BAL fluid showed characteristic intranuclear inclusions by immunofluorescence staining with a monoclonal antibody against CMV immediate early nuclear antigen. Viral cultures of BAL fluid and postmortem lung tissue grew CMV.

Comment

The cytopathic effects induced by CMV infection may not always have the characteristic appearance illustrated by this case. For example, dying cells infected with CMV may appear shrunken and smudged with poorly defined inclusions, resembling inclusions of adenovirus (Figure

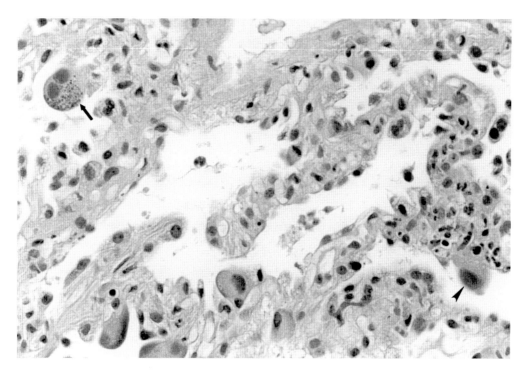

FIGURE 2-23. Section of lung tissue shows enlarged alveolar lining cells with prominent intranuclear inclusions, characteristic of the cytopathic change induced by infection with cytomegalovirus. In addition, one cell has both intranuclear and prominent intracytoplasmic inclusions (*arrow*), and another has an indistinct intranuclear inclusion, resembling the smudge cell of infection with adenovirus (*arrowhead*) (hematoxylin and eosin stain; original magnification, ×100).

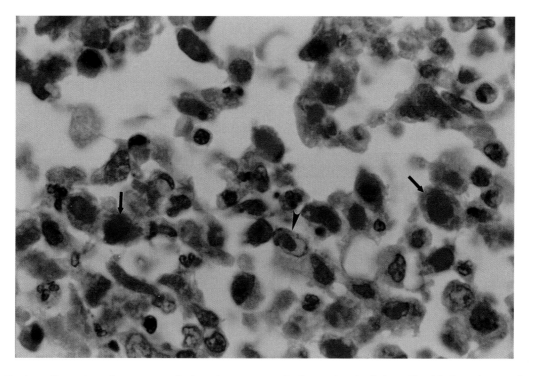

FIGURE 2-24. Section of lung tissue from a case of adenovirus pneumonia shows alveolar lining cells with dense intranuclear inclusions that have indistinct peripheral margins (i.e., smudge cells; *arrows*), typical of cytopathic changes due to adenovirus infection. Near the center of the figure is a cell with an intranuclear inclusion surrounded by a clear zone or halo and an outer margin of clumped chromatin (*arrowhead*), resembling the cytopathic changes induced by infection with cytomegalovirus (hematoxylin and eosin stain; original magnification, ×250).

2-24). When differentiation of infection with CMV and adenovirus is difficult, based on the cytologic changes evident in H and E–stained tissue sections, immunohistochemical studies using commercially available antibodies or in situ hybridization using commercial probes may be useful. Neither immunohistochemical studies nor in situ hybridization, however, is convincingly positive in the absence of viral inclusions, in which case viral culture is necessary for diagnosis.

Because CMV may be present in respiratory secretions without causing disease, diagnosis of CMV pneumonia cannot be based only on detection of the virus in BAL fluid by staining a centrifugation cell culture with CMV-specific fluorescent labeled antibodies. Other criteria that must be fulfilled include the presence of a pulmonary infiltrate documented by chest roentgenogram and histologic evidence of CMV lung infection as demonstrated by characteristic cytopathic changes.

Diagnosis

CMV pneumonia.

ACUTE SUPPURATIVE BRONCHOPNEUMONIA

Clinical History

A 39-year-old man was found unconscious by his wife and transported by ambulance to an emergency department, where he was immediately intubated. His wife stated that her husband had complained of chills and backache for 5 days before admission and had had a cough for the previous 2 days. On physical examination, the patient was cyanotic and unresponsive to painful stimuli. His pupils were dilated and unresponsive to light, and his posture was hyperextended. His temperature was 34.9°C, his pulse was 140–156 beats per minute, his respiratory rate was 18 breaths per minute, and his blood pressure was 100/58 mm Hg. Auscultation of the chest revealed coarse rhonchi, predominantly on the right side. A chest radiograph showed consolidation of the right lung. Pertinent abnormal laboratory test results included a white blood cell count of 2,000 per μl, a hemoglobin concentration of 10.6 g/dl, and elevated liver enzymes. Blood cultures were collected and antibiotics for community-acquired pneumonia were begun. Despite aggressive supportive therapy, the patient died 3 hours after admission.

Pathologic Findings

At autopsy, the lungs weighed 2,050 g combined, and areas of patchy consolidation were scattered throughout the parenchyma of all lobes of the right lung. Histologic exam-ination of H and E–stained sections of areas of consolidation showed alveolar spaces filled with an exudate composed of neutrophils and strands of fibrin (Figure 2-25). These gross and microscopic findings are characteristic of acute bronchopneumonia caused by any one of many pyogenic bacteria.

Differential Diagnoses

The differential diagnoses include *S. pneumoniae* and many other pyogenic bacteria, such as *Streptococcus pyogenes*, *S. aureus*, actinomycetes (*Actinomyces* species and *Nocardia asteroides*), Enterobacteriaceae (especially *K. pneumoniae* and *Escherichia coli*), and various other gram-negative bacilli, especially *P. aeruginosa* but also *H. influenzae* and *Moraxella catarrhalis*.

Microbiology

Gram stain of sections of involved lung tissue in this case showed gram-positive cocci (Figure 2-26), and pre-mortem blood cultures grew *S. pneumoniae*.

Comment

S. pneumoniae is the most common cause of acute, community-acquired bronchopneumonia. The most likely pathogens in this case, based on the limited clin-

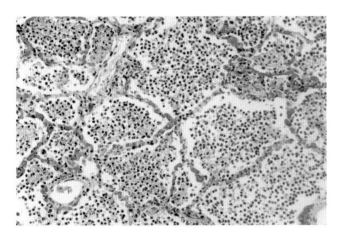

FIGURE 2-25. Section of lung tissue shows alveoli filled with neutrophils and fibrin and congestion of the alveolar capillaries, features consistent with acute bronchopneumonia (hematoxylin and eosin stain; original magnification, ×25).

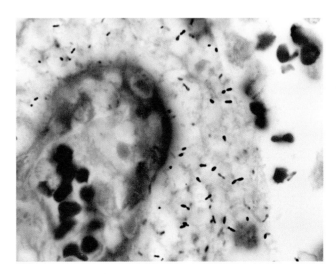

FIGURE 2-26. Section of the lung tissue illustrated in Figure 2.25 shows numerous gram-positive lancet-shaped diplococci, typical of *Streptococcus pneumoniae* (Gram-Weigert stain; original magnification, ×250). Bacterial culture of the involved lung grew *S. pneumoniae*.

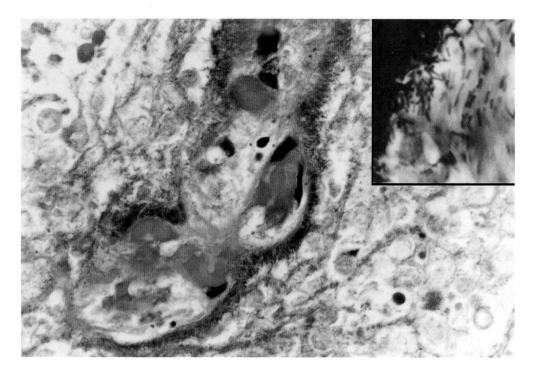

FIGURE 2-27. Photomicrograph of *Pseudomonas aeruginosa* pneumonia demonstrates a dense perivascular bacillary infiltration (hematoxylin and eosin stain; original magnification, ×50). Inset shows myriads of gram-negative bacilli (Brown-Hopps stain; original magnification, ×250).

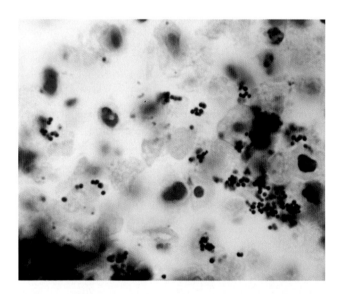

FIGURE 2-28. Section of lung tissue shows gram-positive cocci in clumps, suggestive of staphylococci (Brown-Brenn stain; original magnification, ×250). Cultures of the lung tissue grew *Staphylococcus aureus*.

ical information available and the changes in the liver found at autopsy (i.e., fatty change and bridging fibrosis), are *S. pneumoniae* and *K. pneumoniae*, both of which have a propensity to cause more severe disease in persons who have a history of recent excessive alcohol use. Gram stain may help narrow the list of potential pathogens, but organisms are not always found. Ultimately, identification of the pathogen requires culture. Typical examples of histologic findings in the lungs, cases of bronchopneumonia caused by bacteria other than *S. pneumoniae*, are illustrated in Figures 2-27 (*Pseudomonas* species, frequently associated with a characteristic vasculitis), 2-28 (*S. aureus*), and 2-29 through 2-31 (*Actinomyces* species) and are described in more detail later in this chapter.

Diagnosis

Acute bronchopneumonia due to *S. pneumoniae*.

FIGURE 2-29. Section of lung tissue from a patient with pulmonary actinomycosis shows a sulfur granule associated with a mixed inflammatory infiltrate composed of neutrophils surrounding the granule and aggregates of histiocytes at the periphery (hematoxylin and eosin stain; original magnification, ×50).

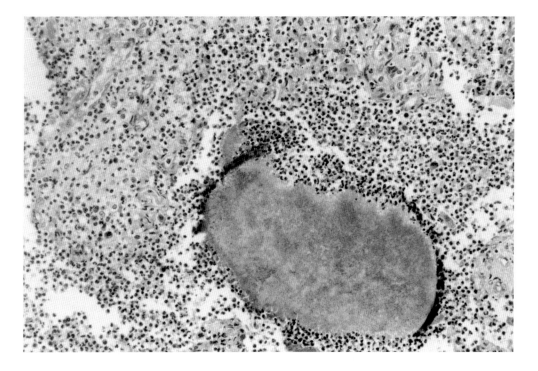

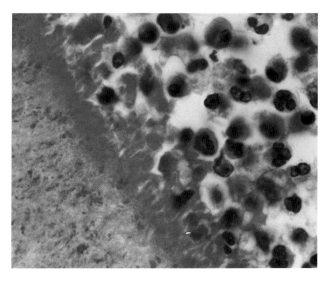

FIGURE 2-30. Higher-power magnification of the section illustrated in Figure 2-29 demonstrates the Splendore-Hoeppli reaction (i.e., elongated, clublike structures radiating centrifugally from a dense eosinophilic band at the periphery of the granule; hematoxylin and eosin stain; original magnification, ×250).

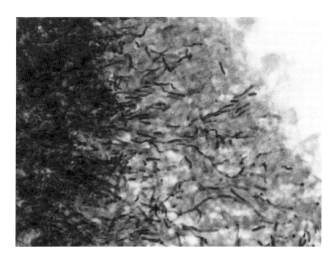

FIGURE 2-31. Section of lung tissue shows the filamentous gram-positive bacilli comprising a sulfur granule (Brown-Brenn stain; original magnification, ×250). Cultures of the lung tissue grew *Actinomyces israelii.*

ACUTE BACTERIAL PNEUMONIA WITH AN EXUDATE OF POLYMORPHONUCLEAR NEUTROPHILS AND MACROPHAGES

Clinical History

The patient was a 67-year-old man with a history of chronic obstructive pulmonary disease. He had had recurrent episodes of pneumococcal pneumonia 6 and 8 years previously. Seven years earlier, he had a pulmonary embolus. He had smoked cigarettes and a pipe for many years.

The final admission was precipitated by the acute onset of severe dyspnea, fever with chills, malaise, and fatigue 1 week earlier. He had a cough productive of brown sputum. At admission, he had a rectal temperature of 39.5°C, blood pressure of 190/100 mm Hg, a pulse of 130 beats per minute, and a labored respiratory rate at 35 breaths per minute. He had rales, rhonchi, and bilateral wheezing, and heart sounds could not be heard. A chest radiograph demonstrated a fluffy white perihilar infiltrate with air bronchograms and patchy infiltrates in the left upper lobe (Figure 2-32). The arterial pH was 7.37, Po_2 was 40 mm Hg, and Pco_2 was 43 mm Hg. The white cell count was 99,000 per µl with 95% mature lymphocytes, and the hematocrit was 36%.

The patient was treated appropriately for pulmonary edema, and empiric therapy for community-acquired bacterial pneumonia was begun. Chronic lymphocytic leukemia was diagnosed, but treatment was not given. After initial improvement, the pulmonary infiltrates and respiratory difficulty increased. Two days after admission, the patient died. The infectious disease physi-cians had noted an unusual incidence of severe bacterial pneumonia at this time that was unresponsive to the usual antimicrobial therapy, including in this patient.

Pathologic Findings

The primary findings were in the lungs. The right lung showed extensive confluent consolidation that was most advanced in the lower lobe (Figure 2-33), where the infil-

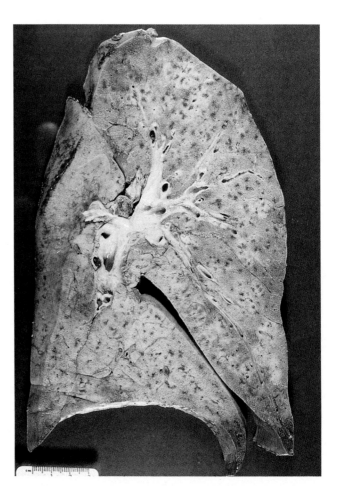

FIGURE 2-33. The lobular location of the inflammatory process in the lung from a smoker is emphasized by the accumulation of carbon pigment around the peripheral bronchioles. The inflammation has become confluent, especially in the lower lobe. Differentiation from a lobar process requires evaluating the overall pattern of disease. Such fine distinctions are even more difficult in radiographs.

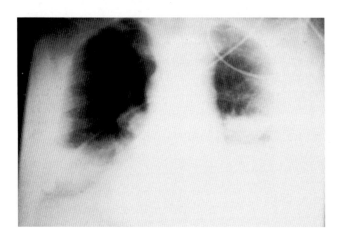

FIGURE 2-32. Chest radiograph shows pulmonary infiltrates, which began in the left upper lobe and progressed to involve both lower lobes. This consolidation could be caused by a large number of pulmonary pathogens.

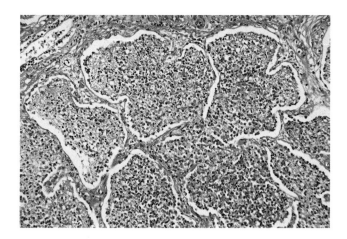

FIGURE 2-34. Section of the lung illustrated in Figure 2-33 shows airspaces packed with mononuclear and polymorphonuclear inflammatory cells, some of which are degenerating. In the background is a proteinaceous exudate. The interstitium is mildly inflamed (hematoxylin and eosin stain; medium-power magnification).

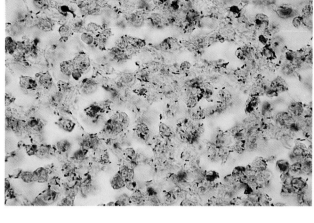

FIGURE 2-35. By staining with a silver impregnation stain, numerous dark brown–black bacilli are seen, both within macrophages and extracellularly. The morphology of the bacilli is obscured by the silver salts that have been deposited on the surface of the bacteria (Dieterle's silver impregnation stain; high-power magnification).

trates involved almost the entire lobe, suggesting a lobar process. In other areas, however, the association of the inflammatory process with bronchioles was clear, indicating that the pneumonia was lobular or focal with confluence of lobular inflammation. The cut section of the lung was granular, and after fixation in formalin, granular fibrinous exudate could be scraped easily from the surface with a scalpel blade.

Microscopically, the airspaces of the involved lung were packed with an exudate of polymorphonuclear neutrophils (PMN) and macrophages (Figure 2-34). Fibrin was abundant in the exudate, and focal microscopic hemorrhage was evident. In some areas, extensive karyolysis and karyorrhexis were present, producing many nuclear fragments and a "dusty" appearance.

Microbiology

Thin, faintly staining gram-negative bacilli were demonstrated in a touch preparation of fresh lung. In sections, the bacteria were demonstrated with the Brown-Hopps stain and with Dieterle's silver impregnation stain (Figure 2-35). The bacteria were extracellular and packed in the cytoplasm of inflammatory cells, especially macrophages. Direct immunofluorescence with polyclonal antisera to the then newly isolated Legionnaires' disease bacillus, performed at the CDC, demonstrated numerous intracellular and extracellular bacteria in formalin-fixed, deparaffinized histologic sections. A culture of postmortem lung tissue yielded a thin, faintly-staining gram-negative bacterium that also reacted with antiserum to the Legionnaires' disease bacillus.

Comment

This early case of Legionnaires' disease demonstrates many features of the infection. It is an acute bacterial pneumonia, which may occur sporadically or, as in this case, as epidemic disease. *Legionella* pneumonia accounts for approximately 2–5% of cases of community-acquired bacterial pneumonia. The frequency of nosocomial infection is similar. In both cases, the focal presence of the bacteria in nature is an important determinant of the incidence. The source of bacteria in the original 1976 Philadelphia epidemic and in this patient remains unknown, but subsequently, most infections have been traced to environmental water sources, both surface water and drinking water. The great majority of human infections are caused by *Legionella pneumophila*, especially serogroups 1 and 6. Other species that are relatively frequently isolated are *Legionella micdadei* (originally known as the *Pittsburgh pneumonia agent*) and *Legionella dumoffii*.

Despite the fact that *Legionella* is a facultative intracellular pathogen, the host response is usually neutrophilic, and granulomas do not develop. Sputum is produced only by approximately one-half of patients, and purulent sputum is distinctly unusual. Many of the infections are characterized as atypical pneumonia because of the absence of sputum production in the presence of extensive radiographic infiltrates. One of the enigmas of this infection is why the intense inflammatory response in the airspaces is not mobilized and expectorated. Pulmonary hemorrhage is common and probably accounts for the brown appearance of the sputum in this case.

Legionella infection cannot be differentiated from other bacterial pneumonias on clinical or pathologic grounds. Pathologic clues to the diagnosis include the intense fibrinous response and the lytic character of the infiltrate, but it should be emphasized that these features are nonspecific. The mainstay of etiologic diagnosis is culture, which is now performed on buffered charcoal yeast extract agar supplemented with α-ketoglutarate. Detec-tion of bacterial antigen in urine is a viable additional method for diagnosis of infections caused by serogroup 1 *L. pneumophila*. Serologic diagnosis requires acute and convalescent specimens and is therefore retrospective.

Diagnosis

Legionnaires' disease.

NECROTIZING BRONCHOPNEUMONIA

Clinical History

A 37-year-old man with acquired immunodeficiency syndrome (AIDS) was admitted with complaints of cough productive of blood-tinged sputum, fever, chills, and night sweats. On physical examination, his temperature was 38.2° C, his respiratory rate was 32 breaths per minute, his pulse rate was 140 beats per minute, and his blood pressure was 156/76 mm Hg. Rales and wheezes were heard on auscultation of the right middle and upper lung fields. The remainder of the examination was noncontributory. Pertinent abnormal laboratory test results included a hemoglobin concentration of 9.4 g/dl and a white blood cell count of 8,000 per μl (48% segmented neutrophils, 32% band forms, 11% lymphocytes, 9% monocytes). A chest radiograph showed bilateral, confluent alveolar opacities, air bronchograms, and focal cavities, most prominent on the right. The differential diagnoses included community-acquired bacterial pneumonia, nocardiosis, tuberculosis, and pulmonary infection with one of the nontuberculous mycobacteria (e.g., *Mycobacterium kansasii*) or a dimorphic fungus (e.g., *Histoplasma capsulatum* or *Coccidioides immitis*).

Sputum was collected for bacterial, mycobacterial, and fungal stains and cultures, and for cytopathology. Empiric antimicrobial therapy directed against the common bacterial causes of community-acquired pneumonia was then initiated. No predominant organism was detected in the sputum smear stained with Gram stain; stains for

mycobacteria and fungi were negative. Many neutrophils were seen in the cytology preparation stained by the Papanicolaou stain, and a preparation stained by the Gram-Weigert method showed a few beaded, filamentous, branching gram-positive bacteria. The filamentous bacilli stained with the modified Kinyoun carbol fuchsin stain (Figure 2-36). Antimicrobial agents effective against *Nocardia* were added to the therapeutic regimen, but the patient's condition worsened and he died 3 days later.

Pathologic Findings

At autopsy, the predominant findings were in the lungs. Patchy areas of consolidation were present in all lobes, and cavities were found in the upper and lower lobes bilaterally (Figure 2-37). Histologic examination of H and E–stained sections of consolidated lung showed a marked intra-alveolar infiltrate composed primarily of neutrophils and

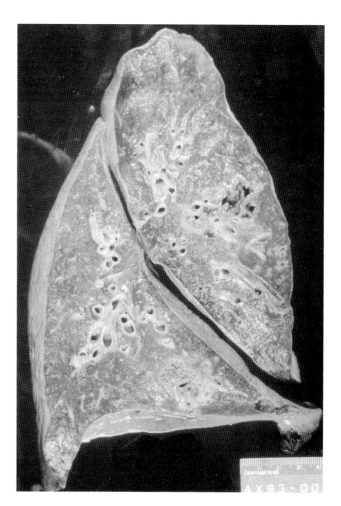

FIGURE 2-37. Photograph of lung shows cavitary pneumonia caused by *Nocardia asteroides*.

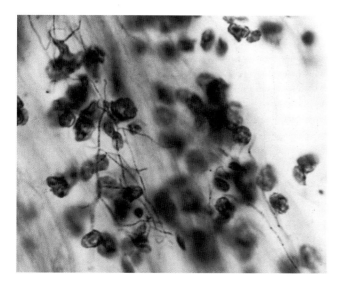

FIGURE 2-36. Cytologic preparation of sputum demonstrates weakly acid-fast organisms showing filamentous, branching bacilli, consistent with *Nocardia* species (modified Kinyoun carbol fuchsin stain; original magnification, ×250).

foci of liquefactive necrosis (Figure 2-38). These gross and microscopic features are consistent with necrotizing bronchopneumonia. The Gram-Weigert stain of postmortem lung tissue showed beaded, filamentous gram-positive bacilli (Figure 2-39), similar in appearance to bacilli observed in the premortem cytologic preparation of sputum.

Differential Diagnoses

The pathogens most likely to cause necrotizing bronchopneumonia are the pyogenic bacteria listed in the pre-

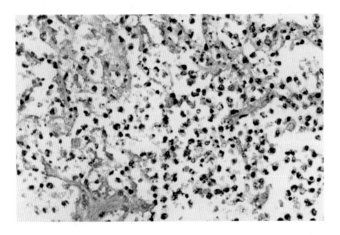

FIGURE 2-38. Section of consolidated lung tissue shows an infiltrate of neutrophils and fibrinous exudate (hematoxylin and eosin stain; original magnification, ×100).

vious case. *Mycobacterium tuberculosis* may be associated with an acute inflammatory response in persons with AIDS and therefore should also be included. Other organisms to consider in an immunocompromised host are *Aspergillus* species and the zygomycetes; however, these are uncommon pathogens in AIDS patients, and hyphal elements of these organisms generally are visible in H and E–stained sections.

Microbiology

Cultures of the premortem sputum specimen and postmortem lung tissue grew *N. asteroides*.

Comment

Based on this differential diagnosis, tissue Gram stain and an acid-fast stain should be performed initially, and depending on the likelihood of a fungal infection, a methenamine silver stain may also be done. A positive result with any of these stains only helps categorize the organism present (e.g., gram-positive cocci, gram-positive branching filamentous bacilli, gram-negative bacilli, AFB, or septate hyphae); culture is essential for identification.

In regard to the etiologic organism, features presented in cytologic preparations and tissue—beaded, filamentous, branching gram-positive bacilli—are most consistent with an actinomycete. Bacilli of *Mycobacterium fortuitum-chelonae* complex may appear similar, although in general the beaded appearance is less promi-

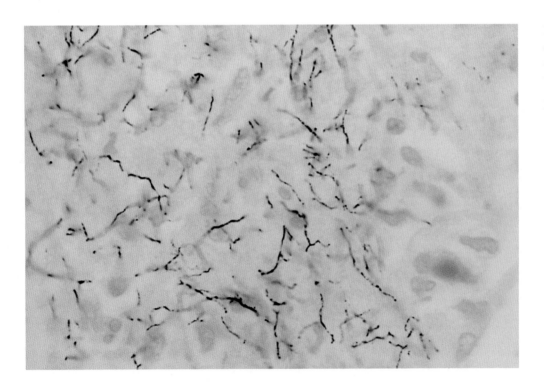

FIGURE 2-39. Section of consolidated lung tissue shows beaded, filamentous, branching gram-positive bacilli, consistent with *Nocardia* species. (Gram-Weigert stain; original magnification, ×250).

nent, and the branching fragments are shorter (Figure 2-40). To help differentiate these organisms, standard and modified Kinyoun carbol fuchsin stains are useful. The filamentous bacilli in this case were stained by the modified Kinyoun carbol fuchsin stain, identifying them as *Nocardia* species rather than *Actinomyces* species, which are not stained. The bacilli did not stain with the standard Kinyoun carbol fuchsin stain, however, which differentiates *Nocardia* species (negative) from mycobacteria (positive). It should be noted, however, that some strains of *M. fortuitum-chelonae* complex stain preferentially with the modified acid-fast stains. In tissue sections from this case, the bacilli did not stain with the modified Fite's method. However, this result is not an uncommon occurrence for *Nocardia* in tissue and therefore cannot be used as a criterion for exclusion from the differential diagnosis.

Diagnosis

Necrotizing bronchopneumonia caused by *N. asteroides.*

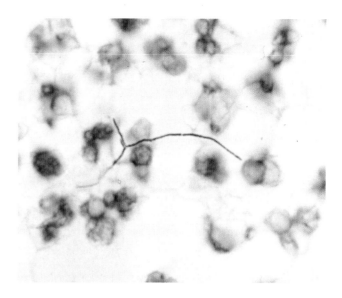

FIGURE 2-40. Smear prepared from material aspirated from an enlarged cervical lymph node of a patient with acquired immunodeficiency syndrome shows filamentous, branching acid-fast bacilli (modified Kinyoun carbol fuchsin stain; original magnification, ×250). Mycobacterial cultures grew *Mycobacterium fortuitum.*

PNEUMONIA CONTAINING HISTIOCYTIC AGGREGATES

Clinical History

A 33-year-old man with AIDS was admitted for persistent cough occasionally productive of blood-tinged sputum. On physical examination, he was tachypneic and in moderate respiratory distress. His temperature was 38°C, his pulse rate was 122 beats per minute, and his respiratory rate was 48 breaths per minute. Auscultation of the chest revealed rales in the left upper lung field. The remainder of the examination was noncontributory. Pertinent laboratory test results included a hemoglobin concentration of 10.8 g/dl, a white blood cell count of 8,200

per μl (75% segmented neutrophils, 4% band forms, 12% lymphocytes, 9% monocytes), and a platelet count of 42,000 per μl. Chest radiograph demonstrated bilateral interstitial infiltrates and a cavitary lesion in the left upper lobe. Computed tomography of the chest showed a cavity in the anterior segment of the left lung (Figure 2-41), air bronchograms, and bilateral pleural effusions. The differential diagnoses included infectious diseases associated with cavitary lung disease in an AIDS patient, such as tuberculosis, nontuberculous mycobacteria (e.g., *M. kansasii*, *Mycobacterium avium* complex), *P. carinii*, nocardiosis, bacterial pneumonia, and histoplasmosis.

The patient was treated with antimicrobial agents appropriate for community-acquired pneumonia and *P. carinii* prophylaxis. A sputum specimen was collected for bacterial, fungal, and mycobacterial stains and cultures. Many gram-positive coccobacilli were seen in the Gram stain smear; no fungal elements or AFB were visualized in the KOH preparation and auramine O–stained smear, respectively. His respiratory condition deteriorated; therefore, bronchoscopy with BAL was performed the following day. BAL fluid was submitted for fungal, mycobacterial, and viral studies and for cytologic evaluation. Cytologic preparations stained with the Papanicolaou stain showed a diffuse infiltrate of granular to foamy histiocytes without definite granuloma formation; no organisms were visualized. Giemsa-stained preparations revealed many intra- and extracellular coccobacilli that appeared to be surrounded by a halo (Figure 2-42), and preparations stained by the

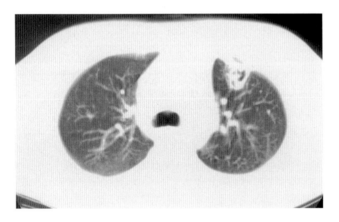

FIGURE 2-41. Computed tomography scan of the thorax shows a thick-walled cavity in the anterior portion of the left lung.

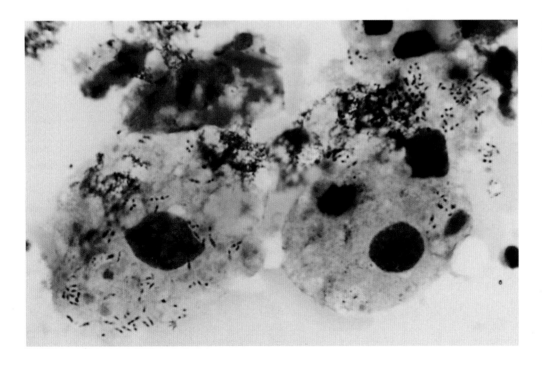

FIGURE 2-42. Cytologic preparation of bronchoalveolar lavage fluid shows alveolar macrophages and numerous intra- and extracellular coccobacilli surrounded by a halo, causing some organisms to appear as beaded bacilli (Giemsa stain; original magnification, ×250).

Gram-Weigert method showed that the bacteria were gram-positive (Figure 2-43). These features of the bacteria (i.e., gram-positive coccobacilli surrounded by a halo), are highly suggestive of *Rhodococcus* species. Antimicrobial therapy was altered appropriately; the patient's condition worsened, however, and he died 5 days later.

Pathologic Findings

At autopsy, the most important findings were in the lungs, which had a combined weight of 1,450 g. In the left lung, multiple small, focally necrotic nodules up to 1 cm in diameter were scattered throughout the parenchyma, and a 2-cm cavity was found in the anterior segment of the upper lobe. Histologic examination of H and E–stained sections of the nodules showed large aggregates of histiocytes with focal areas of necrosis and rare collections of neutrophils (Figure 2-44). On closer examination, occasional laminated, calcified bodies (Figure 2-45) that stained positively for iron and calcium, characteristic of the Michaelis-Gutman bodies of malakoplakia, were found. Sections stained by the Gram-Weigert method showed numerous gram-positive coccobacilli (Figure 2-46), which also stained by the Fite-Faraco acid-fast method for demonstrating weakly acid-fast organisms (Figure 2-47).

Differential Diagnoses

This pattern of inflammation (i.e., histiocytic aggregates) may be associated with infections caused by *M. avium* complex, *Mycobacterium genavense*, *Rhodococcus equi*, *H. capsulatum*, and *Cryptococcus neoformans*.

Microbiology

R. equi was isolated from cultures of both premortem sputum and postmortem lung tissue.

Comment

Based on the differential diagnosis, tissue Gram, methenamine silver, Ziehl-Neelsen, and Fite-Faraco stains should be performed to help identify the responsible pathogen. The staining characteristics observed in this

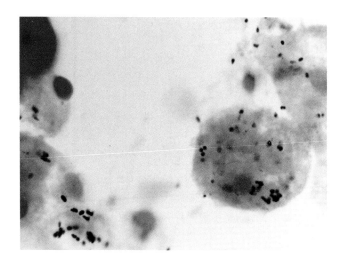

FIGURE 2-43. Gram-Weigert stain of the preparation illustrated in Figure 2-42 shows that the bacteria are gram-positive coccobacilli (Gram-Weigert stain; original magnification, ×250).

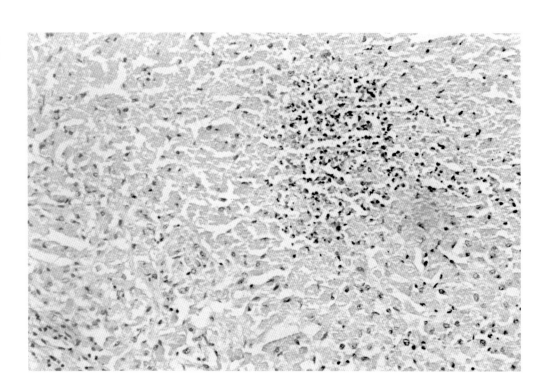

FIGURE 2-44. Section of a pulmonary nodule shows a diffuse infiltrate of foamy histiocytes with foci of necrosis and a rare aggregate of neutrophils (hematoxylin and eosin stain; original magnification, ×250).

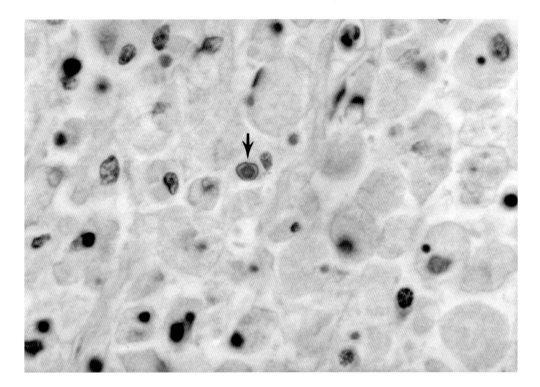

FIGURE 2-45. Section of a pulmonary nodule shows occasional oval structures consistent with Michaelis-Gutman bodies (*arrow*; hematoxylin and eosin stain; original magnification, ×250).

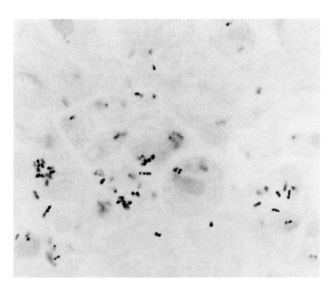

FIGURE 2-46. Section of a pulmonary nodule shows many gram-positive coccobacilli, predominantly within macrophages (Gram-Weigert stain; original magnification, ×250). Cultures of the tissue grew *Rhodococcus equi*.

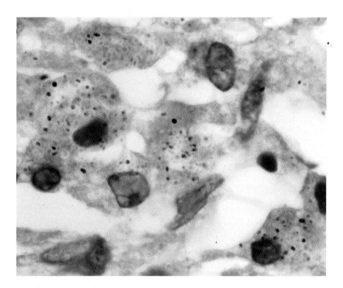

FIGURE 2-47. Section of a pulmonary nodule shows numerous weakly acid-fast coccoid and coccobacillary organisms that appear to be surrounded by a narrow halo (Fite-Faraco acid-fast stain; original magnification, ×250). Cultures of the tissue grew *Rhodococcus equi*.

case are consistent with a diagnosis of *R. equi*, although identification requires culture. The inflammatory response to *R. equi* varies. In addition to aggregates of histiocytes, infection with *R. equi* may be associated with acute, neutrophilic inflammation or a mixed suppurative and granulomatous infiltrate, depending on the duration

of the infection and the immune competence of the patient.

Diagnosis

Rhodococcus pneumonia.

CAVITATING PNEUMONIA
WITH CASEATING GRANULOMAS

Clinical History

An 85-year-old man presented to an emergency department with a 1-week history of progressive shortness of breath, cough productive of yellow sputum, and fever. Past alcohol and injection drug use were uncertain; serologic status for infection with human immunodeficiency virus was unknown. On physical examination, he was in respiratory distress with a respiratory rate of 32 breaths per minute. His temperature was 38.2°C, and his pulse rate was 172 beats per minute. Auscultation of the lung fields revealed decreased breath sounds, bilateral rales, and expiratory wheezes, and there was dullness to percussion. A chest radiograph showed infiltrates in the right lower and left upper lobes. Pertinent laboratory test results included a white blood cell count of 14,200 per µl (61% segmented neutrophils, 30% band forms) and LDH of 956 IU/liter.

Admitting diagnosis was pneumonia, and the differential diagnoses of potential pathogens included *S. pneumoniae*, *H. influenzae*, and *L. pneumophila*.

Empiric broad-spectrum antimicrobial therapy was begun. Two days after admission, he was found unresponsive and in cardiac arrest. He was resuscitated and transferred to the medical intensive care unit, where his course was complicated by recurrent respiratory failure, hypotension, and coagulopathy. Despite aggressive therapy, he died 4 days after admission.

Pathologic Findings

Autopsy examination revealed bilateral lower lobar consolidation, cavitation of the right middle lobe (Figure 2-48), and caseating granulomas in the parabronchial lymph nodes. Sections of the lung lesions stained with hematoxylin and eosin showed caseating and noncaseating granulomas (Figures 2-49 and 2-50). Examination of sections stained by the Ziehl-Neelsen method showed few beaded AFB within macrophages and extracellularly, in the center of the caseation necrosis (Figure 2-51).

Differential Diagnoses

The differential diagnoses associated with caseating granulomas include infection with *M. tuberculosis*, nontuberculous mycobacteria, dimorphic fungi, and *C. neoformans*.

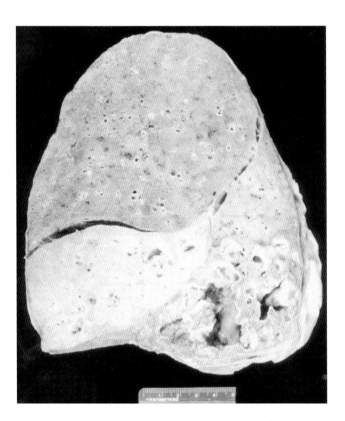

FIGURE 2-48. Lung with consolidation and cavity formation caused by *Mycobacterium tuberculosis*.

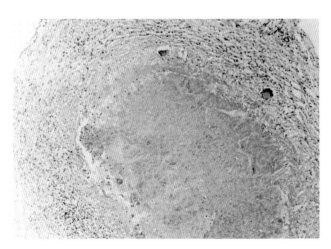

FIGURE 2-49. Section of lung shows a caseating granuloma, characterized by a central area of caseation surrounded by epithelioid histiocytes, lymphocytes, plasma cells, fibroblasts, and a few multinucleated giant cells (hematoxylin and eosin stain; original magnification, ×25). Postmortem mycobacterial cultures of lung tissue grew *Mycobacterium tuberculosis*.

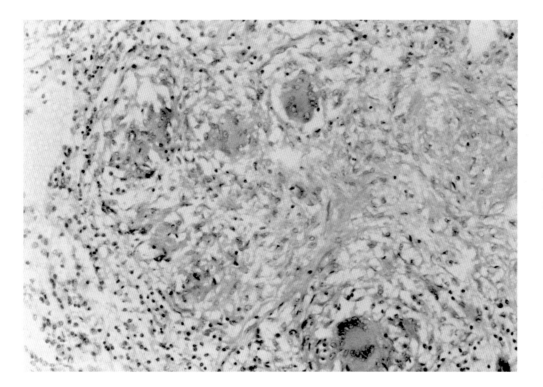

FIGURE 2-50. Section of lung from the same case illustrated in Figure 2-49 shows a noncaseating granuloma, characterized by a well-circumscribed aggregate of epithelioid histiocytes, lymphocytes, and a few multinucleated giant cells (hematoxylin and eosin stain; original magnification, ×50).

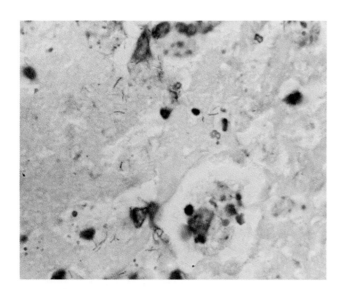

FIGURE 2-51. Section of lung shows occasional beaded acid-fast bacilli, found predominantly in the center of the areas of caseation (Ziehl-Neelsen stain; original magnification, ×250).

Microbiology

Postmortem culture of lung tissue from this case grew *M. tuberculosis*.

Comment

Based on the differential diagnoses, further studies should include special stains for detection of AFB and fungi. With regard to mycobacteria, *M. tuberculosis* is the most likely pathogen; however, certain nontuberculous mycobacteria, especially *M. kansasii* and *M. avium* complex, must be considered. The fungi to include in the differential depend on geographic location and travel history. For example, *H. capsulatum* and *Blastomyces dermatitidis* are endemic in the Ohio, Mississippi, and Missouri River valleys, whereas *C. immitis* is endemic in the southwestern United States. Another possible, but less likely, fungal pathogen is *C. neoformans*, which elicits a variety of inflammatory responses, based on the state of the organism and the immune competency of the host (see Miliary Lesions in the Immunocompromised Patient). Nonencapsulated strains of *C.*

neoformans in an immune competent host are sometimes associated with caseating granulomas.

AFB were present, and their morphology and location were consistent with, but not diagnostic of, *M. tuberculosis*. Bacilli of *M. kansasii* tend to be larger, with prominent crossbars (Figure 2-52). Stains for AFB, however, are not adequate for identification of mycobacteria to the species level. For public health reasons, differentiation of *M. tuberculosis* from other mycobacterial species is an extremely important responsibility of the microbiology laboratory. A diagnosis of tuberculosis triggers contact investigation, whereas this effort is not necessary for infections with nontuberculous mycobacteria. The only method for specific diagnosis is culture of the involved tissue for mycobacteria.

Diagnosis

Pulmonary tuberculosis.

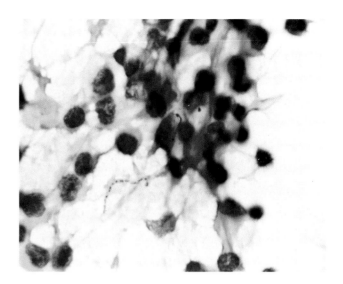

FIGURE 2-52. Cytologic preparation of bronchoalveolar lavage fluid shows long acid-fast bacilli with prominent crossbars, most suggestive of *Mycobacterium kansasii* (Kinyoun carbol fuchsin stain; original magnification, ×250). Mycobacterial cultures of the fluid grew *M. kansasii*.

DIFFUSE INTERSTITIAL PULMONARY INFILTRATES WITH CASEATING GRANULOMAS

Clinical History

A 39-year-old man, diagnosed with human immunodeficiency virus infection 5 years earlier, was admitted for evaluation of fever, anorexia, and weight loss for 1 month. His social history included injection drug use and alcohol abuse. On physical examination, his temperature was 39.5°C, his pulse rate was 130 beats per minute, and his respiratory rate was 20 breaths per minute. Auscultation of his chest revealed basilar crackles bilaterally; the remainder of the examination was noncontributory. Pertinent abnormal laboratory test results included a hemoglobin concentration of 10.7 g/dl, the presence of 27 nucleated red blood cells per 1,000 white blood cells in the peripheral blood smear, and prolonged prothrombin and partial thromboplastin times. Blood for bacterial culture was collected, and empiric broad-spectrum antimicrobic therapy was initiated.

Two days after admission, the patient developed severe shortness of breath and tachycardia. A chest radiograph showed diffuse interstitial infiltrates. The differential diagnosis included tuberculosis, histoplasmosis, and pneumocystosis. Collection of a sputum specimen for mycobac-

terial and fungal stains and cultures was ordered, but the patient was unable to produce an expectorated sputum sample. His respiratory condition worsened, requiring intubation and mechanical ventilation. The next day, intracellular, budding yeast cells were observed in a Wright-stained smear of peripheral blood (Figure 2-53), suggesting the diagnosis of disseminated histoplasmosis. Antifungal therapy was added to the antibiotic regimen, and aggressive supportive care was continued, but he died 3 days later.

Pathologic Findings

Autopsy examination confirmed the suspected diagnosis of disseminated histoplasmosis, involving the lungs, liver, spleen, and thoracic and abdominal lymph nodes. The lungs weighed 2,590 g, and scattered throughout the parenchyma of all lobes were numerous, variably-sized gray nodules, some of which had foci of caseous necrosis, features most suggestive of miliary tuberculosis, histoplasmosis, or coccidioidomycosis. Histologic examination of H and E–stained sections of these pulmonary nodules showed granulomas with central caseous necrosis. Sections stained by the methenamine silver method showed many intra- and extracellular budding yeast cells, 2–4 µm in diameter, both in the granulomas and free in the alveolar spaces (Figure 2-54).

Differential Diagnoses

The differential diagnoses are identical to those listed for the previous case: mycobacteria, dimorphic fungi (depending on the geographic location), and *C. neoformans*.

Microbiology

Culture of postmortem lung tissue grew *H. capsulatum*.

Comment

Based on the differential diagnoses, further studies should include special stains for AFB, which in this case did not reveal any organisms, and for fungi. The morphology of the yeast cells observed in sections stained by the methenamine silver method is most consistent with *H. capsulatum*, but cells of *Candida (Torulopsis) glabrata*, which is a rare cause of invasive, disseminated disease, are similar. Microforms of *B. dermatitidis* may, at first glance, resemble yeast cells of *H. capsulatum*

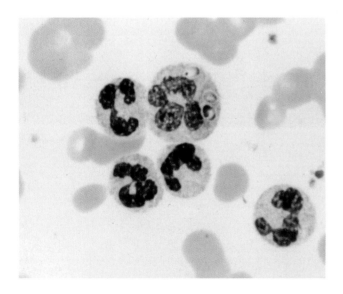

FIGURE 2-53. Smear of peripheral blood shows a neutrophil with intracellular yeast forms 2–3 µm in maximal diameter surrounded by a narrow clear zone, characteristic of *Histoplasma capsulatum* (Wright-Giemsa stain; original magnification, ×250). Fungal blood cultures grew *H. capsulatum*.

FIGURE 2-54. Section of lung tissue shows an alveolar space containing histiocytes laden with round to oval single and budding yeast cells of *Histoplasma capsulatum* (Gomori's methenamine silver stain; original magnification, ×250).

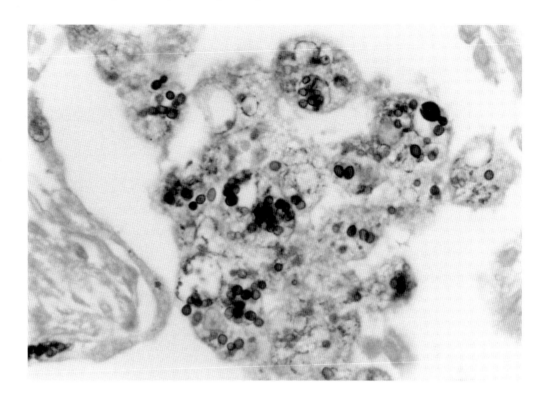

FIGURE 2-55A. Section of a skin biopsy from a case of penicilliosis marneffei shows many oval intracellular and extracellular yeast forms 2–4 μm in diameter (hematoxylin and eosin stain; original magnification, ×250).

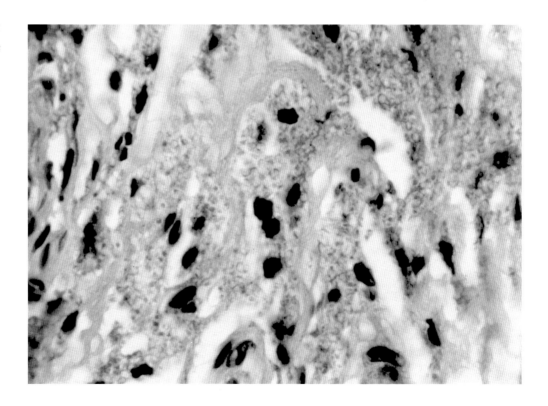

because of their small size (2–4 μm). Morphologically, however, these small forms are typical of *B. dermatitidis*, and they almost always are part of a spectrum of sizes ranging from small to the larger yeast forms characteris-tic of this fungus. Yeast forms of *Penicillium marneffei* also are similar in size and shape to those of *H. capsula-tum*, but on close inspection some cells of *P. marneffei* have a dividing septum (Figures 2-55A and 2-55B), thus

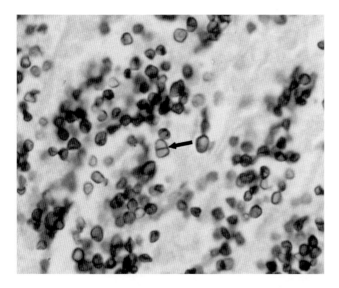

FIGURE 2-55B. A section of the tissue illustrated in Figure 2-55A shows a few yeast cells that are dividing by fission, as indicated by the prominent septum (*arrow*). This feature distinguishes *Penicillium marneffei* from *Histoplasma capsulatum*, cells of which multiply by budding (Gomori's methenamine silver stain; original magnification, ×250).

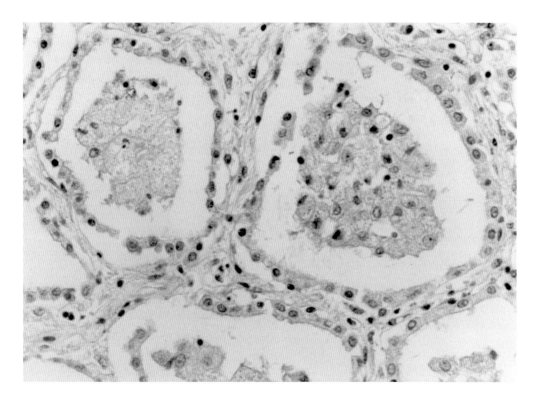

FIGURE 2-56A. Section of lung from a patient with acquired immunodeficiency syndrome who died from disseminated histoplasmosis shows alveolar spaces filled with vacuolated histiocytes, somewhat resembling the response sometimes observed in *Pneumocystis carinii* infection (hematoxylin and eosin stain; original magnification, ×100).

Infections of the Respiratory Tract

FIGURE 2-56B. The section illustrated in Figure 2-56A reveals numerous small (3–4 μm) intracellular yeast cells, some budding with necks, typical of *Histoplasma capsulatum*, which was recovered from the fungal culture of lung tissue taken at autopsy (Gomori's methenamine silver; original magnification, ×250).

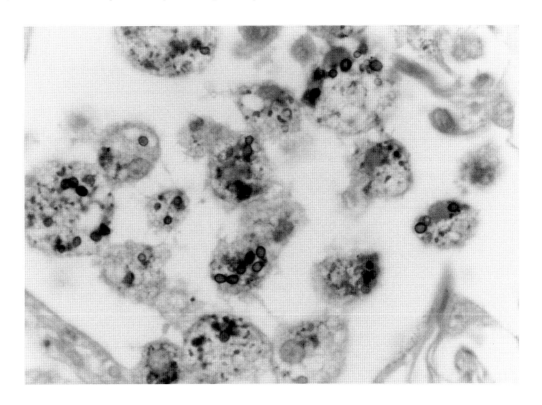

distinguishing them from budding cells of *H. capsulatum*. Additionally, the histopathology of pulmonary histoplasmosis may resemble that of *P. carinii* pneumonia in sections stained with H and E (Figure 2-56A). In such cases, staining the sections with a silver stain is helpful diagnostically if budding yeast forms consistent with those of

H. capsulatum are observed (Figure 2-56B). Culture is essential for accurate diagnosis.

Diagnosis

Miliary histoplasmosis.

PNEUMONIA WITH MIXED SUPPURATIVE AND GRANULOMATOUS INFLAMMATION

Clinical History

A 24-year-old man from rural southeast Louisiana, and no history of travel elsewhere, was admitted for evaluation of productive cough, fever, and chills that had not resolved after a 1-week outpatient course of antimicrobial therapy for presumed community-acquired bacterial pneumonia. On physical examination, his temperature was 38°C, his pulse rate was 97 beats per minute, and his respiratory rate was 16 breaths per minute. Auscultation of the chest revealed decreased breath sounds, rhonchi, and egophony in the right lower lung field. The remainder of the examination was noncontributory. Pertinent abnormal laboratory test results included a hemoglobin concentration of 12.3 g/dl and a white blood cell count of 17,000 per μl (74% segmented neutrophils, 1% band forms, 14% lymphocytes, 11% monocytes). Chest radiograph showed opacification of the posterior and medial portions of the right lower lobe (Figure 2-57). The differential diagnoses, based on clinical presentation and geographic location, included community-acquired pneumonia caused by a bacterium resistant to the usual antimicrobial agents, Legionnaires' disease, tuberculosis, histoplasmosis (endemic in the Ohio, Mississippi, and Missouri River valleys), blastomycosis (endemic in the Ohio and Mississippi River valleys), and postobstructive pneumonia associated with an endobronchial neoplasm.

Sputum specimens were collected for bacterial, fungal, and mycobacterial stains and cultures. No predominant organism was detected in the Gram stain smear, no AFB was visualized in the smear stained with auramine O,

and no fungal elements were seen in the KOH preparation. Bronchoscopy with bronchial brushing and BAL was performed. In the Papanicolaou-stained smears of the brushings, occasional spherical to oval yeast cells, 10–12 μm in diameter, with thick, hyaline, refractile cell walls, centrally retracted cytoplasm, and single broad-based buds were present (Figure 2-58). These features are highly suggestive of *B. dermatitidis*.

The patient left the hospital against medical advice before the cytopathology results were available. Two weeks later, he was readmitted in respiratory failure. Chest radiograph showed bilateral diffuse alveolar infiltrates. Despite appropriate antifungal therapy and supportive care, he died shortly after admission.

Pathologic Findings

At autopsy, the predominant findings were in the lungs, which showed diffuse consolidation of all lobes. Histologic examination of H and E–stained sections of areas of pulmonary consolidation showed a mixed suppurative and granulomatous inflammatory infiltrate composed primarily of neutrophils admixed with epithelioid histiocytes (Figure 2-59). These sections also showed thick-walled

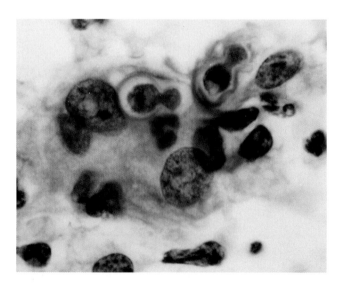

FIGURE 2-58. Cytologic preparation of material collected by bronchial brushing shows an epithelioid histiocyte that has phagocytized two budding yeast cells. The yeast forms have a thick cell wall, centripetal retraction of the cytoplasm, and broad-based buds, characteristic of *Blastomyces dermatitidis* (Papanicolaou stain; original magnification, ×250).

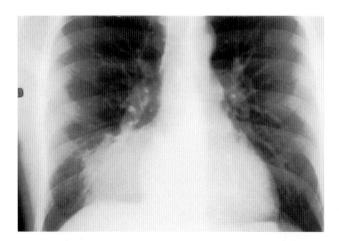

FIGURE 2-57. Chest radiograph shows consolidation of the posterior and medial portions of the right lower lung field.

FIGURE 2-59. Section from an area of pulmonary consolidation shows a mixed suppurative and granulomatous infiltrate composed predominantly of neutrophils with scattered epithelioid histiocytes (hematoxylin and eosin stain; original magnification, ×50).

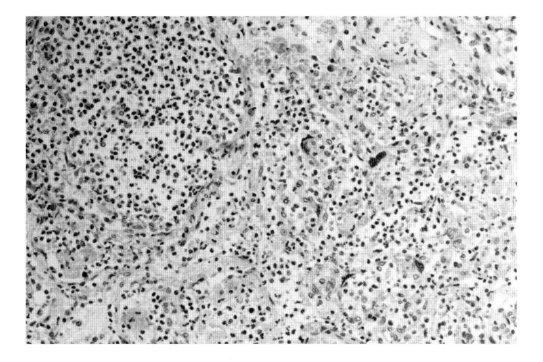

yeast cells with broad-based buds and centrally retracted cytoplasm (Figure 2-60), features that are characteristic of *B. dermatitidis*.

Differential Diagnoses

The differential diagnoses include infections caused by several fungi (e.g., *B. dermatitidis*, *C. immitis*, *Paracoccidioides brasiliensis*, *Sporothrix schenckii*, and various dematiaceous fungi) and by some nontuberculous mycobacteria.

Microbiology

Cultures of premortem sputum and postmortem lung tissue grew *B. dermatitidis*.

Comment

In cases of mixed suppurative and granulomatous inflammation caused by a fungus, the H and E stain typically allows detection of yeast cells of *B. dermatitidis*, *C. immitis*, and *P. brasiliensis* and hyphae of dematiaceous fungi and is the optimal stain for demonstrating the multiple nuclei of *B. dermatitidis*. In this case, examination of H and E–stained sections revealed typical yeast forms of *B. dermatitidis*, although occasionally yeast cells of other fungi may have a similar appearance. For example, immature spherules of *C. immitis* (Figure 2-61) may resemble nonbudding or apparently budding yeast cells of *B. dermatitidis* with poorly stained inner contents. In such cases, however, a careful search usually reveals typical endosporulation forms of *C. immitis*

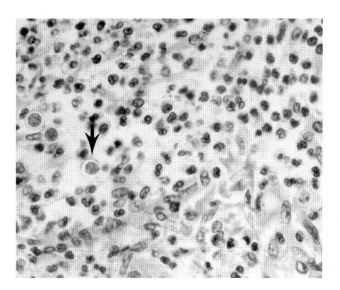

FIGURE 2-60. Higher-power magnification of the section illustrated in Figure 2-59 shows round to oval yeast forms 10–12 μm in diameter, one of which is budding (*arrow*). The size of the yeast cells, the thickness of the refractile cell wall, and the centrally retracted cytoplasm are characteristic of *Blastomyces dermatitidis* (hematoxylin and eosin stain; original magnification, ×100).

(Figure 2-62). In addition, yeast cells of *P. brasiliensis* that do not demonstrate multiple budding occasionally may be confused with *B. dermatitidis* at first glance, but more thorough examination usually shows variation in size of the cells and multiple buds with narrow necks, typical of *P. brasiliensis*.

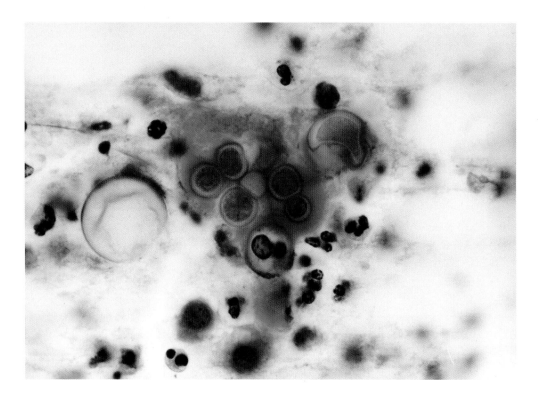

FIGURE 2-61. Cytologic preparation of a fine needle aspiration of a subcutaneous abscess from a patient with coccidioidomycosis shows a large empty spherule of *Coccidioides immitis* and a cluster of smaller immature spherules, resembling yeast forms of *Blastomyces dermatitidis* (Papanicolaou stain; original magnification, ×250). Cultures of the material grew *C. immitis*.

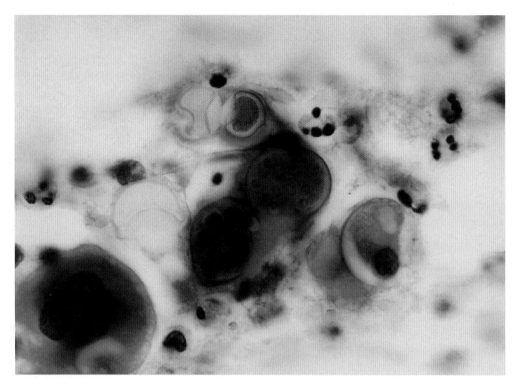

FIGURE 2-62. A different area of the cytologic preparation described in Figure 2-61 shows mature spherules with endospores, characteristic of *Coccidioides immitis* (Papanicolaou stain; original magnification, ×250).

In cases in which the H and E–stained sections fail to demonstrate organisms, special stains for fungal elements and AFB (see Chapter 1) should be performed. Special stains also are useful when only a few yeast cells can be found, as is expected with more chronic infections, in which the granulomatous component predominates (Figure 2-63). The periodic acid-Schiff stain accentuates the important diagnostic features of yeast cells of *B. dermatitidis* (Figure 2-64) and *C. immitis*, but these characteristics are more difficult to recognize in sections stained with a methenamine silver stain. In contrast, the morphology of cells of *P. brasiliensis* is shown best with a

FIGURE 2-63. Section of lung tissue from a patient with chronic pulmonary blastomycosis shows a mixed inflammatory response with a predominantly granulomatous component (hematoxylin and eosin stain; original magnification, ×250).

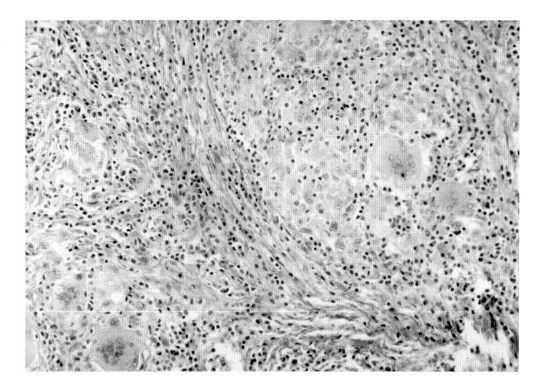

methenamine silver stain; classically, yeast cells vary from 4 to 60 μm in diameter, although most are 5–30 μm, and demonstrate multiple budding with either large, teardrop-shaped blastoconidia or small, oval, or tubular blastoconidia attached to parent cells by narrow necks. Yeast cells of *S. schenckii*, which are difficult to find in H and E–stained sections, sometimes can be demonstrated with either the periodic acid-Schiff stain with diastase digestion or a methenamine silver stain. In addition to special stains, which may not be diagnostic in all cases, cultures for fungi always should be done when a fungal infection is suspected based on tissue histopathology.

Diagnosis

Pulmonary blastomycosis.

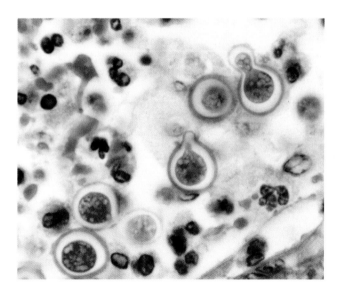

FIGURE 2-64. Section of lung tissue accentuates the features of yeast forms of *Blastomyces dermatitidis*: thick cell wall, centrally retracted cytoplasm, and broad-based buds (periodic acid-Schiff stain; original magnification, ×250).

MILIARY LESIONS IN THE IMMUNOCOMPROMISED PATIENT

Clinical History

A 49-year-old man was admitted for evaluation of a headache, which had lasted for 2 weeks and was only partially relieved by analgesics, and recent onset of altered mental status. He had received a cadaveric renal transplant 1 year earlier for renal failure secondary to polycystic kidney disease and subsequently had been maintained on prednisone and other immunosuppressive agents. On physical examination, he was afebrile, his respiratory rate was 15 breaths per minute, and his pulse rate was 80 beats per minute. He was lethargic but able to follow commands. The remainder of the examination was noncontributory. Pertinent abnormal laboratory test results included a hemoglobin concentration of 12.1 g/dl, white blood cell count of 12,800 per μl (81% segmented neutrophils, 15% band forms, 4% lymphocytes), blood urea nitrogen of 92 mg/dl, and creatine of 4.7 mg/dl. Chest radiograph showed bilateral reticulonodular infiltrates. The differential diagnoses based on the data included pathologic processes associated with both pulmonary and central nervous system disease in an immunocompromised host and included tuberculosis, *C. neoformans* infection, histoplasmosis, coccidioidomycosis, and malignancy.

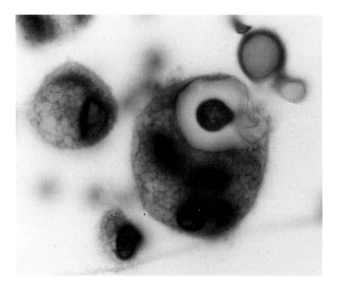

FIGURE 2-65. Cytologic preparation of bronchoalveolar lavage fluid shows lavender-appearing, budding yeast cells with a "fuzzy" outline, suggestive of *Cryptococcus neoformans* (Papanicolaou stain; original magnification, ×250). Fungal cultures of the fluid grew *C. neoformans*.

Lumbar puncture and bronchoscopy with BAL were performed. The cerebrospinal fluid (CSF) white blood cell count was 30 per μl (93% lymphocytes, 7% monocytes). A portion of the CSF and BAL fluid was submitted to the clinical microbiology laboratory for bacterial, fungal, and mycobacterial studies. No organisms were detected in smears of either specimen stained by Gram stain or with auramine O. CSF and BAL fluid also were submitted to the cytology laboratory. Papanicolaou-stained smears of both specimens showed a few macrophages and several pink to lavender yeast cells that varied from 3 to 15 μm in diameter and had a "fuzzy" outline (Figure 2-65), features suggestive of *C. neoformans*. The patient was treated with appropriate antifungal therapy, but his condition deteriorated, and he died 1 month after admission.

Pathologic Findings

The predominant findings at autopsy were in the lungs, which had firm, yellow to gray nodules 0.5 cm in maximum diameter throughout the parenchyma bilaterally (Figure 2-66). H and E–stained sections of the pulmonary lesions showed poorly formed granulomas composed of foamy histiocytes, occasional giant cells, and irregularly shaped vacuoles resembling soap bubbles (Figure 2-67). Within these "soap bubbles," intra- and extracellular, spherical to oval refractile structures 3–10 μm in diameter, often surrounded by halos, were present (Figure 2-68). These structures were somewhat difficult to visualize with the H and E stain but were readily recognized as encapsulated yeast cells in sections stained with the mucicarmine stain (Figure 2-69).

Differential Diagnoses

The gross appearance of the lungs at autopsy is consistent with miliary tuberculosis, disseminated fungal infection, hematogenously disseminated bacterial abscesses, and malignancy.

Microbiology

The CSF cryptococcal antigen was positive (titer, 1:1,024). Cultures of both premortem CSF and BAL fluid specimens grew *C. neoformans*.

Comment

In this case, yeast cells were observed in tissue sections stained with H and E; because their appearance was sug-

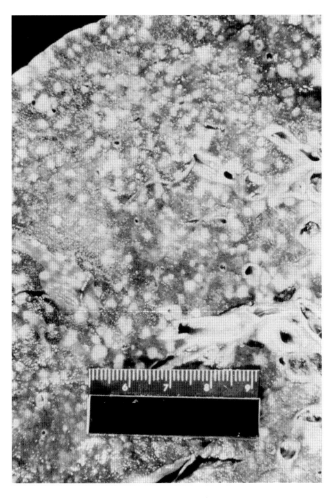

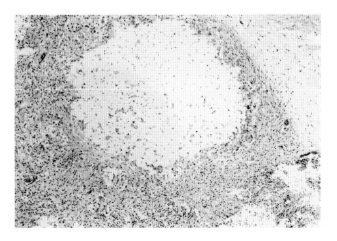

FIGURE 2-66. Photograph of lung shows diffuse, miliary lesions caused by *Cryptococcus neoformans*.

FIGURE 2-67. Section of a pulmonary nodule shows a "soap bubble" lesion, characterized by aggregates of foamy to granular macrophages surrounding a central lucent area (hematoxylin and eosin stain; original magnification, ×25).

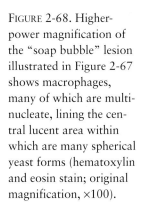

FIGURE 2-68. Higher-power magnification of the "soap bubble" lesion illustrated in Figure 2-67 shows macrophages, many of which are multinucleate, lining the central lucent area within which are many spherical yeast forms (hematoxylin and eosin stain; original magnification, ×100).

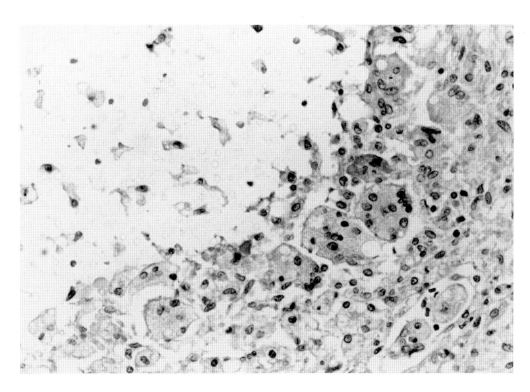

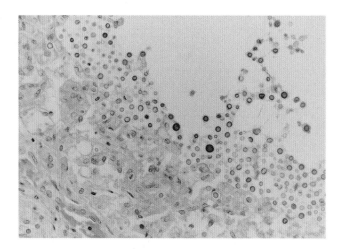

FIGURE 2-69. Section of the "soap bubble" lesion shows numerous encapsulated intra- and extracellular yeast forms, characteristic of *Cryptococcus neoformans* (Meyer's mucicarmine stain; original magnification, ×100).

gestive of *C. neoformans*, a mucicarmine stain was performed. The intense capsular staining of these yeast cells with mucicarmine is a feature almost diagnostic of *C. neoformans*. *Trichosporon beigelii* also stains with mucicarmine but morphologically is quite different from *C. neoformans*; *B. dermatitidis* may stain weakly positive.

The pathology of cryptococcosis varies depending on the nature of the infecting organism and the host immune response, although neutrophils are generally rare. Frequently, the inflammatory response is minimal, especially in severely immunocompromised patients infected with an encapsulated strain of *C. neoformans*. In such patients, yeast cells may infiltrate blood vessels and disseminate throughout the body (Figure 2-70). In contrast, unencapsulated variants of *C. neoformans* are

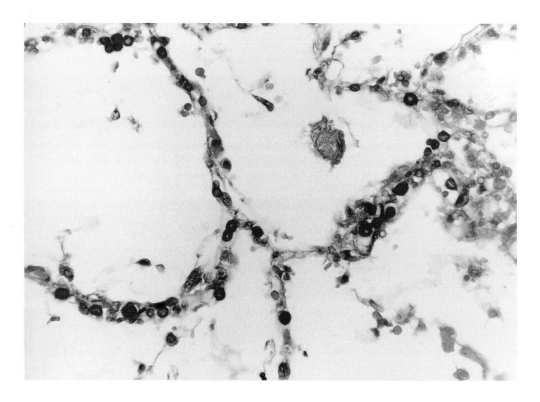

FIGURE 2-70. Section of lung tissue from an human immunodeficiency virus–infected patient with disseminated cryptococcosis (confirmed by culture) shows many yeast forms within the pulmonary capillaries and only rare organisms within the alveolar spaces (Meyer's mucicarmine; original magnification, ×100).

more likely than encapsulated strains to elicit a granulo-matous response, particularly in immune competent hosts. These unencapsulated variants do not stain with mucicarmine but do stain with the Fontana-Masson stain (Figure 2-71), a feature that is useful for identification.

Diagnosis

Disseminated cryptococcosis.

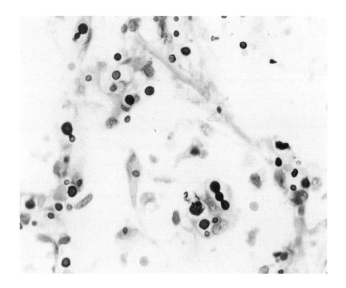

FIGURE 2-71. Section of lung tissue from an human immunode-ficiency virus–infected patient with disseminated cryptococcosis (confirmed by culture) shows budding and nonbudding yeast cells (Fontana-Masson stain; original magnification, ×50).

PULMONARY INTERSTITIAL INFILTRATES IN THE IMMUNOCOMPROMISED PATIENT

Clinical History

A 41-year-old man diagnosed with AIDS 5 years earlier presented to a clinic with complaints of chest pain, dysarthria, and weakness. Medications included aerosolized pentamidine as prophylaxis for *P. carinii* pneumonia and intravenous immunoglobulin G for chronic anemia due to infection with parvovirus B19. On physical examination, his temperature was 36.2°C, his pulse rate was 62 beats per minute, and his respiratory rate was 18 breaths per minute. When asked questions, he was slow to respond, and at times his speech was difficult to understand. Pertinent laboratory test results included a white blood cell count of 2,800 per µl (54% segmented neutrophils, 11% band forms, 7% myelocytes) and a hemoglobin concentration of 11.4 g/dl. An MRI study of the head showed a ring-enhancing lesion in the left temporal lobe, and a chest radiograph showed bilateral pulmonary infiltrates, attributed to pulmonary edema. He was admitted to the hospital for evaluation of the abnormal results of the MRI.

The differential diagnosis of the temporal lesion on admission included toxoplasmosis, lymphoma, and tuberculous abscess (pulmonary tuberculosis 4 years earlier had been treated appropriately). Based on these possibilities, empiric therapy for toxoplasmosis and for tuberculosis was initiated. While the evaluation of the temporal lesion was progressing, he became febrile (temperature, 38.3°C) and increasingly short of breath. The chest radiograph was basically unchanged from admission. Routine sputum cultures (i.e., for aerobic bacteria) grew normal flora with a moderate amount of *S. aureus*. Sputum obtained for fungal and mycobacterial smears and cultures contained no visible fungal elements or AFB. Bronchoscopy with BAL was performed. A portion of the lavage fluid was submitted to the clinical microbiology laboratory to be evaluated for bacteria, fungi, mycobacteria, and viruses. Appropriate cultures were performed; smears stained by Gram stain and auramine O revealed no organisms. Fluid also was submitted for cytologic examination. Cytocentrifuge preparations stained with the Papanicolaou, Giemsa, and methenamine silver stains, illustrated in Figures 2-72 through 2-74, showed trophozoites (Giemsa) and cysts (methenamine silver) of *P. carinii*. Despite appropriate antimicrobial therapy and continued supportive care, the patient died the next day.

Pathologic Findings

At autopsy, the lungs weighed 1,800 g combined, and the parenchyma was firm throughout. Microscopic examination of tissue sections stained with H and E revealed widening of the alveolar septa with an infiltrate of mononuclear cells and a mass of foamy eosinophilic material within many of the alveolar spaces (Figure 2-75), suggestive of *P. carinii* infection. Methenamine silver–stained sections showed round cysts of *P. carinii* 5–6 µm in diameter (Figure 2-76). The only other significant autopsy finding was in the brain. Sections of the lesion in the left temporal lobe, which measured 1 cm in greatest diameter and corresponded to the lesion recognized by MRI, showed a primary B-cell lymphoma.

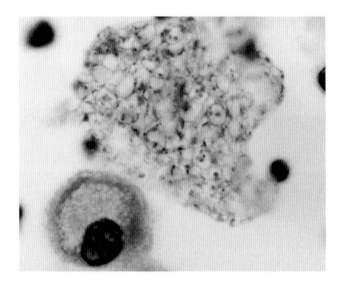

FIGURE 2-72. Cytologic preparation of bronchoalveolar lavage fluid shows a mass of foamy material, typical of *Pneumocystis carinii* infection (Papanicolaou stain; original magnification, ×250).

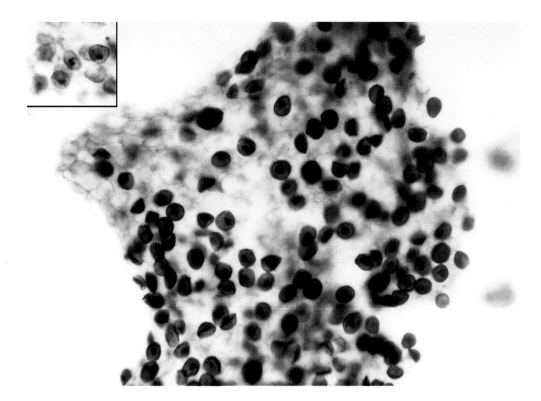

FIGURE 2-73. Cytologic preparation of bronchoalveolar lavage fluid shows round and cup-shaped forms with a prominent density representing thickening of the cyst wall, consistent with cysts of *Pneumocystis carinii* (Gomori's methenamine silver stain; original magnification, ×250). Inset shows a "double-dot" form, which when present helps differentiate *P. carinii* cysts from non-budding yeast forms, especially those of *Histoplasma capsulatum* (Gomori's methenamine silver stain; original magnification, ×250).

Differential Diagnoses

The differential diagnoses include other fungi that can produce nonbudding yeast forms in tissue, such as *Candida* species and *H. capsulatum*.

Comment

Cysts of *P. carinii* may appear similar to nonbudding yeast cells. Features that favor the diagnosis of *P. carinii* are the presence of cup-shaped or hat-shaped forms and, in sections stained with a silver stain, wrinkled forms with a small round- to comma-shaped thickening of the wall found either on the side or in the center, depending on the orientation. If the diagnosis is in doubt, however, antibodies against *P. carinii* are commercially available for use in immunohistochemical stains. Use of these antibodies is more costly than nonspecific stains, which in most cases detects trophozoites or cysts; therefore, limiting use of immunohistology or immunocytology to specific situations is reasonable. Immunohistology or immunocytology is most helpful in the diagnosis of *P. carinii* pneumonia when the host response to the infection is atypical, when few organisms are present, and when distinguishing *P. carinii* cysts from nonbudding yeast forms, especially cells of *H. capsulatum* (Figure 2-77), is difficult. Immunostaining also

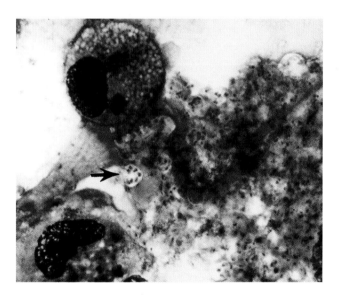

FIGURE 2-74. Cytologic preparation of bronchoalveolar lavage fluid demonstrates a mass of extracellular *Pneumocystis carinii* trophozoites and cysts, each containing up to eight trophozoites. Trophozoites have a magenta nucleus and blue cytoplasm; cysts, which do not stain by Romanowsky methods such as Giemsa, appear as clear circles containing organisms (*arrow*; Giemsa stain; original magnification, ×250).

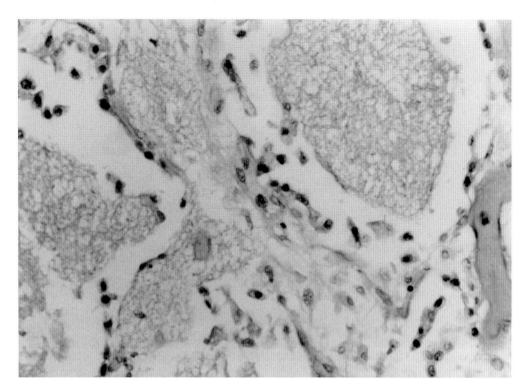

FIGURE 2-75. Section of lung tissue shows acellular, frothy intra-alveolar material resembling seafoam. No inflammatory cells are present within the foamy material, and very few are present in the interstitium. These features are characteristic of *Pneumocystis carinii* pneumonia in immunocompromised patients, such as those with acquired immunodeficiency virus (hematoxylin and eosin stain; original magnification, ×100).

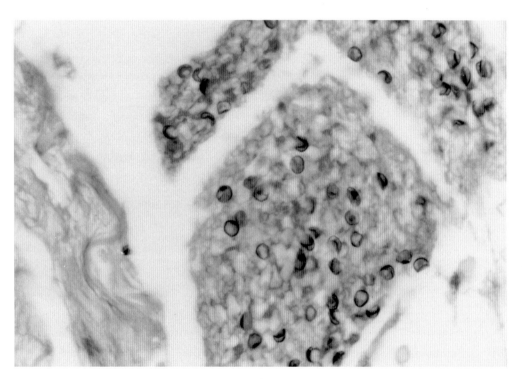

FIGURE 2-76. Section of lung tissue shows characteristic, 5–6 μm diameter cysts of *Pneumocystis carinii*. Cysts vary in shape; some are round, whereas others are cup-shaped. Several demonstrate the typical thickening of the wall, found either in the center or along the side (Gomori's methenamine silver stain; original magnification, ×250).

may be useful when examining tissues from extrapulmonary sites in cases of suspected disseminated or localized extrapulmonary *P. carinii* infection.

Occasionally, the host response to *P. carinii* is unusual, including granuloma formation or features of diffuse alveolar damage (Figure 2-78).

Diagnosis

P. carinii pneumonia.

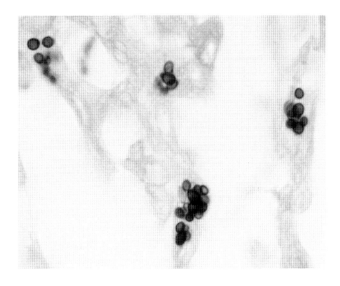

FIGURE 2-77. Section of lung tissue shows nonbudding yeast forms of *Histoplasma capsulatum*, which are similar in size and shape to cysts of *Pneumocystis carinii* but lack the prominent central thickening (Gomori's methenamine silver stain; original magnification, ×250).

FIGURE 2-78. Section of lung tissue shows masses of foamy material within alveoli (*Pneumocystis carinii* organisms) associated with changes of diffuse alveolar damage, including type II pneumocyte hyperplasia, focal hyaline membrane formation, and a focus of incipient fibrosis (hematoxylin and eosin stain; original magnification, ×100).

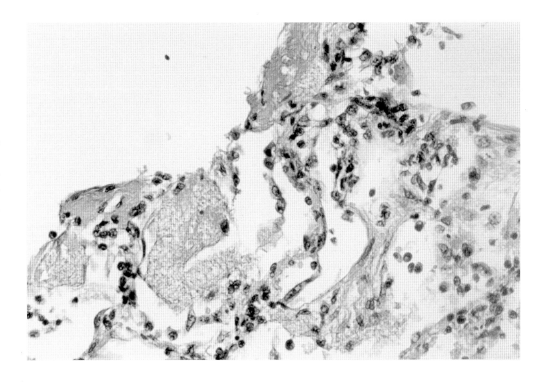

RECURRENT HEMOPTYSIS AND RADIOLOGIC PULMONARY LESION

Clinical History

A 39-year-old woman, who had an episode of hemoptysis 20 years earlier, experienced occasional mild to moderate hemoptysis for 4 days before presentation to the emergency room. At that time, she complained of coughing up 2–3 cups of blood that day. She was afebrile and did not have chills, night sweats, weight loss, or chest pain. Results of the physical examination were normal. Purified protein derivative (tuberculin) skin test elicited a 15-mm zone of dermal induration and erythema. She was mildly anemic (hematocrit, 35%). Chest radiograph showed a right upper lobe opacity that was revealed to be a fluid-containing cavity by CT scan. Bronchoscopy demonstrated a cavity in the right upper lobe, and material collected from the cavity contained branching, septate hyphae identified by cytopathology. Smears of three sputum samples did not contain any detectable AFB.

She was treated prophylactically for tuberculosis. Her hemoptysis decreased remarkably, and she was discharged. Six weeks later, she was readmitted for right upper lobectomy. She appeared healthy and had a stable hematocrit (37%). The surgical procedure was performed without complication, and she recovered uneventfully.

Pathologic Findings

The resected right upper lobe showed apical fibrosis and a thick-walled (1–3 mm) cavity, measuring 2.5 cm × 3 cm × 5 cm, near the apex. It was filled to near capacity by yellowish-gray, friable material. Histologic examination of sections of the cavity wall showed that it was lined by multifocally eroded respiratory epithelium, beneath which was a dense infiltrate of lymphocytes, macrophages, and plasma cells. The cavity contained a blood clot and masses of septate hyphae that had parallel walls and dichotomous branching at a 45 degree angle (Figures 2-79 and 2-80). In the center of the mass, the nonviable hyphae were eosinophilic, and at the periphery they were basophilic. No evidence of fungal invasion of tissue was present, and no conidiophores were observed.

Microbiology

One of the two fungal cultures of sputum samples collected during the first hospitalization yielded *Aspergillus fumigatus*. A bronchial washing specimen from the right upper lobe contained hyphae consistent with *Aspergillus* in a KOH preparation and by Papanicolaou-stained cytology, but the fungal culture was negative.

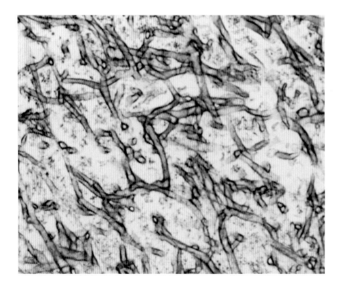

FIGURE 2-79. Section of a pulmonary aspergilloma stained by periodic acid-Schiff method demonstrates a colony of fungi with numerous septate hyphae (hematoxylin and eosin stain; original magnification, ×100).

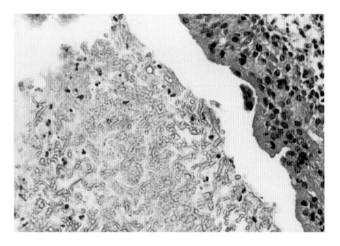

FIGURE 2-80. Section of lung shows a pulmonary aspergilloma in a cavity that is lined by chronically inflamed respiratory epithelium and contains distorted and intact septate hyphae with dichotomous branching (hematoxylin and eosin stain; original magnification, ×250).

Comment

The clinical differential diagnosis included bronchogenic carcinoma, tuberculosis, pneumonia of other etiology, and fungus ball. Often, a radiologic diagnosis of fungus ball can be made by positional changes of the patient demonstrating that a freely moveable structure is present within a cavity. This patient's hemoptysis 20 years ago was most likely due to tuberculosis. Her recent severe hemoptysis was associated with aspergilloma and was the reason for surgical resection. Fungus balls represent colonization of a preexisting space that has impaired ability to clear the spores, such as those inhaled into cavities caused by tuberculosis, sarcoidosis, or histoplasmosis, or bronchiectasis; beyond an obstruction (e.g., neoplasm); or into the nasal sinuses. Mycobacteria are seldom found in cavitary lesions colonized by *Aspergillus*. The large, intracavitary fungal colony contains dead eosinophilic, sometimes distorted hyphae in the center; viable basophilic hyphae at the periphery; and occasionally conidiophores and conidia (so-called fruiting heads), the only structures by which the fungal genus and species can be identified morphologically. The genus *Aspergillus* was named for the microscopic resemblance of the conidiophore and conidia to the aspergillum, a perforated globe for the sprinkling of holy water. *Aspergillum* is the Latin word meaning "to sprinkle." Although septate hyphae usually represent *Aspergillus fumigatus*, *Aspergillus niger*, or *Aspergillus flavus*, their morphology is indistinguishable from *Pseudallescheria boydii* and *Fusarium* species, and the nonviable, distorted hyphae may resemble zygomycetes. The finding of birefringent oxalate crystals (Figure 2-81) in the wall of the cavity is characteristic of *Aspergillus*, particularly *A. niger*. Fungus ball can be caused not only by *Aspergillus* but also by *Pseudallescheria*, *Sporothrix*, *Coccidioides*, and other fungi.

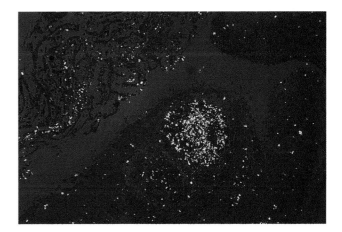

FIGURE 2-81. Polarized illumination of the wall of an aspergilloma caused by *Aspergillus niger* contains numerous brightly birefringent oxalate crystals.

Sometimes, the lesions of invasive pulmonary aspergillosis are confused with aspergillomas when the vascular invasion of both the pulmonary arteries and the bronchial arteries causes ischemic necrosis that undergoes cavitation. Important differences are the invasion of tissue and the presence of necrotic lung in the cavity of cavitary invasive aspergillosis. Occasionally, even fruiting heads are present owing to the high oxygen concentration in the cavitary lesion.

Diagnosis

Aspergillus pulmonary fungus ball.

COIN LESION

Clinical History

A 50-year-old man presented to his primary care physician with complaints of nonproductive cough, low-grade fever, and left-sided chest pain for 1 week. He had a 20-pack-year history of smoking cigarettes, but he had stopped smoking 10 years previously. Results of the physical examination and laboratory tests were normal, with the exception of a slightly increased eosinophil count. A posteroanterior chest roentgenogram revealed a well-circumscribed pleura-based nodule in the left lower lung field that measured approximately 2 cm × 2 cm. He was treated as an outpatient with empiric oral antimicrobial therapy. One month later, his symptoms had resolved, but the findings on a chest radiograph were unchanged. Conventional CT of the lung lesion showed neither cavitation nor calcification; the borders of the nodule were smooth, and the lateral edge was contiguous with the pleural surface. Bronchoscopy was performed, and washings from the region of the nodule were submitted for cytologic studies and for fungal and mycobacterial cultures. The cytologic findings were normal, and all cultures were negative. Because of the patient's age, smoking history, and his concern about the lesion, a left thoracotomy and a wedge resection were performed.

Pathologic Findings

Palpation of the resected lung segment revealed a firm nodule at the center. On cut section, a well-circumscribed, uniformly yellow, necrotic nodule 2 cm in maximum diameter was surrounded by normal lung parenchyma. Microscopic

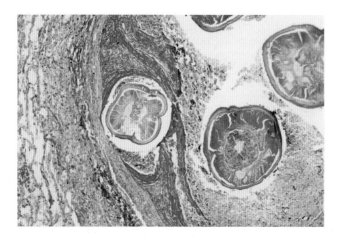

FIGURE 2-82. A section of tissue from the nodule shows thrombosis of a branch of the pulmonary artery and several cross sections of a worm within the necrotic debris (hematoxylin and eosin stain; original magnification, ×25).

examination of sections from this nodule showed an organizing pulmonary infarct with thrombosis of the pulmonary artery and sections of a nematode within the lumen of the necrotic artery (Figure 2-82). Examination of the nematode under higher-power magnification (Figure 2-83) revealed a thick cuticle, well-developed muscle cells, an intestine, and a genital tube, features consistent with a diagnosis of *Dirofilaria* species.

Differential Diagnoses

Differential diagnoses include dirofilariasis, neoplasm, and granulomatous infections, such as histoplasmosis, cryptococcosis, coccidioidomycosis, brucellosis, tuberculosis, or one of the nontuberculous mycobacteria. The gross features of the lesion are consistent with these same entities, except neoplasm, and with pulmonary infarction due to thromboembolism and limited Wegener's granulomatosis. Diagnosis of dirofilariasis requires recognition of the worm, which may be difficult in older, organized lesions in which the worm has died and deteriorated.

Comment

Human pulmonary dirofilariasis is diagnosed most commonly in areas where high concentrations of *Dirofilaria immitis*, the dog heartworm, are found. *D. immitis* has a nearly worldwide distribution; in the United States, it has been found in every state, but the highest concentrations, and consequently most human cases, occur in the south, the eastern seaboard, and the Mississippi and Ohio River basins. The histopathology of the lesion depends on its age. Generally, in the center of the lesion, a small- to medium-sized branch of the pulmonary artery that contains a thrombus in different stages of organization and one or several cross sections of the worm are present. In early lesions, a marked granulomatous inflammatory reaction occurs, composed of histiocytes, foreign body giant cells, eosinophils, lymphocytes, and plasma cells at the periphery and moderate to severe arteritis involving adjacent branches of the occluded vessel. The degree of tissue eosinophilia varies from minimal to extensive, resembling hypersensitivity pneumonitis. Older lesions appear as organized infarcts, usually well circumscribed, and ultimately form a collagenous nodule with or without calcification. Definitive diagnosis is not possible in the absence of a worm.

Recent lesions contain relatively well-preserved worms, whereas in older lesions the worms are necrotic with various degrees of degeneration and calcification. On cut section, *Dirofilaria* species have uniform features.

FIGURE 2-83. Higher-power magnification of the section illustrated in Figure 2-81 shows the typical features of *Dirofilaria* species (i.e., a thick cuticle, well-formed muscle cells, and the genital tube; hematoxylin and eosin stain; original magnification, ×50).

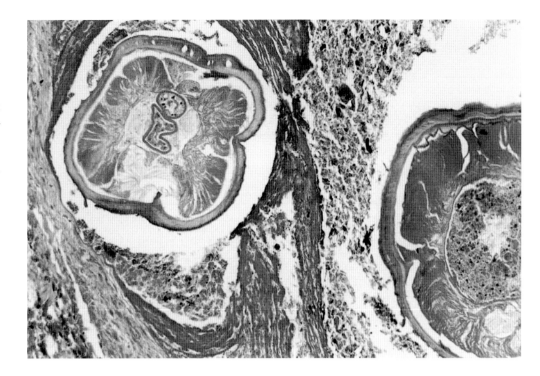

The parasite varies from 100 to 600 μm in diameter, depending on the species and sex of the worm. The maximum diameter of *D. immitis*, the most common species infecting humans, ranges from 140 to 200 μm for males and up to 300 μm for females. The cuticle is thick, layered, and, depending on the species, has either a smooth surface (e.g., *D. immitis*) or longitudinal ridges, which on cross section appear as rounded or sharply elevated structures. A ridge that varies in size and shape, depending on the species and sex of the worm, is found on the inner layer of the cuticle. The muscle cells are well developed, and the sexual organs generally are immature.

Diagnosis

Pulmonary coin lesion due to *Dirofilaria* species.

RECOMMENDED READING

General

Chandler FW, Watts JC. Pathologic Diagnosis of Fungal Infections. Chicago: ASCP Press, 1980;13, 55, 123, 149, 265, 279.

Tang Y-W, Procop GW, Zheng X, et al. Histologic parameters predictive of mycobacterial infection. Am J Clin Pathol 1998;109:331.

Ulbright TM, Katzenstein AL. Solitary necrotizing granulomas of the lung: differentiating features and etiology. Am J Surg Pathol 1980;4:13.

Fungal Sinusitis

Gwattney JM Jr. Acute community-acquired sinusitis. Clin Infect Dis 1996;23:1209.

Iwen PC, Rupp ME, Hinrichs SH. Invasive mold sinusitis: 17 cases in immunocompromised patients and review of the literature. Clin Infect Dis 1997;24:1178.

Kinsella JR, Bradfield JJ, Gourley WK, Calhoun KH. Allergic fungal sinusitis. Clin Otolaryngol 1996; 21:389.

Meyer RD, Gaultier CR, Yamashita JT, et al. Fungal sinusitis in patients with AIDS: report of 4 cases and review of the literature. Medicine (Baltimore) 1994;73:69.

Stammberger H, Jakse R, Beaufort F. Aspergillosis of the paranasal sinuses: x-ray diagnosis, histopathology, and clinical aspects. Ann Otol Rhinol Laryngol 1984;93:251.

Washburn RG, Kennedy DW, Begley MG, et al. Chronic fungal sinusitis in apparently normal hosts. Medicine (Baltimore) 1988;67:231.

Respiratory Syncytial Virus

Aherne W, Bird T, Court SMD, et al. Pathological changes in virus infections of the lower respiratory tract in children. J Clin Pathol 1970;23:7.

Gardner PS, Turk DC, Aherne WA, et al. Deaths associated with respiratory tract infection in childhood. BMJ 1967;4:316.

Groothuis JR, Gutierrez KM, Lauer BA. Respiratory syncytial virus infection in children with bronchopulmonary dyplasia. Pediatrics 1988;82:199.

Halstead DC, Todd S, Fritch G. Evaluation of five methods for respiratory syncytial virus detection. J Clin Microbiol 1990;28:1021.

Henderson FW, Clyde WA Jr, Collier AM, et al. The etiologic and epidemiologic spectrum of bronchiolitis in pediatric practice. J Pediatr 1979;95:183.

Kellogg JA. Culture vs. direct antigen assays for detection of microbial pathogens from lower respiratory tract specimens suspected of containing the respiratory syncytial virus. Arch Pathol Lab Med 1991; 115:451.

Influenza Virus

Hers JFP, Masurel N, Mulder J. Bacteriology and histopathology of the respiratory tract and lungs in fatal Asian influenza. Lancet 1958;29:1141.

Oseasohn R, Adelson L, Kaji M. Clinicopathologic study of the thirty-three fatal cases of Asian influenza. N Engl J Med 1959;260:509.

Yeldandi AV, Colby TV. Pathologic features of lung biopsy specimens from influenza pneumonia cases. Hum Pathol 1994;25:47.

Herpes Simplex Virus

Graham BS, Snell JD Jr. Herpes simplex virus infection of the adult lower respiratory tract. Medicine 1983; 62:384.

Ramsey PG, Fife KH, Hackman RC, et al. Herpes simplex virus pneumonia: clinical, virologic, and pathologic features in 20 patients. Ann Intern Med 1982;97:813.

Hantavirus

Butler JC, Peters CJ. Hantavirus and hantavirus pulmonary syndrome. Clin Infect Dis 1994;19:387.

Duchin JS, Koster FT, Peters CJ, et al. Hantavirus pulmonary syndrome: a clinical description of 17 patients with a newly recognized disease. N Engl J Med 1994;330:949.

Nolte KB, Feddersen RM, Foucar K, et al. Hantavirus pulmonary syndrome in the United States: a pathological description of a disease caused by a new agent. Hum Pathol 1995;26:110.

Zaki SR, Greer PW, Coffield LM, et al. Hantavirus pulmonary syndrome. Pathogenesis of an emerging infectious disease. Am J Pathol 1995;146:552.

Cytomegalovirus

Rimsza LM, Vela EE, Frutiger YM, et al. Rapid automated combined in situ hybridization and immunohistochemistry for sensitive detection of cytomegalovirus in paraffin-embedded tissue biopsies. Am J Clin Pathol 1996;106:544.

Rodriguez-Barradas MC, Stool E, Musher DM, et al. Diagnosing and treating cytomegalovirus pneumonia in patients with AIDS. Clin Infect Dis 1996;23:76.

Weiss RL, Snow GW, Schumann GB, Hammond ME. Diagnosis of cytomegalovirus pneumonitis on bronchoalveolar lavage fluid: comparison of cytology, immunofluorescence, and in situ hybridization with viral isolation. Diagn Cytopathol 1991;7:243.

Woods GL, Thompson AB, Rennard SL, Linder J. Detection of cytomegalovirus in bronchoalveolar lavage specimens. Spin amplification and staining with a monoclonal antibody to the early nuclear antigen for diagnosis of cytomegalovirus pneumonia. Chest 1990;98:568.

Bacterial Pneumonia

Bartlett JG, Mundy LH. Community-acquired pneumonia. N Engl J Med 1995;333:1618.

Lerner AM, Jankauskas K. The classic bacterial pneumonias. Dis Mon 1975;2:1.

Marrie TJ. Community-acquired pneumonia. Clin Infect Dis 1994;18:501.

Actinomycosis

Brown JR. Human actinomycosis—a study of 181 subjects. Hum Pathol 1973;4:319.

Hotchi M, Schwartz J. Characterization of actinomycotic granules by architecture and staining methods. Arch Pathol 1972;93:392.

Legionella

Winn WC Jr. Legionnaires' disease: historical perspective. Clin Microbiol Rev 1988;1:60.

Winn WC Jr., Myerowitz RL. The pathology of the *Legionella* pneumonias. A review of 74 cases and the literature. Hum Pathol 1981;12:401.

Nocardia

Beaman BL, Beaman L. Nocardia species: host-parasite relationships. Clin Microbiol Rev 1994;7:213.

Beaman BL, Burnside J, Edwards B, Causey W. Nocardial infections in the United States, 1972–1974. J Infect Dis 1976;134:286.

Lerner PL. Nocardiosis. Clin Infect Dis 1996;22:891.

Scully RE, Marks EJ, McNeely WF, McNeely BU. Weekly clinicopathological exercise—pulmonary nocardiosis. N Engl J Med 1991;325:1155.

Rhodococcus

Harvey RL, Sunstrum JC. *Rhodococcus equi* infection in patients with and without human immunodeficiency virus infection. Rev Infect Dis 1991; 13:139.

Kwon KY, Colby TV. *Rhodococcus equi* pneumonia and pulmonary malakoplakia in acquired immunodeficiency syndrome: pathologic features. Arch Pathol Lab Med 1994;118:744.

Prescott JF. *Rhodococcus equi*: an animal and human pathogen. Clin Microbiol Rev 1991;4:20.

Mycobacteria

Bloom BR, Murray CJL. Tuberculosis: commentary on a reemergent killer. Science 1992;257:1055.

Dannenberg AM Jr. Delayed-type hypersensitivity and cell-mediated immunity in the pathogenesis of tuberculosis. Immunol Today 1991;12:228.

Kim JH, Langston AA, Gallis HA. Miliary tuberculosis: epidemiology, clinical manifestations, diagnosis, and outcome. Rev Infect Dis 1990;12:583.

Sepkowitz KA, Raffalli J, Riley L, et al. Tuberculosis in the AIDS era. Clin Microbiol Rev 1995;8:180.

Woods GL, Washington JA II. Mycobacteria other than *Mycobacterium tuberculosis*: review of microbiologic and clinical aspects. Rev Infect Dis 1987;9:275.

Histoplasma capsulatum

Goodwin RA Jr., Des Prez RM. Pathogenesis and clinical spectrum of histoplasmosis. Southern Med J 1973;66:13.

Goodwin RA Jr., Des Prez RM. Histoplasmosis. Am Rev Respir Dis 1978;117:929.

Wheat LJ, Slama TG, Zeckel ML. Histoplasmosis in the acquired immune deficiency syndrome. Am J Med 1985;78:203.

Blastomyces dermatitidis

Hardin HF, Scott DF. Blastomycosis. Occurrence of filamentous forms *in vivo*. Am J Clin Pathol 1974; 62:104.

Sarosi GA, Davies SF. Blastomycosis. Am Rev Respir Dis 1979;120:911.

Tan G, Kaufman L, Petersen EM, et al. Disseminated atypical blastomycosis in two patients with AIDS. Clin Infect Dis 1993;16:107.

Tenenbaum MJ, Greenspan J, Kerkering TM. Blastomycosis. Crit Rev Microbiol 1982;9:139.

Tuttle JG, Lichtwardt HE, Altshuler CH. Systemic North American blastomycosis. Report of a case with small forms of blastomycetes. Am J Clin Pathol 1953;23:890.

Watts JC, Chandler FW, Mihalov ML, et al. Giant forms of *Blastomyces dermatitidis* in the pulmonary lesions of blastomycosis: potential confusion with *Coccidioides immitis*. Am J Clin Pathol 1990;93:575.

Coccidioides immitis

Drutz DJ, Catazaro A. Coccidioidomycosis. Am Rev Respir Dis 1978;117:559.

Pappagianis D, Zimmer BL. Serology of coccidioidomycosis. Clin Micro Rev 1990;3:247.

Singh VR, Smith DK, Lawrence J, et al. Coccidioidomycosis in patients infected with human immunodeficiency virus: review of 91 cases at a single institution. Clin Infect Dis 1996;23:563.

Stevens DA. Coccidioidomycosis. N Engl J Med 1995; 332:1077.

Cryptococcus neoformans

Cameron ML, Bartlett JA, Gallis HA, Waskin HA. Manifestations of pulmonary cryptococcosis in patients with acquired immunodeficiency syndrome. Rev Infect Dis 1991;13:64.

Meyohas MC, Roux P, Bollens D, et al. Pulmonary cryptococcosis: localized and disseminated infections in 27 patients with AIDS. Clin Infect Dis 1995;21:628.

Pneumocystis carinii

Amin MB, Mezger E, Zarbo RJ. Detection of Pneumocystis carinii. Comparative study of monoclonal antibody and silver staining. Am J Clin Pathol 1992;98:13.

Foley NM, Griffiths MH, Miller RF. Histologically atypical Pneumocystis carinii pneumonia. Thorax 1993; 48:996.

Liu YC, Tomashefski JF Jr., Tomford JW, et al. Necrotizing Pneumocystis carinii vasculitis associated with lung necrosis and cavitation in a patient with acquired immunodeficiency syndrome. Arch Pathol Lab Med 1989;113:494.

Luna MA, Cleary KR. Spectrum of pathologic manifestations of Pneumocystis carinii pneumonia in patients with neoplastic diseases. Semin Diagn Pathol 1989; 6:262.

Nayar R, Tabbara SO. Detecting Pneumocystis carinii by immunohistochemistry. Lab Med 1996;27:547.

Saldana MJ, Mones JM. Cavitation and other atypical manifestations of Pneumocystis carinii pneumonia. Semin Diagn Pathol 1989;6:273.

Saldana MJ, Mones JM. Pulmonary pathology in AIDS: atypical Pneumocystis carinii infection and lymphoid interstitial pneumonia. Thorax 1994; 49:S46.

Travis WD, Pittaluga S, Lipschik GY, et al. Atypical pathologic manifestations of Pneumocystis carinii pneumonia in the acquired immune deficiency syndrome. Review of 123 lung biopsies from 76 patients with emphasis on cysts, vascular invasion, vasculitis, and granulomas. Am J Surg Pathol 1990; 14:615.

Weber WR, Askin FB, Dehner LP. Lung biopsy in Pneumocystis carinii pneumonia. A histopathologic study of typical and atypical features. Am J Clin Pathol 1977;67:11.

Aspergillus

Bardana EJ. The clinical spectrum of aspergillosis—Part 2: classification and description of saprophytic, allergic, and invasive variants of human disease. Crit Rev Clin Lab Sci 1981;13:85.

Denning DW. Invasive aspergillosis. Clin Infect Dis 1998;26:781.

Khoo SH, Denning DW. Invasive aspergillosis in patients with AIDS. Clin Infect Dis 1994;19:S41.

Rinaldi MG. Invasive aspergillosis. Rev Infect Dis 1983; 5:1061.

Scully RE, Mark EJ, McNeely WF, McNeely BU. Weekly clinicopathological exercise—aspergilloma. N Engl J Med 1990;323:1329.

Yousem SA. The histological spectrum of chronic necrotizing forms of pulmonary aspergillosis. Hum Pathol 1997;28:650.

CHAPTER
3

Infections of the Gastrointestinal Tract

An infectious disease begins with an encounter between an infectious agent and a susceptible human host. A large percentage of those encounters occur in the gastrointestinal tract, which is 25 linear feet of prime epithelial target without any of the protective coating provided by the squamous epithelium of the skin.

The normal gastrointestinal tract is a welcoming home to a vast array of microbial species that not only live peacefully with their innkeeper but also pay their way by providing essential services. These duties include enzymatic processing of waste products, such as bile, and helping exclude pathogenic organisms from the tract. Things go awry when the normal defenses have been overwhelmed by large numbers of microbial species or invading pathogens, a pathogen is particularly virulent, or the normal defenses have been damaged by potent immunosuppressive iatrogenic and natural factors.

The relationships between pathogens and the gastrointestinal tract are quite varied. In some instances, a pathogen needs only elaborate potent toxins as it multiplies in the gut, as occurs with botulism and food poisoning caused by *Staphylococcus aureus*, *Bacillus cereus*, and other organisms. Cholera represents a slightly more complicated scenario; the bacteria must first attach to the bowel mucosa before they produce their enterotoxin toxins. Other organisms, exemplified by certain nematodes, such as *Trichuris trichiura* and *Enterobacter vermicularis*; protozoa such as *Cryptosporidium*; and bacteria, such as *Helicobacter pylori*, *Salmonella* species, *Shigella* species, and *Campylobacter jejuni*, produce local damage to the gastrointestinal tract without causing distant or systemic infection.

The gastrointestinal tract is also a portal of entry for pathogens that produce systemic disease. The classic example of systemic infection from a gastrointestinal source is typhoid fever, but this scenario may also be found among fungal, viral, and parasitic organisms. The gastrointestinal tract itself may or may not suffer ill effects.

Less frequently, the alimentary tract is subject to infection, such as when a pathogen from a distant source reaches the bowel through the blood stream or lymphatics. Examples include infections caused by *Histoplasma capsulatum* and *Schistosoma mansoni*.

Bacteria are now known to produce intestinal lesions that were previously considered noninfectious. The most dramatic example of this phenomenon is *Helicobacter pylori*, which produces chronic gastritis, duodenal and gastric ulcers, lymphoproliferative disease, and possibly gastric carcinoma.

The morphologic expression of infection in the gastrointestinal tract is extremely varied. Most infections in immunocompetent individuals are self-limited and are diagnosed by examination of feces in a clinical microbiology laboratory without the need for biopsy and histologic analysis. Therefore, relatively little is known about the histopathology of many of these infections. If the toxin elaborated by a bacterium does not affect the gastrointestinal tract (e.g., botulinum toxin) or has no cytolytic activity (e.g., cholera toxin), the epithelium of the bowel may appear normal morphologically. If an active infection with a pyogenic organism is present (e.g., *Shigella*, *Salmonella*, *Yersinia*, or *Campylobacter*) or if a cytotoxin is elaborated (e.g., *Clostridium difficile*), acute inflammation with or without necrosis may result. If the organism normally elicits a granulomatous response (e.g., *Mycobacterium tuberculosis*, *H. capsulatum*, or *Salmonella typhi*), the response in the gut is also granulomatous. Viral infections tend to affect only the surface epithelium and elicit only a scant mononuclear inflammatory infiltrate. Exceptions to these rules exist, however. *Yersinia* infections in the bowel tend to be acutely inflammatory, although they are often centered in lymphoid tissue, whereas the characteristic stellate granulomas are usually found in regional lymph nodes. Herpes simplex virus (HSV) causes ulceration and acute inflammation in the esophagus, and disseminated cytomegalovirus (CMV) infection prominently afflicts vascular endothelium, often producing necrosis and ulceration.

Virtually the entire spectrum of interactions between infectious agents and hosts or victims may be studied in the gastrointestinal tract. The variety of the processes is impressive, and their complexity increases as more is learned about new agents of infection.

OROPHARYNGEAL ULCERS

Clinical History

A 51-year-old man from east Texas presented to an emergency department with complaints of dysphagia, low-grade fever, and weight loss of 25 pounds during the previous 6 weeks. On physical examination, he was afebrile, his pulse rate was 106 beats per minute, his respiratory rate was 16 breaths per minute, and his blood pressure was 100/70 mmHg. A few small gingival ulcers (0.5 mm in diameter) and white plaques on the tonsillar pillars were present within the oral cavity. Pertinent laboratory test results pertained to elevated serum alkaline phosphatase and lactate dehydrogenase (LDH) levels. The differential diagnoses included a malignancy and chronic histoplasmosis. He was referred to oral surgery for biopsy of the gingival ulcers; tissue was submitted for histologic studies and fungal culture.

Pathologic Findings

Sections of the biopsy specimens stained with hematoxylin and eosin (H and E) showed marked acanthosis of the squamous epithelium (Figure 3-1), and throughout the submucosa aggregates of histiocytes filled with small, round yeast cells that appeared to be surrounded by a halo or clear space were present (Figure 3-2A). Gomori's methenamine silver stain allowed numerous single and budding yeast cells to be more easily identified (Figure 3-2B).

Differential Diagnoses

The differential diagnoses of intracellular yeast cells (2–4 μm in diameter) include *H. capsulatum*, microforms of *Blastomyces dermatitidis*, *Candida glabrata*, *Penicillium marneffei*, and *Pneumocystis carinii*. In addition to yeast cells, amastigotes of *Leishmania* species and *Trypanosoma cruzi* (when within histiocytes) have a similar appearance; depending on the residence and travel history of the patient and the site of the lesions, they should be considered among the potential pathogens.

Microbiology

Fungal culture of the biopsy specimen grew *H. capsulatum*.

Comment

This case is a classic example of subacute (intermediate type) disseminated histoplasmosis for two reasons: (1) the clinical presentation of a patient who lives in or has traveled to an area endemic for *H. capsulatum* and (2) the histopathology of the lesions. Oropharyngeal ulcers, which typically are deep and have rolled edges but may have any appearance, occur in over 25% of adult patients with subacute disseminated histoplasmosis, and should suggest the diagnosis when present.

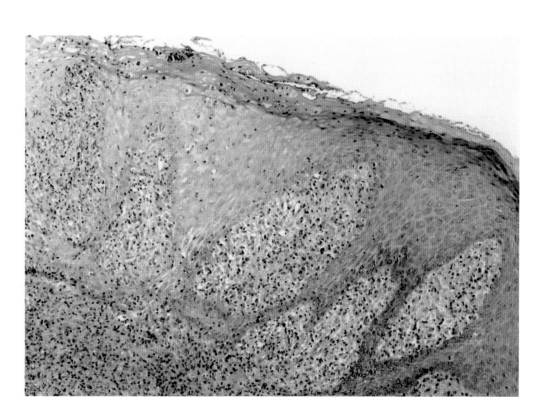

FIGURE 3-1. Section of the oral mucosal lesion shows marked acanthosis of the squamous epithelium and clusters of histiocytes within the submucosa (hematoxylin and eosin stain; original magnification, ×25).

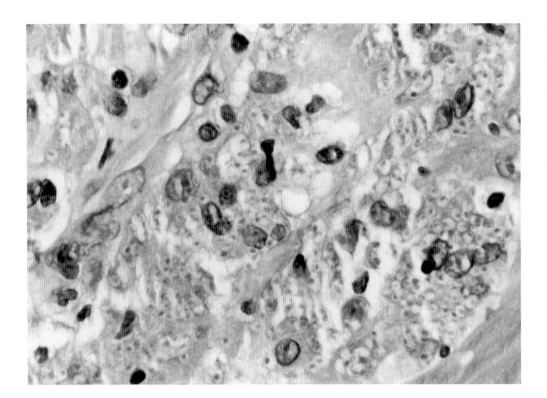

FIGURE 3-2A. Higher-power magnification of the section illustrated in Figure 3-1 demonstrates that the histiocytes are filled with numerous small, round yeast cells characteristic of *Histoplasma capsulatum* (hematoxylin and eosin stain; original magnification, ×250).

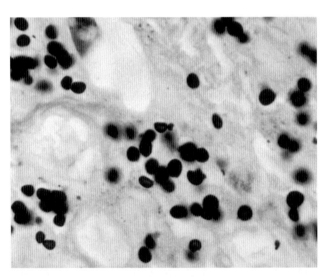

FIGURE 3-2B. By staining a section of the oral lesion illustrated in Figure 3-1 with a silver stain, the histoplasma yeast cells, several of which are budding, are more readily visible (Gomori's methenamine silver stain; original magnification, ×250).

The following are helpful diagnostic features used to identify other organisms that may resemble *H. capsulatum* in tissue sections. The intracellular microforms of *B. dermatitidis* are similar in size to yeast cells of *H. capsulatum*, but the former are multinucleate, have thicker walls and broad-based buds, and generally are mixed with larger, more typical *B. dermatitidis* cells 8–15 μm in diameter. Although yeast cells of *C. glabrata* are of comparable size to those of *H. capsulatum*, those of *C. glabrata* often are slightly larger and tend to be more variable in size. In addition, in sections stained with H and E, *C. glabrata* cells stain entirely; they do not exhibit the halo or pseudocapsule effect that is typical of *H. capsulatum*. *P. marneffei*, an organism indigenous to southeast Asia, is very similar in size and shape to *H. capsulatum* but divides by fission with a septum separating the developing daughter cells rather than by budding. Cysts of *P. carinii* may be confused with yeast cells of *H. capsulatum*, especially in sections of lung stained with methenamine silver; however, *P. carinii* cysts are predominantly extracellular and also do not reproduce by budding. Amastigotes of *Leishmania* species and *T. cruzi* are differentiated from cells of *H. capsulatum* by the presence of small, bar-shaped kinetoplasts that stain with hematoxylin. They typically do not stain with methenamine silver.

Diagnosis

Oropharyngeal ulcer of subacute disseminated histoplasmosis.

INFLAMMATORY MASS OF THE JAW WITH GRANULES

Clinical History

A 25-year-old man presented to the outpatient clinic with the complaint of swelling in the right sub-mandibular area. Seven months earlier, his mandibular third molars had been removed; afterward, he experienced continued edema and swelling of the right jaw. Five months after the procedure, a sequestrum involving the right jaw was removed. On physical examination, the patient was afebrile and had a pulse rate of 80 beats per minute, a respiratory rate of 18 breaths per minute, and blood pressure of 122/60 mm Hg. Examination of the oral cavity showed good dentition with no swelling, exudate, or other indication of infection. Inferior to the angle of the right jaw was a firm, tender mass measuring 4.2 cm × 3.5 cm. Laboratory test results were within normal limits. The patient was admitted for evaluation of this mass. The day after admission, fine needle aspiration of the mass was per-

formed. Material obtained was submitted for aerobic and anaerobic cultures and for cytologic studies.

Pathologic Findings

Examination of cytologic preparations showed sulfur granules, characteristic of actinomycosis (Figure 3-3). Appropriate antimicrobial therapy was initiated. One week after the patient was admitted, the mass was surgically excised. Histologic examination of sections of the excised mass showed granulation tissue with acute and chronic inflammation and one sulfur granule surrounded by neutrophils (Figure 3-4).

Differential Diagnoses

The differential diagnoses of granules include (in addition to actinomycosis) *Nocardia*; eumycotic mycetoma,

FIGURE 3-3A. Cytologic preparation of material aspirated from a mass at the angle of the right jaw shows a microcolony (granule) of filamentous bacteria surrounded by neutrophils and occasional histiocytes (Papanicolaou stain; original magnification, ×100).

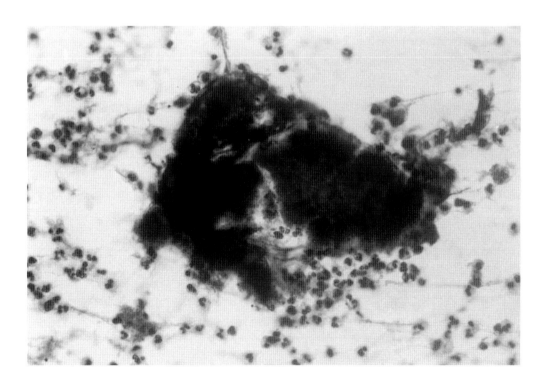

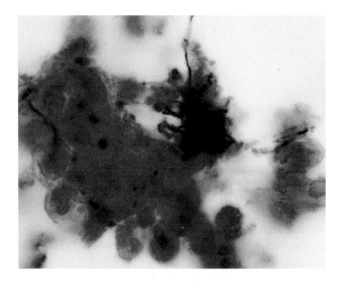

FIGURE 3-3B. Gram stain of the material illustrated in **A** shows beaded, gram-positive, filamentous bacilli extending centrifugally from the center of the microcolony, features consistent with actinomycosis (Gram-Weigert stain; original magnification, ×250). Cultures eventually grew *Actinomyces meyeri* and *Actinomyces odontolyticus.*

which may be caused by many different fungi; and botry-omycosis, most commonly caused by *S. aureus* and less often by *Pseudomonas* species, *Escherichia coli, Proteus vulgaris,* and *Streptococcus* species.

Microbiology

Anaerobic cultures of the aspirated material eventually grew *Actinomyces meyeri* and *Actinomyces odontolyticus.*

Comment

To help classify the granule, special stains for fungi (e.g., methenamine silver, which also stains filamentous bacteria, such as *Nocardia* and *Actinomyces*) and bacteria (e.g., Brown-Brenn, Brown-Hopps, or Gram-Weigert) must be performed. The granules of eumycotic mycetomas are composed of branched, septate, sometimes brown-pigmented hyphae. Actinomycotic granules, however, including those caused by *Nocardia,* consist of delicate, branched, gram-positive filaments approximately 1 µm wide. In the United States, *Nocardia* usually do not form dense microcolonies or granules but rather a network that contains an admixture of inflammatory cells within the branches. To distinguish actinomycetes from bacilli of *Nocardia,* a modified acid-fast stain should be performed. Nocardiae are weakly acid-fast; actinomycetes are not. Granules of botryomycosis are composed either of gram-positive cocci or gram-negative bacilli.

Diagnosis

Oral actinomycosis.

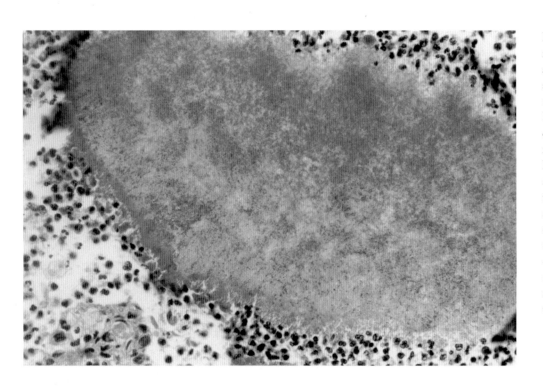

FIGURE 3-4. Section of a mass excised from the angle of the right jaw shows a microcolony (granule) of filamentous bacteria bordered by clublike eosinophilic material (Splendore-Hoeppli phenomenon) and surrounded by neutrophils. These features are consistent with a diagnosis of actinomycosis, which ultimately was confirmed by culture (hematoxylin and eosin stain; original magnification, ×100).

ESOPHAGITIS

Clinical History

A 35-year-old man diagnosed with the acquired immun-odeficiency syndrome (AIDS) 1 year earlier presented to an outpatient clinic with complaints of dysphagia, odynophagia, and chest pain for 3 weeks. Physical examination was noncontributory, except for oral thrush. Esophagoscopy revealed ulcers in the distal third of the esophagus. The differential diagnosis of infectious agents that cause ulcerative esophagitis in patients infected with human immunodeficiency virus (HIV) include *Candida*, CMV, and HSV. Brushings of the ulcers were collected for cytologic studies and viral culture, and several biopsy specimens were submitted for histologic evaluation.

Pathologic Findings

The brushings and biopsy samples showed changes consistent with cytopathic effects induced by infection with HSV (Figures 3-5 and 3-6).

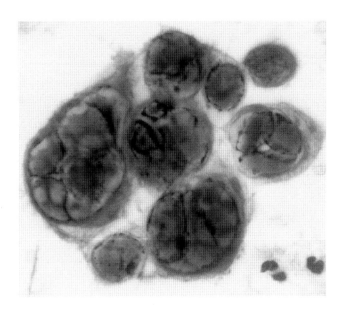

Figure 3-5. Cytologic preparation of esophageal brushings shows a cluster of epithelial cells that demonstrate cytopathic changes characteristic of infection with herpes simplex virus (i.e., multinucleation and margination of the nuclear chromatin that cause a ground-glass appearance; Papanicolaou stain; original magnification, ×250).

Figure 3-6. Biopsy of an esophageal ulcer shows epithelial cells that illustrate cytopathic effects of infection with herpes simplex virus: intranuclear inclusions and margination of the nuclear chromatin (hematoxylin and eosin stain; original magnification, ×100).

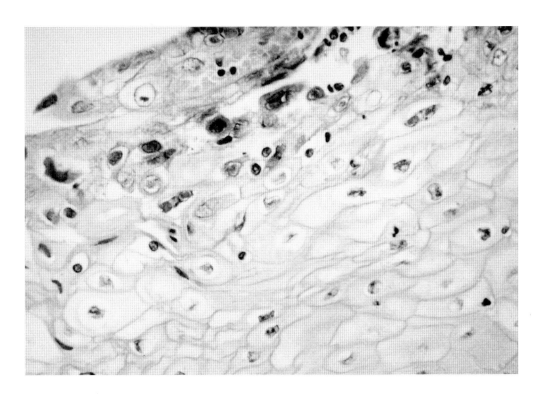

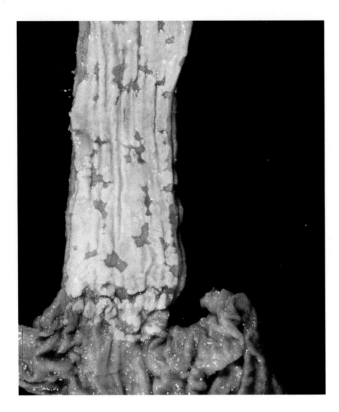

FIGURE 3-7. Photograph of an esophagus with multiple irregularly shaped ulcers caused by herpes simplex virus.

Microbiology

After incubation for 3 days, viral cultures of the esophageal brushings grew HSV type 1.

Comment

Esophagitis due to infection with HSV, CMV, or *Candida* is the most common of upper gastrointestinal tract disease in patients with AIDS. The gross appearance of the esophageal lesions is not diagnostic, but certain findings are more common for each of these infectious agents. For example, HSV typically produces multiple, deep esophageal ulcers (Figure 3-7), whereas CMV causes numerous large, shallow, erythematous ulcerations, although single ulcers may occur. *Candida* esophagitis, however, is characterized by the combination of diffuse ulcerations and friable, cheesy plaques that produce a cobblestone appearance.

HSV infects the squamous epithelial cells. In contrast, CMV typically involves the endothelium of blood vessels, causing ischemic ulcers (see Small Intestinal Ulcers with Perforation in a Patient with Acquired

FIGURE 3-8. Cytologic preparation of esophageal brushings shows candidal pseudohyphae and a few yeast cells, admixed with squamous epithelial cells and bacteria (Papanicolaou stain; original magnification, ×250).

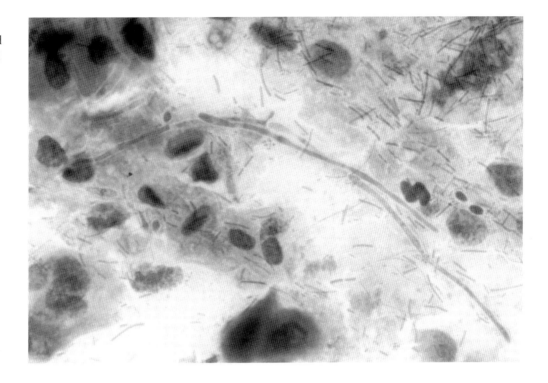

Immunodeficiency Syndrome). Therefore, cells with cytopathic changes due to CMV are not often found in cytologic preparations of esophageal brushings of the squamous epithelium. The cytologic and histopathologic findings of *Candida* esophagitis, which were not present in this patient, are illustrated in Figures 3-8 and 3-9.

Diagnosis

HSV esophagitis.

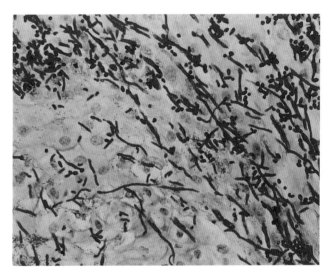

FIGURE 3-9. Section of an esophageal biopsy specimen shows pseudohyphae, hyphae, and budding and nonbudding yeast cells, findings that are consistent with candidal esophagitis (Periodic acid-Schiff–hematoxylin and eosin stain; original magnification, ×100).

ACTIVE CHRONIC GASTRITIS

Clinical History

A 65-year-old woman was referred to a gastroenterology clinic by her physician for evaluation of heme-positive stools and complaints of epigastric fullness and heartburn after a heavy meal. Physical examination was noncontributory. On esophagogastroduodenoscopic examination, the esophagus and duodenum appeared normal, but focal mucosal erythema and edema of the gastric cardia and fundus were present. Mucosal biopsies of the abnormal-appearing cardia were submitted for histologic examination.

Pathologic Findings

H and E–stained sections of the mucosal biopsies showed a mixed acute and chronic inflammatory cell infiltrate in the lamina propria and focal areas of disintegration and loss of the apical mucin-containing portions of the epithelial cells (Figure 3-10). Under higher-power magnification, curved bacteria were visible in the mucous layer on the epithelial surface (Figure 3-11). Immunohistochemical analysis of the tissue sections that used a monoclonal antibody specific for *H. pylori* identified the bacterium as *H. pylori.*

Comment

The differential diagnosis in this case is that of spiral bacteria in gastric mucosal biopsies. The most common pathogen is *H. pylori.* Another possible pathogen producing gastritis in humans is *Helicobacter heilmanii* (also known as *Gastrospirillum hominis*). *H. pylori* is a spiral or curved bacillus that causes active chronic gastritis and duodenal ulcers and more recently has been associated with gastric carcinoma and lymphoproliferative disorders. Characteristic histopathologic changes associated with active chronic gastritis are a mixed acute and chronic inflammatory cell infiltrate in the lamina propria, as was seen in this case; an infiltrate of neutrophils within the epithelium; and degenerative changes of the gastric epithelium, most commonly disintegration and loss of apical mucus with formation of epithelial pits. Other epithelial changes include microerosion, conventional erosion, and ulceration. In some cases of *H. pylori* infection, the inflammation in the lamina propria is predominantly chronic, and granulomatous gastritis has been described. Therefore, when any of these changes are observed in H and E–stained sections of gastric biopsies, close examination of the mucous layer on the crypt epithelium under high-power magnification for curved bacilli is warranted. Although bacilli of *H. pylori*

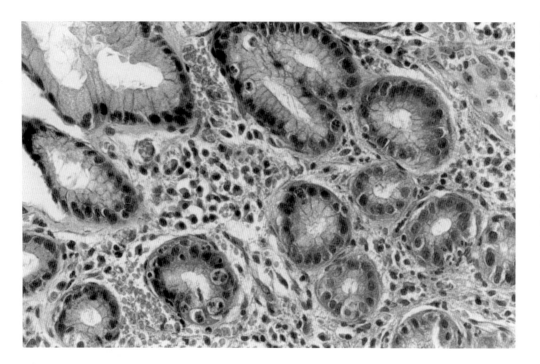

FIGURE 3-10. Section of a gastric biopsy specimen from a patient with *Helicobacter pylori* gastritis shows chronic active infection characterized by an infiltrate of mononuclear cells and neutrophils in lamina propria and neutrophils within the glandular epithelium (hematoxylin and eosin stain; original magnification, ×100).

FIGURE 3-11. Section of a gastric biopsy specimen shows numerous slender, spiral-shaped bacilli in the gastric mucus adherent to the epithelial surface (hematoxylin and eosin stain; original magnification, ×250). *Inset*: The bacilli are more readily detected in tissue sections by immunohistochemical staining using monoclonal antibodies to *H. pylori* (Dako stain; original magnification, ×100).

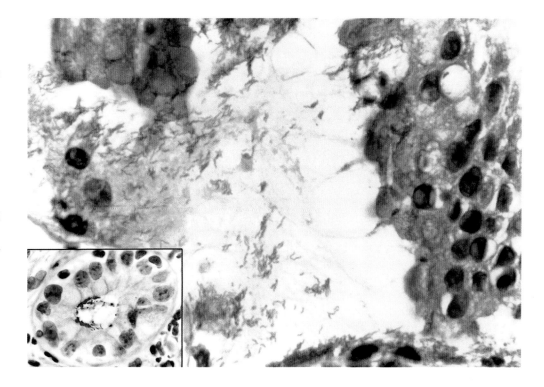

are seen in H and E–stained sections, other stains, particularly Warthin-Starry or Steiner silver stains (Figure 3-12), demonstrate the bacilli more dramatically. *H. pylori* also is visualized with modified Giemsa stain, acridine orange, Wright-Giemsa stain, or toluidine blue, but none of these appears to be as sensitive as the Warthin-Starry stain. Moreover, none of these stains adequately allows simultaneous detection of *H. pylori* bacilli and histopathologic evaluation of the features of the gastric mucosa. To overcome the latter problem, a single tissue section can be stained with a combination of the Steiner, H and E, and alcian blue stains; this technique is as sensitive as the Warthin-Starry stain for detecting the bacteria. Alternatively, an H and E counterstain can be performed on the section first stained with the Warthin-Starry or Steiner silver stains. Other methods for diagnosis of *H. pylori* gastritis include culture, serologic tests, and a urea breath test.

Diagnosis

H. pylori gastritis.

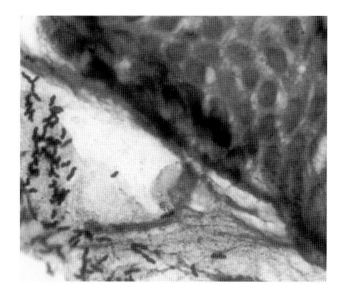

FIGURE 3-12. Staining sections of the biopsy shown in Figure 3-10 with a silver impregnation method accentuates the spiral-shaped bacilli of *Helicobacter pylori* (Steiner–hematoxylin and eosin stain; original magnification, ×250).

AFEBRILE SUBACUTE ABDOMINAL DISTRESS

Clinical History

A 33-year-old man was evaluated as an outpatient for a 2-month history of nausea (without vomiting), dysphagia, abdominal pain, early satiety, and weight loss of 15 pounds. He had been evaluated at another institution, where stool cultures revealed no pathogens and radiographic studies of his upper gastrointestinal tract were reported to be within normal limits. On physical examination, he was afebrile and had a pulse rate of 84 beats per minute, a respiratory rate of 20 breaths per minute, and a blood pressure of 120/69 mm Hg. The remainder of the examination was noncontributory.

Diagnostic evaluation included collection of three stool specimens on separate days to be examined for ova and parasites; no pathogens were visualized in the stained smears. Outpatient esophagogastroduodenoscopy revealed a 1-cm hiatal hernia of the distal esophagus and nonspecific inflammation of the duodenal bulb and duodenum, characterized by diffuse mucosal erythema.

Pathologic Findings

Biopsies of the endoscopically abnormal duodenal mucosa showed histologically normal villous architecture with clusters of cells lining the mucosal surface (Figure 3-13A). The absence of inflammation and the location of the cell clusters are typical of infection with *Giardia lamblia*. Close examination of the morphology of the parasites on the villous surface (Figure 3-13B) confirms the diagnosis of giardiasis.

Comment

The most common finding in biopsies of the small intestine in giardiasis is the presence of varying numbers of parasites within the crypts and on the surface of the villi; tissue invasion is rare. In tissue, only trophozoites are seen; cysts are not present. The appearance of the organisms varies based on the plane of sectioning. When cut longitudinally, trophozoites are elongated and slender. In

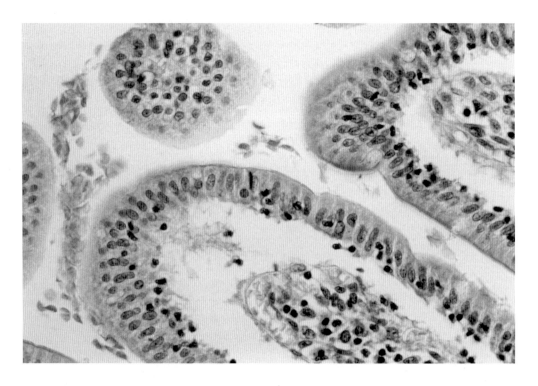

FIGURE 3-13A. Section of a duodenal biopsy shows normal villous architecture with clusters of *Giardia* lining the mucosal surface (hematoxylin and eosin stain; original magnification, ×100).

FIGURE 3-13B. Higher-power magnification of the section illustrated in **A** shows pear-shaped organisms with two nuclei, features diagnostic of *Giardia lamblia* trophozoites (Iron hematoxylin stain; original magnification, ×250).

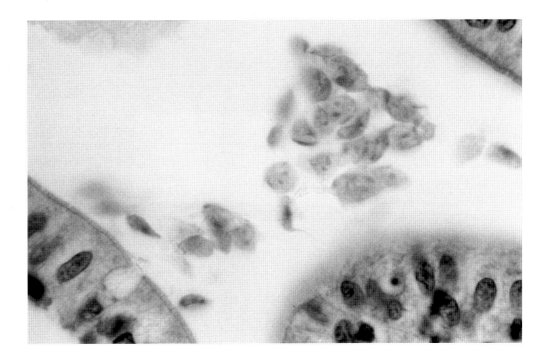

coronal sections, they resemble the trophozoites seen microscopically in smears of stool samples; in cross sections, they appear as small, concave organisms. The histologic changes of the mucosa in persons with giardiasis generally do not correlate well with the presence or absence of symptoms or the severity of the disease. In endemic areas, biopsies of older children and adults with giardiasis usually reveal a normal intestinal structure. In nonendemic areas, some biopsies from infected patients are normal structurally, whereas others have various changes that include loss of the brush border, epithelial cell damage, slight flattening of the villi, increased goblet cells, and a mixed inflammatory cell infiltrate of neutrophils and mononuclear cells in the lamina propria.

In most cases, the diagnosis of giardiasis is made in the clinical microbiology laboratory by microscopic detection of *G. lamblia* trophozoites and cysts in stool specimens. Diagnosis may require examination of several stool specimens collected at 2- to 3-day intervals, because elimination of parasites is cyclic in some infected persons, with periods of positive stools alternating with negative specimens. Invasive techniques, such as biopsy, are reserved for unusual cases in which examination of multiple stool samples fails to reveal the parasites.

Diagnosis

Giardiasis.

ENTEROCOLITIS ACCOMPANIED BY PULMONARY DISEASE

Clinical History

A 29-year-old man, known for 7 years to be infected with HIV, was admitted for evaluation of fever; chills; productive cough; hemoptysis; nausea; vomiting; and sharp, diffuse abdominal pain for 2 weeks. On physical examination, he appeared ill and was in moderate distress. His temperature was 37.8°C, his pulse rate was 126 beats per minute, his respiratory rate was 22 breaths per minute, and his blood pressure was 110/56 mm Hg. Auscultation of the chest revealed rales at the bases and decreased breath sounds. Abdominal examination showed moderate diffuse tenderness; his stool test for occult blood was negative. The chest radiograph was reported as possibly having diffuse interstitial infiltrates. Pertinent abnormal laboratory test results included a hemoglobin concentration of 10.1 g/dl and a serum LDH of 641 IU/liter.

Esophagogastroduodenoscopy and sigmoidoscopy, performed the day after admission, revealed diffuse mucosal erythema of the pyloric channel, duodenum, and sigmoid colon. Appropriate therapy was initiated. Two days later, the patient experienced bleeding from the upper gastrointestinal tract and severe respiratory distress that required intubation and mechanical ventilation. Material aspirated by tracheal suction was submitted for cytologic and microbiologic studies. Despite continued antiparasitic therapy and aggressive supportive care, the patient died 15 days after admission. Permission for autopsy examination was denied.

Pathologic Findings

Sections of biopsies of abnormal-appearing duodenum and colon showed nematodes, characteristic of *Strongyloides stercoralis* (Figures 3-14 and 3-15).

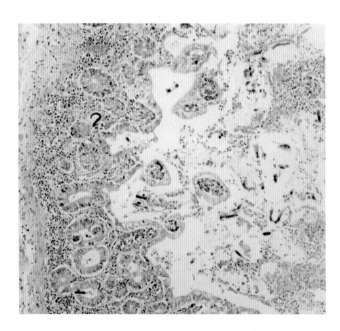

FIGURE 3-14. Section of duodenum shows mucosal ulceration, flattened villi, and larvae, consistent with *Strongyloides stercoralis*, within glands and free within the lumen (hematoxylin and eosin stain; original magnification, ×25).

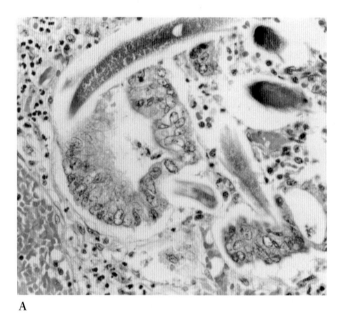

A

FIGURE 3-15. Higher-power magnification of the section illustrated in Figure 3-14 shows (**A**) adult worms within the intestinal mucosa and (**B**) the larval forms of *S. stercoralis* within the intestinal crypts (hematoxylin and eosin stain; original magnification, ×100).

FIGURE 3-15. (continued)

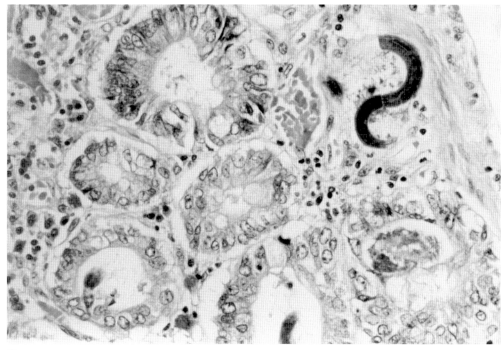

B

Microbiology

The smear of the material from the tracheal aspirate prepared for ova and parasite examination and the cytologic preparation revealed nematode larvae typical of *S. stercoralis* (Figure 3-16).

Comment

The diagnosis of strongyloidiasis is usually made in the microbiology laboratory by finding rhabditoid larvae (which must be differentiated from rhabditoid larvae of hookworms developing in stool samples that have been left at room temperature) in stool specimens. Hookworms also may be seen in tissue sections, where the worms are found attached to the mucosa throughout the small intestine. In contrast, all stages of the parasite are seen in the duodenum in strongyloidiasis (i.e., female worms, eggs, and larvae in different stages of development).

In immune competent hosts, the gross pathologic changes associated with strongyloidiasis are minimal. The duodenal mucosa appears normal or only slightly edematous. Sections of duodenum and colon typically show normal mucosal architecture with a minimal inflammatory cellular infiltrate, composed predominantly of mononuclear cells with a few neutrophils and eosinophils. Female worms are located deep in the crypts, accompanied by eggs, and larvae are found in the interstitium. In cross and oblique sections, females measure up to 35 μm in diameter, and often internal structures, such as the intestine, gonads, and immature eggs in the uterus

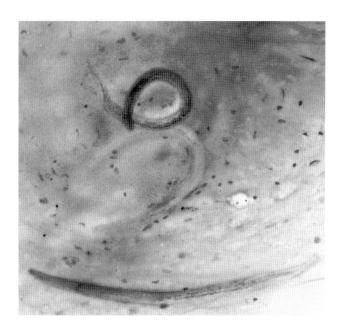

FIGURE 3-16. Cytologic preparation of material aspirated by tracheal suction shows larval forms consistent with the filariform stage of *Strongyloides stercoralis* (Gram stain; original magnification, ×250).

are visualized. Eggs that have recently been laid appear as basophilic or eosinophilic granular masses within a very thin shell, measuring 33 μm × 52 μm. Hatched rhabditoid larvae are approximately 14 μm in diameter and typically are found in the mucosa near the lumen.

In immunocompromised hosts with hyperinfection or overwhelming strongyloidiasis, several organ systems are involved. The small intestine may appear normal or show signs of duodenitis, whereas ulcerations measuring up to 20 mm in diameter are found throughout the colon. Consolidation and hemorrhage are present in all lobes of the lung due to transit of the larvae through the pulmonary circulation to the alveoli. Because of the migration through the lungs, strongyloidiasis may be diagnosed by detection of larvae in sputum specimens or, as occurred in this patient, by finding strongyloides larvae in the trachea en route from the alveoli to the mouth. Petechiae, edema, and focal necrosis are found in the brain. In tissue sections, the inflammatory infiltrate depends on the host's immune status, but often consists of mononuclear cells, neutrophils, occasional histiocytes and giant cells, and a few eosinophils. Dead larvae associated with granulomatous inflammation have been described in the liver and brain.

Diagnosis

Strongyloidiasis.

ENTEROCOLITIS IN A PATIENT WITH ACQUIRED IMMUNODEFICIENCY SYNDROME

Clinical History

A 56-year-old man, diagnosed with AIDS 2 years earlier, presented to an outpatient clinic with complaints of weight loss and a 2-week history of abdominal pain and cramping unrelieved by antacids and an increased frequency of bowel movements (approximately eight soft stools per day, all of small volume). On physical examination, he was afebrile and had a pulse rate of 105 beats per minute and a blood pressure of 109/69 mm Hg. Small perirectal ulcerations were present, and his stool contained no occult blood. The remainder of the examination was noncontributory. The differential diagnoses included infections caused by organisms associated with chronic diarrhea in a patient with AIDS, including *Cryptosporidium*, microsporidia, *Cyclospora cayetanensis*, *Mycobacterium avium* complex (MAC), CMV, *G. lamblia*, *Entamoeba histolytica*, and *C. difficile*.

Stool specimens were submitted to the microbiology laboratory to be examined for ova and parasites using stains for cryptosporidia and microsporidia, *C. difficile* toxin assay, and mycobacterial and viral cultures. Esophagogastroduodenoscopy and colonoscopy also were performed and revealed abnormalities of the duodenal and rectal mucosa, respectively. Biopsies of the abnormal areas were submitted for histologic examination.

Pathologic Findings

Sections of the duodenum stained with H and E showed flattening of the villi and an infiltrate of the lamina propria composed predominantly of lymphocytes with occasional plasma cells. Sections of the rectal biopsy also showed a moderate chronic inflammatory cellular infiltrate in the lamina propria. In sections of both biopsy specimens, rows of small, basophilic spherical structures were present at the epithelial cell surface of several glands (Figure 3-17). The inflammatory response and the size, shape, and location of the structures are consistent with a diagnosis of cryptosporidiosis.

Comment

The small intestine is the main target of cryptosporidia, but the organism may infect the large intestine, biliary tree, pancreas, gallbladder, and respiratory tract. With light infections, the tissue architecture is often normal, but heavy infections usually are associated with an inflammatory infiltrate of lymphocytes and plasma cells with occasional neutrophils, causing distortion of the normal mucosal architecture. Cryptosporidia, which appear as spheric structures

2–4 μm in diameter, are found in rows or clusters along the microvillous border of the enteric epithelial cells. Organisms can be detected with an H and E stain, but they have a more prominent appearance and thus are more easily visualized in sections stained by Fite's method (Figure 3-18). Although appearing to be attached to the surface of the enterocyte, electron microscopy reveals that they reside intracellularly just beneath the enterocyte cell membrane.

Microsporidia cause clinical manifestations identical to those associated with cryptosporidia, and they infect the same cell types. Moreover, the histologic findings associated with microsporidiosis resemble those of cryptosporidiosis, with the exception of the location of the organisms. With light microsporidial infections, the tissue architecture is often normal, whereas with heavy infections, villi are shortened and blunted, epithelial cells are necrotic, and the lamina propria contains lymphocytes and plasma cells. Microsporidia are located in the cytoplasm of enterocytes or other ciliated cells between the microvillous border and the nucleus. Although organisms can be seen in H and E–stained tissue sections, their detection requires careful search. The tissue diagnosis of microsporidiosis is most easily made by staining with a Brown-Brenn or Brown-Hopps method, the former of which stains the microsporidial spores (Figure 3-19). Microsporidia may also be detected in tissue with a Warthin-Starry or modified trichrome stain.

The clinical disease caused by *C. cayetanensis*, a relatively newly identified intestinal pathogen of humans, is also similar to cryptosporidiosis in patients with AIDS. The light microscopic findings associated with cyclospora

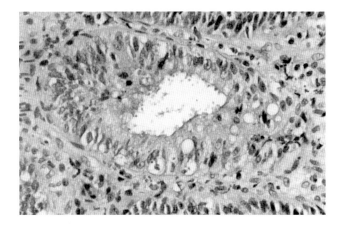

FIGURE 3-17. Section of a rectal biopsy shows small, spherical structures lining the crypt epithelium, features typical of cryptosporidiosis (hematoxylin and eosin stain; original magnification, ×50).

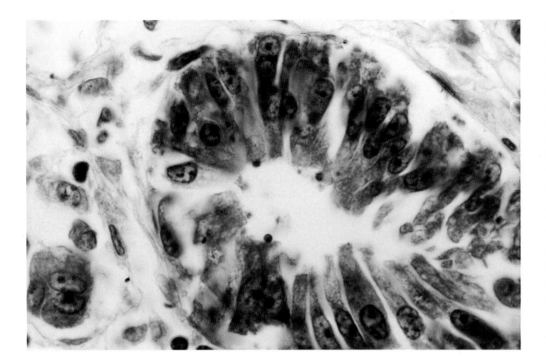

FIGURE 3-18. Section of small intestine stained by the modified Kinyoun method shows deep blue spheric cysts of *Cryptosporidium* at the luminal surface of the bowel epithelium. In tissue, these cysts do not stain with modified acid-fast stains (unlike the oocysts passed in feces), but their visualization is enhanced by the methylene blue counterstain (modified Kinyoun carbol fuchsin stain; original magnification, ×250).

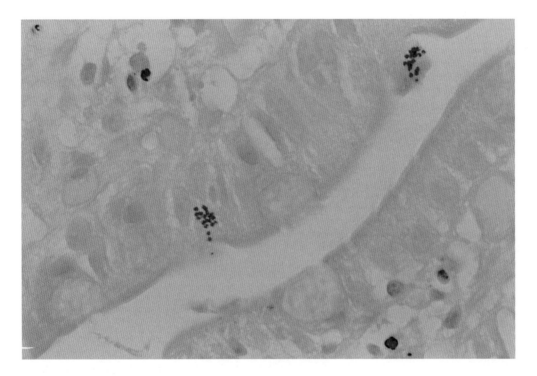

FIGURE 3-19. Section of a biopsy of the small intestine, stained with a tissue Gram stain, shows gram-variable spheric structures within the enterocyte cytoplasm. This feature is consistent with infection caused by microsporidia, such as *Enterocytozoon bieneusi* (Brown-Brenn stain; original magnification, ×250).

infection are reported to resemble those associated with microsporidiosis, but published descriptions are limited. Histologic findings in sections of duodenum stained with H and E include expansion of the lamina propria by an infiltrate of lymphocytes and plasma cells and the presence of *Cyclospora* organisms, which appear as basophilic, round to oval structures 4–10 μm in diameter surrounded by a clear zone within enterocytes. The organisms are located between the nucleus and the microvillous border,

predominantly in the villi of the duodenal mucosa; they have not been found in deep portions of the crypts and have not been identified in sites outside the duodenum. Organisms have not been detected in sections stained by a Giemsa stain or methenamine silver methods.

Diagnosis

Cryptosporidiosis.

SMALL INTESTINAL ULCERS WITH PERFORATION IN A PATIENT WITH ACQUIRED IMMUNODEFICIENCY SYNDROME

Clinical History

A 48-year-old man, known for 3 years to be infected with HIV, was admitted for evaluation of poor appetite, weakness, and diarrhea of several weeks' duration. On physical examination, he was afebrile and had a pulse rate of 89 beats per minute, a respiratory rate of 20 breaths per minute, and blood pressure of 112/68 mm Hg. Abdominal examination revealed tenderness, most pronounced in the left lower quadrant. His stool contained no occult blood. The remainder of the examination was noncontributory. Chest radiograph showed mild changes, reported as interstitial infiltrates versus old scarring. The differential diagnoses included infections associated with chronic diarrhea in persons infected with HIV, as discussed in the previous case. Stool specimens were examined for ova and parasites, including stains for cryptosporidia and microsporidia, detection of *C. difficile* toxin, and mycobacterial stains and culture. No parasites or acid-fast bacilli (AFB) were visualized in stained smears, and *C. difficile* toxin was not detected.

Over the next 2 days, the patient experienced increasing nausea and vomiting and became hypotensive, requiring transfer to the intensive care unit. Abdominal examination revealed distension, decreased bowel sounds, generalized tenderness (most severe in the right lower quadrant), and occult blood in the stool. Abdominal radiograph showed distended loops of small bowel and marked dilatation of the stomach, consistent with small bowel obstruction. The patient underwent immediate exploratory laparotomy, which revealed several areas of necrotic jejunum, one of which had perforated. Four segments of seemingly necrotic small intestine 1.5–3.0 cm long were resected and submitted for histologic studies. After the operation, the patient developed renal failure and severe respiratory distress, requiring intubation and ventilator support. Despite appropriate antiviral therapy and aggressive supportive care, he died 2 weeks later.

Pathologic Findings

The serosal surfaces of the resected segments of small intestine were covered with a green, fibrinous exudate, and the mucosa was covered by a green pseudomembrane. A perforation measuring 0.4 cm in diameter was found in the center of one segment. H and E–stained sections of all segments showed severe CMV enteritis, characterized by extensive CMV infection of the vascular endothelium and smooth muscle cells (Figure 3-20). Autopsy documented disseminated CMV involving the small intestine, lungs, adrenal glands, liver, and kidneys.

Comment

CMV colitis occurs in up to 10% of patients with AIDS. Symptoms are nonspecific and include diarrhea, abdominal pain, weight loss, anorexia, and fever. Colonoscopy typically demonstrates nonspecific, diffuse mucosal ulcerations. The diagnosis of CMV enteritis is based on the presence of CMV-induced cytopathic changes in sections of involved tissue, as illustrated in Figure 3-21, or vasculitis and nonspecific inflammation plus detection of CMV in the involved tissue by viral culture. Potential complications of CMV colitis are colonic perforation, as occurred in this case; hemorrhage; and peritonitis.

Infectious agents that may cause intestinal ulceration in addition to CMV are *Entamoeba histolytica*, *Balantidium coli*, *S. typhi*, *M. tuberculosis*, and *H. capsulatum*, the latter two of which are discussed in the next case. The classic lesion produced by *E. histolytica* is a flask-shaped ulcer involving the mucosa and sub-

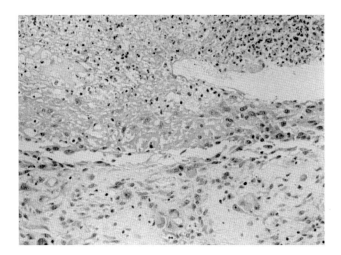

FIGURE 3-20. Section of resected small intestine from a patient with cytomegalovirus enteritis shows marked necrosis of the mucosa and submucosa. A fibrinopurulent exudate covers the luminal surface of the intestine, and in the underlying tissue, proliferating fibroblasts, a few chronic inflammatory cells, and enlarged vascular endothelial cells and smooth muscle cells are present (hematoxylin and eosin stain; original magnification, ×50).

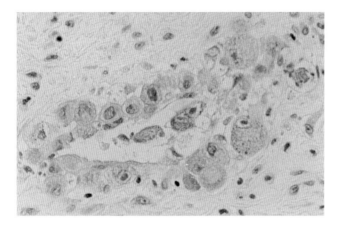

FIGURE 3-21. Higher-power magnification of the section shown in Figure 3-20 shows that the enlarged vascular endothelial cells have intranuclear inclusions surrounded by a clear halo and intracytoplasmic inclusions, characteristic of cytomegalovirus cytopathic effect (hematoxylin and eosin stain; original magnification, ×100).

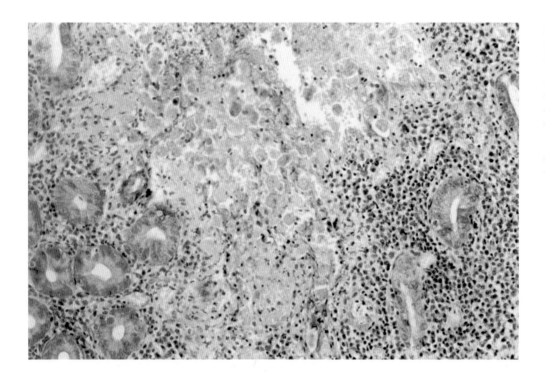

FIGURE 3-22A. Section of rectum shows mucosal ulceration, a mild chronic inflammatory infiltrate, and numerous protozoa of *Entamoeba histolytica* within the lamina propria (hematoxylin and eosin stain; original magnification, ×50).

mucosa of the colon. The ulcer bed contains degenerating neutrophils, epithelial cells, and fibrin and is surrounded by an inflammatory cell infiltrate of neutrophils and lymphocytes. Amoebae are found at the edge of the ulcers in the zone between dead and viable tissue. In tissue sections stained by the hematoxylin and eosin method, amebic trophozoites measure 15–25 μm in diameter and have uniformly vacuolated cytoplasm,

sometimes with ingested red blood cells (Figure 3-22). Trophozoites may resemble histiocytes, but differentiating the two usually is not difficult if the nuclear structures of both cells are compared. The histiocyte nucleus is more convoluted, has a variable chromatin pattern, and appears in almost all sections of the histiocyte; the trophozoite nucleus has a homogeneous chromatin distribution, is round and smaller, and is thus not present

FIGURE 3-22B. Higher-power magnification better demonstrates the morphologic features of *Entamoeba histolytica* trophozoites in tissue: a nucleus that is smaller than that of a histiocyte nucleus, finely vacuolated cytoplasm, and erythrophagocytosis (*arrows*; hematoxylin and eosin stain; original magnification, ×250).

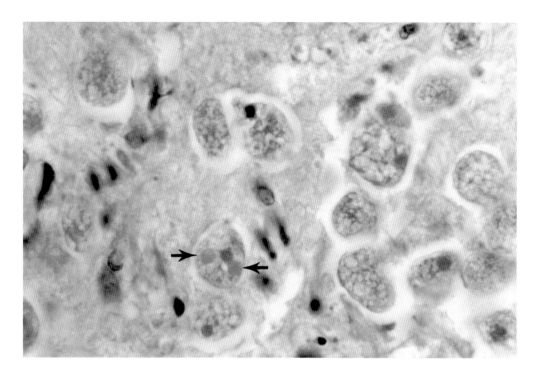

in many planes of section. Amoebae stain positively with the periodic acid–Schiff (PAS) stain and are easier to detect on low-power magnification in sections stained by this method. However, histiocytes also are PAS-positive, and this stain obscures the morphologic features of the amoebae. Therefore, the PAS stain can be used, if needed, to locate the area in which the parasites are found; the H and E stain should be used to study the parasite morphology. In transmural lesions, trophozoites migrate through the muscle layers until they reach the peritoneal surface, producing necrosis of the surrounding tissues. Organisms also invade blood vessels, causing lysis of the vessel wall and formation of thrombi with subsequent ischemia and tissue necrosis.

In acute balantidiasis, ulcers that vary in size and appear similar to those of amoebiasis generally are found throughout the entire colon. Ulcers may extend to the deeper layers of the colon, with subsequent perforation, but they typically do not extend laterally in the submucosa. Histopathologically, the ulcer of *B. coli* appears as a shallow indentation with a wide opening filled with necrotic debris. *B. coli* trophozoites, which measure up to 200 μm in diameter, are found at the edge and bottom of the ulcer (Figure 3-23) accompanied by an infiltrate of lymphocytes, plasma cells, and a few neutrophils. If the small blood vessels are involved, thrombosis occurs in the submucosa, and the ulcer usually extends deeply to the muscularis propria and may perforate. Dissemination of *B. coli* to the small intestine, stomach, and esophagus has been reported in immunocompromised persons but is rare.

Classic gastrointestinal lesions of typhoid fever involve the terminal ileum. Peyer's patches become

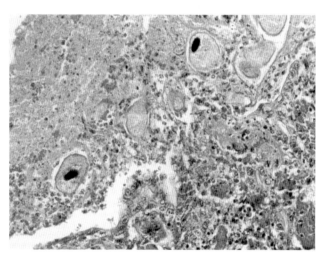

FIGURE 3-23A. Section of a colonic ulcer from a patient with acute balantidiasis shows necrosis of the mucosa and several large protozoa of *Balantidium coli*, each with dark-staining, reniform nucleus and peripheral cilia, within the necrotic debris (hematoxylin and eosin stain; original magnification, ×50).

enlarged, producing plaquelike elevations up to 8 cm in diameter. During the second week of illness, the mucosa overlying these areas is shed, resulting in oval ulcers with their long axes in the direction of enteric flow. The appearance of these ulcers resembles those seen with *Yersinia* infections (discussed in Granulomatous Inflammation of the Mid–Gastrointestinal Tract and Draining

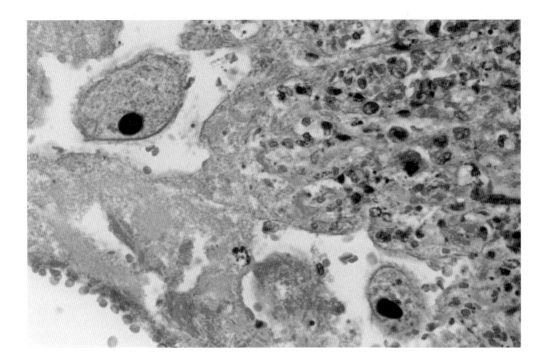

FIGURE 3-23B. Higher-power magnification of the section illustrated in **A** shows extensive coagulative necrosis, a sparse infiltrate of neutrophils, and *Balantidium coli* protozoa with prominent macronuclei (hematoxylin and eosin stain; original magnification, ×250).

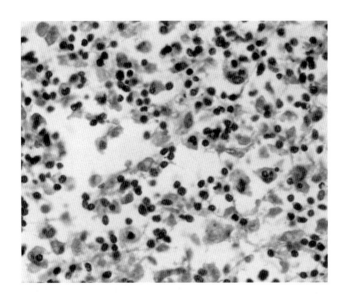

FIGURE 3-24. Section of an ulcerated lesion of the ileum from a patient with typhoid fever shows an infiltrate of mononuclear cells, predominantly macrophages and lymphocytes (hematoxylin and eosin stain; original magnification, ×100).

Lymph Nodes), but differs from the ulcers of tuberculosis, which are circular or transverse. Histopathologically, lesions of typhoid fever (Figure 3-24) comprise nodular aggregates of macrophages (granulomas) containing nuclear debris and sometimes bacteria and erythrocytes within Peyer's patches. Admixed with the macrophages are lymphocytes and plasma cells; neutrophils are seen on the ulcerated mucosal surface.

Diagnosis

CMV enteritis.

ENTERIC DISEASE WITH CASEATING GRANULOMAS

Clinical History

A 48-year-old man who had a history of injection drug use presented to an emergency department with complaints of productive cough and shortness of breath for 1 week; abdominal pain, nausea, and vomiting for 3 days; and weight loss of 20 pounds over the previous 2 months. On physical examination, he was afebrile and had a pulse rate of 104 beats per minute, a respiratory rate of 23 breaths per minute, and blood pressure of 94/56 mm Hg. Auscultation of the chest revealed decreased breath sounds bilaterally. His inguinal and left cervical lymph nodes were enlarged. His stool was heme-positive. Chest radiograph showed bilateral, diffuse, reticulonodular infiltrates. Pertinent abnormal laboratory test results included a hemoglobin concentration of 9.5 g/dl, a white blood cell count of 3,700 per μl with a left shift, elevation of the serum alkaline phosphatase and LDH, and the presence of antibodies to HIV. The admitting differential diagnoses included disseminated tuberculosis, bacterial pneumonia, *P. carinii* pneumonia, and lymphoma. Antimicrobial therapy appropriate for community-acquired pneumonia was initiated.

Sputum specimens were collected for bacterial, fungal, and mycobacterial studies. No predominant organism was detected in the Gram-stained smear of sputum, and no fungal elements were visualized in the sputum KOH preparation. A few AFB were seen in the sputum smear stained with auramine O, and appropriate antituberculous agents were added to the treatment regimen. On day 5 of his hospitalization, the patient developed severe respiratory distress requiring intubation and ventilator support, and he experienced an episode of bleeding from the upper gastrointestinal tract. Despite aggressive supportive care, he died 2 days later.

Pathologic Findings

Autopsy revealed pulmonary cavitary tuberculosis and disseminated tuberculosis, including involvement of the gastrointestinal tract. In the middle portion of the jejunum, a 1-cm transverse mucosal ulcer covered with a green membrane was found, and at the ileocecal junction, a deeper ulcer that had two areas of perforation and measured 6 cm in diameter was present. Histologic examination of sections of the larger ulcer showed multiple caseating and noncaseating granulomas (Figure 3-25) involving the full thickness of the bowel wall, including the margins of the perforations. Sections stained by the Ziehl-Neelsen method showed beaded AFB (Figure 3-26).

FIGURE 3-25. Section of tissue from the cecum shows a mature granuloma with minimal central necrosis (hematoxylin and eosin stain; original magnification, ×50).

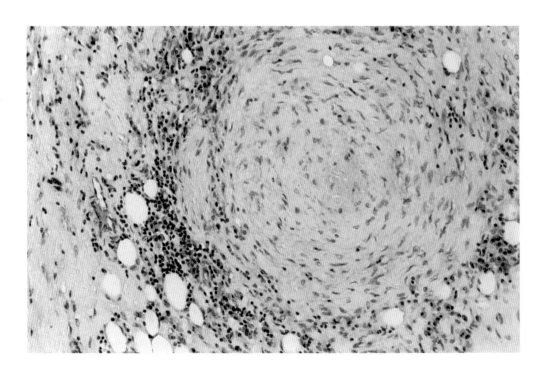

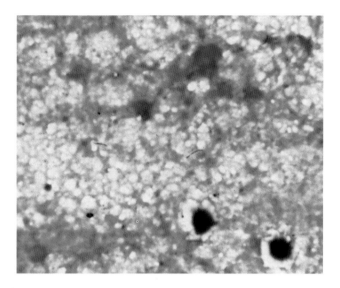

FIGURE 3-26. Section of this tissue stained by the Ziehl-Neelsen method shows a few acid-fast bacilli in the central areas of necrosis (Ziehl-Neelsen stain; original magnification, ×250). Premortem sputum specimens and postmortem lung tissue from this patient grew *Mycobacterium tuberculosis*.

Microbiology

M. tuberculosis was recovered from premortem sputum and postmortem lung tissue.

Comment

In this particular patient, the most probable diagnosis is tuberculosis or, less likely, infection with a nontuberculosis mycobacterium, based on his premortem sputum smear containing AFB. However, if AFB smear data were not available, histoplasmosis also would be included as a possible cause of intestinal perforation associated with caseating granulomas. Thus, based on the differential diagnosis, stains for AFB and fungi should be performed on sections of involved tissue. In this case, AFB were present, but this finding does not allow a specific diagnosis. Culture is necessary for identification of the mycobacterium. In patients with AIDS, *Mycobacterium kansasii*, MAC, or *Mycobacterium genavense* may infect the gastrointestinal tract. The latter two mycobacteria, however, do not elicit formation of mature granulomas; rather, infection with these organisms is associated with diffuse infiltrates of histiocytes with granular cytoplasm. Granulomas may also be observed in the bowel wall in Crohn's disease.

Histologic findings in sections of small intestine from a patient with disseminated histoplasmosis are illustrated in Figure 3-27. In this case, marked necrosis occurs with few intact histiocytes, and the yeast cells appear to be extracellular. More commonly, the host response associated with disseminated histoplasmosis is characterized by aggregates of histiocytes, as is true of disseminated MAC

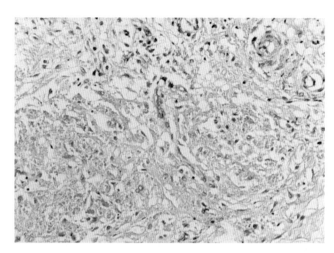

FIGURE 3-27A. Section of an ulcerated lesion in the small intestine shows a well-circumscribed area of necrosis with a few intact histiocytes involving the serosa (hematoxylin and eosin stain; original magnification, ×50).

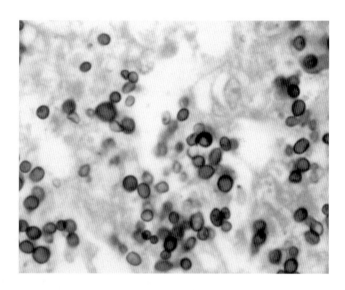

FIGURE 3-27B. Staining with methenamine silver shows many small (3–5 μm) budding yeast cells, most of which appear to be extracellular (methenamine silver stain; original magnification, ×250). The features of these yeast are typical of *Histoplasma capsulatum*, which ultimately grew from the fungal culture of the necrotic tissue.

and *M. genavense*, and the yeast cells of *H. capsulatum* are found intracellularly within histiocytes.

Diagnosis

Tuberculosis.

ENTERIC DISEASE WITH DIFFUSE HISTIOCYTIC INFILTRATES

Clinical History

A 42-year-old man was referred to a gastroenterology clinic for evaluation of weakness, epigastric pain, diarrhea, and weight loss of 20 pounds during the previous 8 months. On physical examination, he was cachectic and afebrile; his pulse rate was 104 beats per minute, and his blood pressure was 97/63 mm Hg. The only pertinent laboratory test result was a hemoglobin concentration of 8.5 g/dl. The result of a serologic test for antibodies to HIV was negative. Chest and abdominal radiographs showed no abnormalities. A single stool examination revealed no ova or parasites. Outpatient esophagogastroduodenoscopy revealed normal esophagus and stomach, but the mucosa of the duodenal bulb and duodenum was diffusely friable and had a white reticular pattern. Duodenal biopsies were performed.

Pathologic Findings

Histologic examination of sections of biopsies of the abnormal-appearing mucosa showed blunted villi with aggregates of foamy histiocytes in the lamina propria (Figure 3-28A). Sections stained by the PAS method showed numerous macrophages containing PAS-positive material in the lamina propria (Figure 3-28B), whereas stains for fungi and AFB were negative.

Differential Diagnoses

Infectious agents associated with aggregates of histiocytes in the gastrointestinal tract include Whipple's disease bacillus (*Tropherema whippleii*), *H. capsulatum*, MAC, and *M. genavense*.

Comment

Of the potential pathogens, MAC and *M. genavense* are extremely unusual in persons not infected with HIV. In addition, the macrophages associated with MAC infection often have a more foamy appearance than the macrophages associated with Whipple's disease. Tissue stains useful for diagnosis are PAS, Gomori methenamine silver, and Ziehl-Neelsen methods. Electron microscopic examination of the tissue is helpful for confirmation of

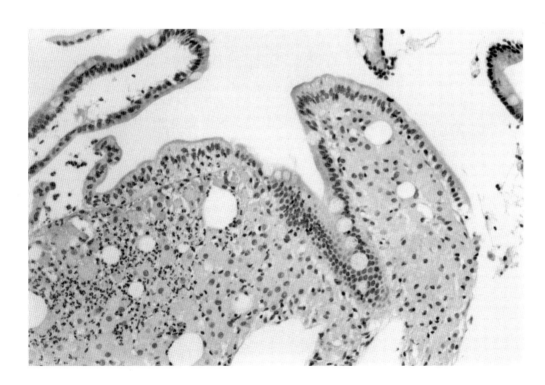

FIGURE 3-28A. Section of duodenal biopsy from a patient with Whipple's disease shows blunted villi and a diffuse infiltrate of granular macrophages with a focal aggregate of neutrophils in the lamina propria (hematoxylin and eosin stain; original magnification, ×250).

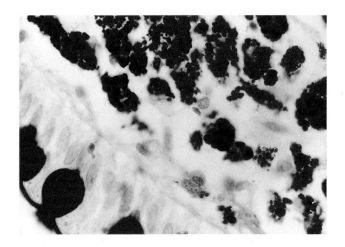

FIGURE 3-28B. Section of tissue illustrated in **A** stained by the periodic acid–Schiff (PAS) method shows macrophages filled with intensely PAS-positive globules, consistent with a diagnosis of Whipple's disease (periodic acid–Schiff stain; original magnification, ×250).

the presence of Whipple bacilli but is not usually necessary, because bacilli are identified by light microscopy in properly prepared specimens. Although the organism has yet to be cultivated, its phylogeny has been determined by DNA sequence analysis of the polymerase chain reaction product of amplification of the 16S rRNA gene.

Findings characteristic of MAC enteritis are illustrated in Figure 3-29. The histologic appearance of infection with *M. genavense* in tissue sections stained with H and E or a stain for AFB cannot be differentiated from that of MAC. Therefore, culture must be performed to differentiate these species.

Diagnosis

Whipple's disease.

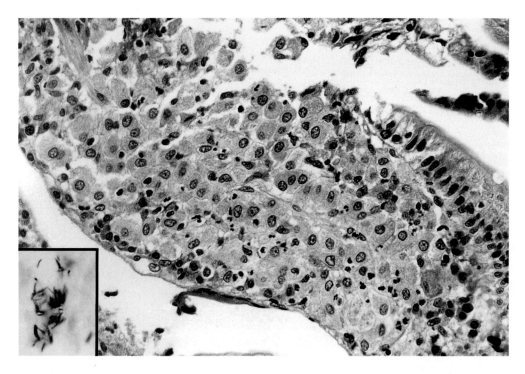

FIGURE 3-29. Section of small intestine from a patient with acquired immunodeficiency syndrome shows a diffuse infiltrate of macrophages in the lamina propria, similar in appearance to the biopsy illustrated in Figure 3-28A (hematoxylin and eosin stain; original magnification, ×100). *Inset:* A section stained by the Ziehl-Neelsen method shows that the macrophages are filled with acid-fast bacilli (Ziehl-Neelsen stain; original magnification, ×250). Mycobacterial cultures of blood from this patient grew *Mycobacterium avium* complex.

GRANULOMATOUS INFLAMMATION OF THE MID–GASTROINTESTINAL TRACT AND DRAINING LYMPH NODES

Clinical History

A 2-year-old girl was admitted to a hospital with persistent abdominal pain, vomiting, and diarrhea. She had had intermittent fever for 12 days. The peripheral white cell count varied between 20,000 and 30,000 cells per µl with a shift to the left. Her temperature was 38.7°C, her pulse rate was 120 beats per minute, and her respiratory rate was 24 breaths per minute. No abdominal masses were palpated. Right-sided abdominal guarding and rectal tenderness on the right were noted. The preoperative diagnosis was acute appendicitis. At the operation, the appendix was erythematous and thickened, as was the distal ileum. Multiple mesenteric lymph nodes were enlarged. Postoperatively, the fever resolved and she recovered uneventfully.

Pathology

No fecaliths were found in her appendix. Multiple areas of suppuration and necrosis were present in the mucosa of the appendix, and the overlying epithelium was focally ulcerated. In several areas, however, the association of the suppuration with submucosal lymphoid tissue was evident as a linear suppurative granuloma extending through the submucosa, whereas the overlying mucosa was intact. The histologic lesion had the appearance of a suppurative granuloma with geographic necrosis. The necrotic tissue contained both mononuclear cells and polymorphonuclear neutrophils (Figure 3-30). Tissue from the distal ileum and the mesenteric lymph nodes showed stellate granulomas (Figure 3-31).

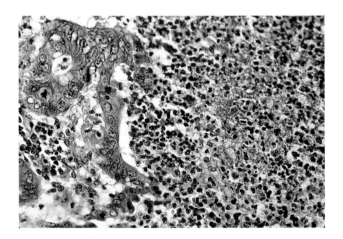

FIGURE 3-30. The inflammatory process containing necrotic material, neutrophils, and macrophages has ruptured from the submucosa through the appendiceal epithelium (hematoxylin and eosin stain; high-power magnification). A culture of the specimen yielded pure growth of *Yersinia enterocolitica* serogroup O:8.

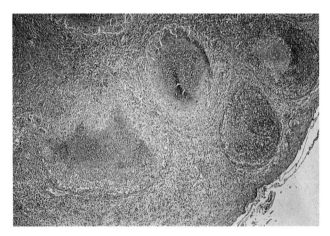

FIGURE 3-31. Biopsy of a mesenteric lymph node shows a well-demarcated stellate granuloma (hematoxylin and eosin stain; low-power magnification).

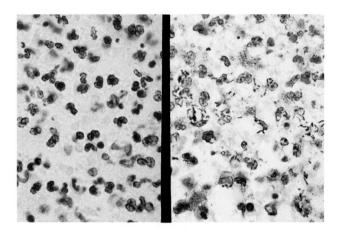

FIGURE 3-32. A Dieterle silver-impregnation stain (left) and a Brown-Hopps stain on an adjacent section (right) demonstrate numerous bacilli of *Yersinia enterocolitica* in inflammatory lesions.

A Brown-Hopps stain of the appendix disclosed no bacteria in the lesions, whereas the Dieterle stain revealed many bacillary organisms in the areas of suppurative necrosis (Figure 3-32). A modified Brown-Hopps stain was performed in another laboratory, revealing numerous gram-negative bacilli in the necrotic tissue. The importance of small, methodologic variations and technical experience in the success of these "standard" stains is illustrated by this dichotomy of results.

Microbiology

A portion of excised appendix, submitted for culture by the surgical pathologist, grew a pure culture of *Yersinia enterocolitica*, serotype O:8, biotype 2.

Commentary

The genus *Yersinia* contains several human pathogens, including *Yersinia pestis*, *Yersinia pseudotuberculosis*, and *Y. enterocolitica*. *Y. pestis* is the cause of classic plague, a suppurative disease of lymph nodes associated with septicemia, and, rarely, primary pulmonary disease. It is transmitted by fleas and maintained in nature in populations of sylvatic rodents and rats. The other two *Yersinia* species most often produce gastrointestinal dis-

ease. They are transmitted in contaminated water or food and do not have a rodent host or insect vector.

Y. enterocolitica and *Y. pseudotuberculosis* produce a clinical syndrome dominated by gastroenteritis, appendicitis, mesenteric adenitis, or a combination of these lesions. *Y. enterocolitica*, by far the more frequent pathogen, usually produces uncomplicated gastroenteritis, especially in young children. Extraintestinal disease, predominantly thyroid disease and nonsuppurative arthritis apparently of immunopathologic origin, occur in Scandinavia more frequently than in the United States. Interesting epidemiologic associations of particular serotypes with disease have been recorded. In the United States, the most frequent isolates are serotype O:8, as represented by this case from northern New England, whereas 50 miles north in Quebec, Canada, the predominant serotype is O:3. Infections with *Y. pseudotuberculosis*, although much less common, are more likely to result in isolated mesenteric lymphadenitis without overt gastroenteritis. A variety of skin lesions, conjunctivitis, and pharyngitis have been ascribed to *Yersinia* species. Rarely, either species can produce fatal septicemic disease in immunocompromised patients and individuals with disorders of iron storage. These bacteria are able to grow at refrigerator temperatures (psychrophiles). This physiologic characteristic is probably responsible for the relatively frequent association of *Yersinia* species with contamination of blood products and septicemic transfusion reactions. At least one outbreak of epidemic disease was produced by contaminated milk that seemed to have been pasteurized with no break in technique, perhaps because of the growth of small numbers of residual bacteria in the stored refrigerated milk.

The histologic response to infection with *Yersinia* species is the suppurative granuloma involving particularly lymphoid tissue. Nonspecific inflammation and ulceration of the gastrointestinal mucosa may also be present. Giant cells, which are rare in suppurative granulomas, are particularly likely to occur in disease produced by *Y. pseudotuberculosis*. The differential diagnosis is suppurative granulomas, which is discussed in Chapter 8. In the clinical situations discussed here, by far the most likely pathogen is yersinia.

Diagnosis

Y. enterocolitica ileitis, appendicitis, and mesenteric adenitis.

RECOMMENDED READING

Histoplasma capsulatum

Goodwin RA Jr, Des Prez RM. Pathogenesis and clinical spectrum of histoplasmosis. Southern Med J 1973; 66:13.

Goodwin RA Jr, Des Perez RM. Histoplasmosis. Am Rev Respir Dis 1978;117:929.

Wheat LJ, Slama TG, Zeckel ML. Histoplasmosis in the acquired immune deficiency syndrome. Am J Med 1985;78:203.

Actinomyces

Brown JR. Human actinomycosis—a study of 181 subjects. Hum Pathol 1973;4:319.

Hotchi M, Schwartz J. Characterization of actinomycotic granules by architecture and staining methods. Arch Pathol 1972;93:392.

Esophagitis

Wheeler RR, Peacock JE Jr, Cruz JM, Richter JE. Esophagitis in the immunocompromised host: role of esophagoscopy in diagnosis. Rev Infect Dis 1987; 9:88.

Wilcox CM, Schwartz DA, Clark WS. Esophageal ulceration in human immunodeficiency virus infection. Ann Intern Med 1995;122:143.

Helicobacter pylori

Dixon MF. Histological responses to *Helicobacter pylori* infection: gastritis, atrophy and preneoplasia. Baillieres Clin Gastroenterol 1995;9:467.

Dixon MF, Genta RM, Yardley JH, et al. Classification and grading of gastritis—the updated Sydney system. Am J Surg Pathol 1996;20:1161.

Dunn BE, Cohen H, Blaser MJ. *Helicobacter pylori*. Clin Microbiol Rev 1997;10:720.

Genta RM, Hamner HW, Graham DY. Gastritis lymphoid follicles in *Helicobacter pylori* infection: frequency, distribution, and response to triple therapy. Hum Pathol 1993;24:577.

Goodwin CS. *Helicobacter pylori* gastritis, peptic ulcer, and gastric cancer: clinical and molecular aspects. Clin Infect Dis 1997;25:1017.

Giardia

Gutierrez Y. Intestinal and Urogenital Flagellates. In Diagnostic Pathology of Parasitic Infections with Clinical Correlations. Philadelphia: Lea and Febiger, 1990; 10–15.

Ortega YR, Adam RD. Giardia: overview and update. Clin Infect Dis 1997;25:545.

Wolfe MS. Giardiasis. Clin Microbiol Rev 1992;5:93.

Strongyloides stercoralis

Genta RM. Global prevalence of strongyloidiasis: critical review with epidemiologic insights into the prevention of disseminated disease. Rev Infect Dis 1989;11:755.

Gutierrez Y. Rhabdita-Strongyloides and Other Free Living Nematodes. In Diagnostic Pathology of Parasitic Infections with Clinical Correlations. Philadelphia: Lea and Febiger, 1990;185–195.

Mahmoud AAF. Strongyloidiasis. Clin Infect Dis 1996; 23:949.

Neva FA. Biology and immunology of human strongyloidiasis. J Infect Dis 1986;153:397.

Cryptosporidium

Current WL, Garcia LS. Cryptosporidiosis. Clin Microbiol Rev 1991;4:325.

Current WL, Garcia LS. Cryptosporidiosis. Clin Lab Med 1991;11:873.

Gutierrez Y. The Intestinal Amebae. In Diagnostic Pathology of Parasitic Infections with Clinical Correlations. Philadelphia: Lea and Febiger, 1990;55–79.

Microsporidia

Giang TT, Kotler DP, Garro ML, Orenstein JM. Tissue diagnosis of intestinal microsporidiosis using the chromotrope-2R modified trichrome stain. Arch Pathol Lab Med 1993;117:1249.

Lamps LW, Bronner MP, Vnencak-Jones CL, et al. Optimal screening and diagnosis of microsporida in tissue sections. A comparison of polarization, special stains, and molecular techniques. Am J Clin Pathol 1998;109:404.

Weber R, Bryan RT, Schwartz DA, Owen RL. Human microsporidial infections. Clin Microbiol Rev 1994; 7:426.

Cyclospora

Sun T, Ilardi CF, Asnis D, et al. Light and electron microscopic identification of cyclospora species in the small intestine. Evidence of the presence of asexual life cycle in human host. Am J Clin Pathol 1996;105:216.

Cytomegalovirus

Drew WL. Nonpulmonary manifestations of cytomegalovirus infection in immunocompromised patients. Clin Microbiol Rev 1992;5:204.

Drew WL. Cytomegalovirus infection in patients with AIDS. Clin Infect Dis 1992;4:608.

Entamoeba histolytica

Gutierrez Y. The Intestinal Amebae. In Diagnostic Pathology of Parasitic Infections with Clinical Correlations. Philadelphia: Lea and Febiger, 1990; 55–79.

Lesh FA. Massive development of amebas in the large intestine. Am J Trop Med Hyg 1975;24:383.

Phillips SC, Mildvan D, William DC, et al. Sexual transmission of enteric protozoa and helminths in a venereal-disease-clinic population. N Engl J Med 1981;305:603.

Sorvillo FJ, Strassburg MA, Seidel J, et al. Amebic infections in asymptomatic homosexual men, lack of evidence of invasive disease. Am J Publ Health 1986;76:1137.

Tuberculosis

Bloom BR, Murray CJL. Tuberculosis: commentary on a reemergent killer. Science 1992;257:1055.

Dannenberg AM Jr. Delayed-type hypersensitivity and cell-mediated immunity in the pathogenesis of tuberculosis. Immunol Today 1991;12:228.

Hoon JR, Dockerty MB, Pemberton J. Ileocecal tuberculosis including a comparison of this disease with nonspecific regional enterocolitis and noncaseous tuberculated enterocolitis. Inter Abstr Surg 1950; 91:417.

Kim JH, Langston AA, Gallis HA. Miliary tuberculosis: epidemiology, clinical manifestations, diagnosis, and outcome. Rev Infect Dis 1990;12:583.

Schulze K, Warner HA, Murray D. Intestinal tuberculosis. Experience at a Canadian teaching institution. Am J Med 1977;63:735.

Sepkowitz KA, Raffalli J, Riley L, et al. Tuberculosis in the AIDS era. Clin Microbiol Rev 1995;8:180.

Woods GL, Washington JA II. Mycobacteria other than Mycobacterium tuberculosis: review of microbiologic and clinical aspects. Rev Infect Dis 1987;9:275.

Whipple's Disease/Mycobacterium avium Complex

Inderlied CB, Kemper CA, Bermudez LEM. The Mycobacterium avium complex. Clin Microbiol Rev 1993; 6:266.

Klatt EC, Jensen DF, Meyer PR. Pathology of Mycobacterium avium-intracellulare infection in acquired immunodeficiency syndrome. Hum Pathol 1987; 18:709.

Lewin KJ, Riddell RH, Weinstein WM. Gastrointestinal Pathology and Its Clinical Implications. New York: Igaku-Shoin, 1992;779–807.

Maschek H, Georgil A, Schmidt RE, et al. Mycobacterium genavense: autopsy findings in three patients. Am J Clin Pathol 1994;101:95.

Roth RI, Owen RL, Keren DF, Volberding PA. Intestinal infection with Mycobacterium avium in acquired immune deficiency syndrome (AIDS): histological and clinical comparison with Whipple's disease. Dig Dis Sci 1985;30:497.

Strom RL, Gruninger RP. AIDS with Mycobacterium avium-intracellulare lesions resembling those of Whipple's disease. N Engl J Med 1983;309:1323.

Wang HH, Tollerud D, Damar D. Another Whipple-like disease in AIDS? N Engl J Med 1986;314:1577.

Weinberger SE, Weiss JW. The diagnosis of Whipple's disease. N Engl J Med 1995;6:390.

Yersinia enterocolitica

Bradford WD, Noce PS, Gutman LT. Pathologic features of enteric infection with Yersinia enterocolitica. Arch Pathol 1974;98:17.

Gleason TH, Patterson SD. The pathology of Yersinia enterocolitica ileocolitis. Am J Surg Pathol 1982;6:347.

Saari TN, Triplett DA. Yersinia pseudotuberculosis mesenteric adenitis. J Pediatr 1974;85:656.

Sternby NH. Morphologic findings in appendix in human Yersinia enterocolitica infection. Contrib Microbiol Immunol 1973;2:141.

CHAPTER 4

Infections of the Liver

The liver is involved in many infectious diseases. In hepatitis A or yellow fever, for example, it is the principal target of infection. Conversely, in miliary tuberculosis or histoplasmosis, hepatic involvement indicates that the liver is one of many organs that contains infectious lesions. Within the liver itself, various anatomic structures and cell types are infected in different processes (e.g., ascending bacterial cholangitis and pylephlebitis involving the bile ducts and portal veins, respectively). In general, the primary target cell of most etiologic agents of granulomatous hepatitis is the Kupffer cell. Viral agents may show some zonal specificity (e.g., yellow fever virus preferentially affects midzonal hepatocytes), whereas Lassa virus and hepatitis B virus (HBV) are much less selective for the lobular location of the infected hepatocytes. In other infections of the liver, a localized, space-occupying lesion, such as an abscess or cyst, is present.

The signs and symptoms of hepatic infections often include a variable combination of jaundice, hepatomegaly, and right upper quadrant tenderness that direct attention to the liver and the common nonspecific symptoms of fever, nausea, vomiting, and anorexia. Hepatic infections are frequently diagnosed by one or more clinical laboratory or radiologic imaging methods. However, some diagnoses still rely on the anatomic pathologist's skill in identifying the etiologic agent in a characteristic lesion. The critical caveat is that few lesions are etiologically pathognomonic, and even the detection of an infectious agent by histochemistry, such as by an acid-fast stain, would lead to a differential diagnosis containing several *Mycobacterium* species. Definitive diagnosis usually requires microbiologic culture or specific immunohistochemical or molecular methods. Nevertheless, the liver has always been a challenging source of diagnostic coups for the pathologist, and it is likely to remain so forever.

ACUTE HEPATITIS

Clinical History

A 10-year-old boy developed abdominal pain and cramping followed the next day by fever and headache. After 5 days of symptomatic treatment, he developed dark urine and jaundice. He was hospitalized the next day. On the second hospital day, he appeared to be having hallucinations and was suspected to be in hepatic failure. He had diffuse abdominal tenderness, markedly increased serum bilirubin (31.8 mg/dl total, 16 mg/dl conjugated), and elevated hepatic enzymes (alanine aminotransferase [ALT], 355 IU/liter; aspartate aminotransferase [AST], 1,435 IU/liter). The patient also developed a pruritic maculopapular rash and hemolytic anemia. A needle biopsy of the liver was performed on day 14 of illness to evaluate the possibility of massive hepatic necrosis.

Pathologic Findings

The liver biopsy revealed the classic features of acute viral hepatitis: lobular disarray caused predominantly by periportal cell injury manifested as swollen cells with clear vacuoles in the cytoplasm (ballooning degeneration), anisocytosis, multifocal necrosis with hepatocellular dropout and mononuclear leukocytic infiltration (Figures 4-1 and 4-2), focal acidophilic necrosis with engulfed Councilman-like bodies in sinusoidal macrophages, and cholestasis (Figure 4-3). Also present were marked sinusoidal lining cell activation, portal inflammation with more lymphocytes and macrophages than plasma cells

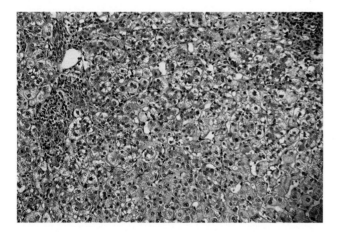

FIGURE 4-1. Low-power magnification photomicrograph of the hepatic biopsy from a patient shows lobular disarray owing to ballooning degeneration of hepatocytes and patchy mononuclear inflammation (hematoxylin and eosin stain; low-power magnification).

and polymorphonuclear neutrophils, minimal to mild steatosis, hepatocellular cholestasis, and a fibrin-ring granuloma (Figure 4-4).

Differential Diagnoses

Acute hepatitis is a condition defined by necrosis and inflammation of the liver. Acute viral hepatitis, although caused by a variety of agents, manifests a syndrome with many similar signs, symptoms, and abnormal laboratory results. Hepatitis A virus (HAV), HBV, hepatitis C virus (HCV), delta hepatitis virus, and hepatitis E virus (HEV) infect the liver predominantly and are the most important etiologic agents to consider. Other viruses, bacteria, drugs, chemicals, and pathologic conditions can also cause illnesses that in some cases resemble acute viral hepatitis. Important examples of the latter include ethanol, anoxia, intrahepatic and extrahepatic biliary obstruction, and Wilson's disease.

Microbiology

Serologic workup revealed immunoglobulin M (IgM) antibodies to HAV, no circulating hepatitis B surface antigen (HB$_s$Ag), no antibodies to hepatitis B core antigen (HB$_c$) or leptospiral antigens, and negative results to a monospot test.

Comment

A liver biopsy is rarely necessary to diagnose acute viral hepatitis, although it is often a useful procedure to evaluate chronic hepatitis, suspected alcohol-associated hepatic disease, and hepatic necrosis in immunocompromised patients. The histopathologic alterations in HAV, HBV, HCV, delta viral hepatitis, HEV, and some forms of drug-induced hepatitis share the basic features seen in the biopsy of this patient. In acute viral hepatitis, it is easier and more sensitive to detect HAV, HBV, and delta hepatitis virus antigens or antibodies in the serum than in a liver biopsy. The most useful serologic tests in the etiologic diagnosis of acute viral hepatitis are IgM anti-HAV, HB$_s$Ag, and IgM anti-HB$_c$. HAV infection is diagnosed in the acute phase by the presence of IgM anti-HAV. Acute HBV infection is diagnosed by the presence of HB$_s$Ag, IgM anti-HB$_c$, or both. After the immune clearance of HB$_s$Ag from the serum, anti-HB$_c$ may be the only detectable antibody to HBV for a variable period until antibodies to hepatitis B surface antigen appear during convalescence. When all of the three tests are negative, non-A, non-B viral hepatitis is a strong possibility. Anti–hepatitis delta virus (HDV) antibodies occur with

FIGURE 4-2. Photomicrograph of viral hepatitis A shows ballooning degeneration of hepatocytes and a focal mononuclear cell infiltrate (hematoxylin and eosin stain; original magnification, ×100).

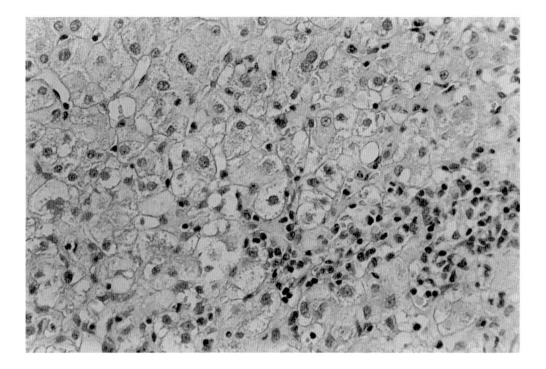

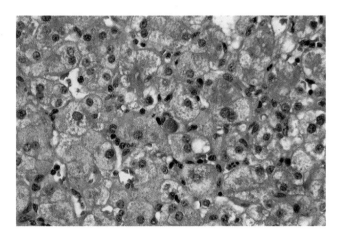

FIGURE 4-3. A different field of the section shown in Figure 4-2 reveals an hepatocyte in the center manifests cell death as an eosinophilic shrunken appearance (Councilman-like body) with adjacent swollen injured cells and cholestasis (hematoxylin and eosin stain; high-power magnification).

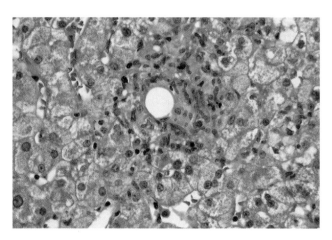

FIGURE 4-4. An unusual, but previously reported, observation in this patient was a ring granuloma, a characteristic lesion of Q fever hepatitis that also occurs with other etiologic agents of hepatic injury including viruses (hematoxylin and eosin stain; high-power magnification).

HB$_s$Ag because HDV requires HBV for its complete synthesis. When HBV and HDV occur as acute coinfections, resolution is the result in more than 95% of cases. In contrast, HDV superinfection in chronic HBV carriers results in chronic hepatitis more than 70% of the time.

Disruption of the limiting plate is observed frequently in HAV using light microscopy, but less than 25% of the limiting plate is involved. Ballooning degeneration of hepatocytes corresponds to ultrastructural dilation of

cisternae of rough endoplasmic reticulum, and acidophilic necrosis appears as condensed, electron-dense cytoplasm. These lesions are presumably the effect of cell-mediated immune attack on antigens of HAV in the liver cell membrane. Chronic hepatitis is not a sequela of hepatitis A.

Diagnosis

Acute hepatitis due to HAV.

ACUTE HEPATITIS IN AN IMMUNOSUPPRESSED PATIENT

Clinical History

A 5-year-old boy received a bone marrow transplant as therapy for mediastinal lymphoblastic lymphoma. He had been immunocompromised for 10 months before transplantation, having been treated with multiple immunosuppressive drugs and radiotherapy. Approximately 5 weeks after transplantation, he developed liver failure and suspected graft versus host disease. Broad-spectrum antibiotics, including amphotericin B, were instituted. He developed bilateral lower lobe pulmonary infiltrates and a pericardial effusion. Nine weeks after transplantation, his condition deteriorated and he died.

Pathologic Findings

Autopsy revealed that the liver had severe, multifocal coagulative necrosis, which was randomly distributed within the lobule (Figure 4-5). Numerous intranuclear inclusions that varied in appearance were present (Figure 4-6); some were acidophilic and angulated, resembling herpes simplex virus (HSV) inclusions, whereas others were large and amphophilic to basophilic with a peri-inclusion halo suggestive of cytomegalovirus (CMV) cytopathology. Smudge cells, in which basophilic material completely filled the nucleus and obliterated the nuclear membrane, were also abundant (see Figure 4-6). Additional findings included single-cell acidophilic Councilman-like bodies and moderate steatosis.

Differential Diagnoses

Acute hepatitis can be caused by viruses other than classic hepatitis viruses, including Epstein-Barr, rubella, rubeola, mumps, coxsackie, and echo viruses. Hepatitis in an immunocompromised patient has a larger differential diagnosis than acute viral hepatitis in immunologically normal hosts. Of particular concern are HSV types 1 and 2, varicella-zoster virus, CMV, and adenoviruses.

Microbiology

The diagnosis of adenoviral infection was not considered until the microscopic slides of autopsy liver were examined. A policy of routinely storing samples of various organs frozen at –70°C until after the autopsy report was finalized could have yielded a definitive diagnosis by viral culture. In this case, in situ hybridization documented the presence of adenoviral DNA in the infected hepatocytes, and the typical appearance of crystalline arrays of icosahedral adenovirus virions was observed ultrastructurally in tissue recovered from the paraffin block (Figure 4-7).

Comment

The diagnosis of adenoviral hepatitis can be achieved definitively by percutaneous needle biopsy of liver. In liver transplant recipients, the diagnosis of adenovirus is important because distinguishing between rejection and hepati-

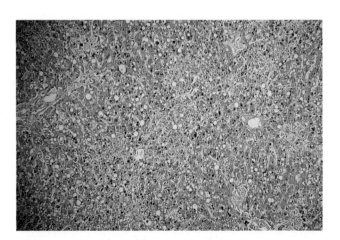

FIGURE 4-5. Low-power magnification photomicrograph of adenoviral hepatitis in an immunocompromised patient shows multiple foci of confluent hepatocellular necrosis. At the margin of the necrotic areas are slightly enlarged cytopathic cells with nuclear changes (hematoxylin and eosin; low-power magnification).

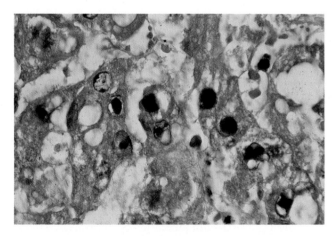

FIGURE 4-6. At higher magnification, cells with intranuclear herpesvirus-like inclusions and fully developed smudge cells are seen (hematoxylin and eosin stain; high-power magnification).

tis on a clinical basis is quite difficult. If immunosuppression is curtailed judiciously, the immune system may clear the viral infection from the liver. However, increased immunosuppression for presumed rejection could allow further progression of the adenoviral disease. Fatality rates are quite high in transplant patients with adenovirus infection (60% for infected bone marrow transplant patients). Disseminated adenoviral infection occurs more frequently in children with transplants than in adults with transplants. Immunocompromised children usually are infected with the same serotypes that are prevalent in the community. In transplant recipients with adenoviral hepatitis, endogenous reactivation is one of the sources of infection. Because adenoviruses cause latent infections with prolonged viral shedding, detection of adenovirus at other sites, such as in the feces or throat, does not indicate that concurrent hepatic disease is due to the virus.

Diagnosis

Adenoviral hepatitis.

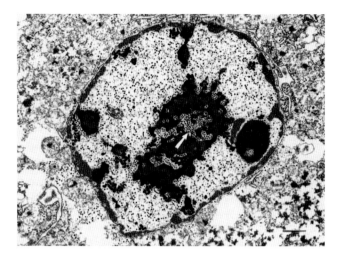

FIGURE 4-7. Electron photomicrograph of an adenovirus-infected hepatocyte demonstrates numerous intranuclear virions, some of which are arranged in a tight array (*arrow*; magnification, ×13,000; *bar* = 1 μm). (Courtesy of Dr. Vsevolod L. Popov.)

CHRONIC HEPATITIS

Clinical History

A 36-year-old man presented to an internal medicine department for his annual physical examination. He was asymptomatic, had no medical problems of which he was aware, took no medicines, was a nonsmoker, and denied excessive alcohol use. Pertinent medical history included receipt of a blood transfusion 14 years previously at the time of a severe electrical injury. In accordance with his physician's protocol, a complete blood cell count and a routine chemistry panel were performed, the latter of which showed elevated aminotransferases (AST five times the upper limit of normal; ALT 10 times the upper limit of normal). Based on these results, serologic tests for infection with HBV and HCV and for autoantibodies were performed. Antibodies against HCV were present, whereas results for antigen and antibody tests for HBV and tests for autoantibodies were negative. A percutaneous liver biopsy was performed before initiation of therapy with alpha interferon.

Pathologic Findings

Hematoxylin and eosin (H and E)–stained sections of the liver biopsy (Figures 4-8 and 4-9) showed a lymphoid infiltrate in the portal tract that extended through the limiting plate and surrounded periportal hepatocytes, some of

which were injured. The epithelium of the small bile duct exhibited reactive changes. In the parenchyma, occasional loose clusters of lymphocytes in the sinusoids; a few acidophil bodies, some of which were associated with inflammatory cells; and some hepatocytes showing mild steatosis were present. Sections stained with the trichrome stain demonstrate portal, periportal, and portal-portal bridging fibrosis (Figure 4-10).

Differential Diagnoses

Based on the histologic findings alone, the differential diagnoses are those of chronic hepatitis and include HBV; HCV; autoimmune chronic hepatitis; alcohol-associated chronic hepatitis; drug-induced chronic hepatitis (acetaminophen, aspirin, dantrolene, diclofenac, fenofibrate, glafenine, isoniazid, methyldopa, nitrofurantoin, oxyphenisatin, papaverine, pemoline, perihexilene maleate, propylthiouracil, sulfonamides, ticrynafen, and tolazamide have been implicated); chronic hepatitis associated with inherited metabolic diseases (e.g., Wilson's disease); and cryptogenic chronic hepatitis.

Microbiology

In this case, antibodies against HCV were present.

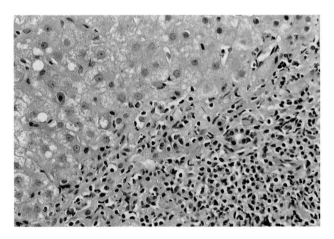

FIGURE 4-8. Section of a liver biopsy from a patient with chronic hepatitis C shows a lymphoid infiltrate in the portal tract that extends through the limiting plate and surrounds periportal hepatocytes, some of which are injured (called *interface necrosis*). Additionally, the epithelium of the small bile duct demonstrates reactive changes, with crowding and irregular spacing of the nuclei, and a few acidophil bodies are present in the parenchyma (hematoxylin and eosin stain; medium-power magnification). (Courtesy of Dr. A. Brian West.)

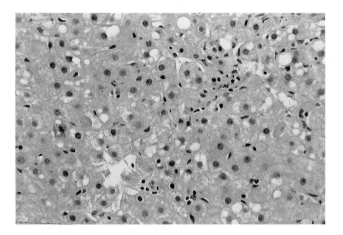

FIGURE 4-9. Section of a liver biopsy from a patient with chronic hepatitis C shows occasional loose clusters of lymphocytes in the sinusoids, a few acidophil bodies, and mild steatosis (hematoxylin and eosin stain; medium-power magnification). (Courtesy of Dr. A. Brian West.)

Comment

Chronic hepatitis is a clinical diagnosis. Characteristic histopathologic features of chronic hepatitis include piecemeal necrosis (the most important), bile duct lesions, portal inflammation, intra-acinar degeneration and necrosis, and periportal and bridging fibrosis. Chronic hepatitis C cannot be distinguished with confidence from chronic hepatitis of other causes based on histologic findings alone. Immunohistochemical studies using HCV antibodies may be performed but are not necessary if the results of serologic tests are available, as in this case.

Of the lesions associated with chronic hepatitis C, the most characteristic are lymphoid aggregates and follicles, bile duct damage, and steatosis, although these features are neither always present nor pathognomonic. The portal infiltrate usually is in the form of a dense, rounded aggregate of lymphocytes often surrounding a small bile duct that may have reactive epithelium and appear injured, although serum alkaline phosphatase levels are normal in most cases. Plasma cells and eosinophils are rare or absent. Lymphocytes may extend into the parenchyma with interface necrosis. Small groups of lymphocytes are present in the sinusoids, and focal hepatocyte necrosis and isolated acidophil bodies may be present. Steatosis is common. Fibrosis frequently is more extensive than expected based on symptoms, serum liver enzyme concentrations, or the severity of the inflammation; in a biopsy, it may be encountered at any point on the pathway, including portal, periportal, portal-portal bridging fibrosis, and cirrhosis.

The current recommendations for reporting chronic hepatitis are to abandon the terms *chronic active, chronic aggressive, chronic persistent,* and *chronic lobular* and to

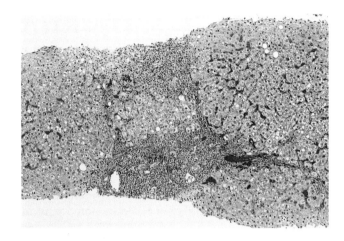

FIGURE 4-10. Section of a liver biopsy from a patient with chronic hepatitis C and stained with the trichrome stain shows portal, periportal, and portal-portal bridging fibrosis and a dense aggregate of lymphocytes surrounding a bile duct in the lower portal tract (trichrome stain; low-power magnification). (Courtesy of Dr. A. Brian West.)

report instead by etiology, stage (fibrosis), and grade (necroinflammatory activity). Thus, in this case, the surgical pathology report should read "chronic hepatitis C (by serologic tests) with portal-portal bridging fibrosis and mild activity."

Diagnosis

Chronic hepatitis C.

FEVER, HEPATIC INJURY, AND A FATAL OUTCOME IN A PATIENT IN WEST AFRICA

Clinical History

A 19-year-old man from a village in Liberia went to Monrovia to purchase goods for his father's store in April during the dry season. One day before arrival in the city, he began to feel ill with fever, malaise, and weakness. On the third day of fever, he noted pain in his back, hips, and knees and a dry, nonproductive cough. He began self-medication with antibiotics and an antimalarial drug. Two days later, he sought medical attention because of severe frontal headache, sore throat, and sharp retrosternal pain and was admitted to the hospital.

Physical examination revealed a temperature of 39.1°C, a pulse rate of 98 beats per minute, a respiratory rate of 24 breaths per minute, blood pressure of 101/77 mm Hg, a red and swollen posterior pharynx, tonsils with patchy yellow exudates, conjunctivitis, and a diffusely tender abdomen. Laboratory data included a white blood cell count of 4,600 cells per µl; hematocrit, 51%; serum aspartate transaminase, 645 IU/liter; and serum urea nitrogen, 31 mg/dl. On the second hospital day, he developed vomiting and diarrhea and the next day suffered complete prostration with bleeding from the gums, edema of the face and neck, stridor, shock, coma, and seizures. He died on the ninth day of illness.

Pathologic Findings

At postmortem examination, few macroscopic findings were present, other than ecchymoses in the gingiva and conjunctivae and scattered cutaneous and serosal petechiae. Histologic examination revealed only focal necrosis of the adrenal cortex, necrosis and fibrin deposition in the marginal zone of the splenic periarteriolar lymphoid sheaths, and multifocal hepatocellular necrosis involving approximately 20% of the hepatic parenchymal cells (Figure 4-11). Foci of 1–10 contiguous hepatocytes randomly distributed in the lobule showed coagulative-type necrosis with nucleolysis, and less frequently, acidophilic cell death resembling Councilman's bodies or apoptosis (Figure 4-12). There was a moderate degree of phagocytosis of dead hepatocytes by macrophages.

Differential Diagnoses

The differential diagnosis of multifocal hepatic necrosis in a patient with a tropical exposure depends in part on the geographic region: Lassa fever, Argentine hemorrhagic fever, Bolivian hemorrhagic fever, Venezuelan hemorrhagic fever, Marburg disease, Ebola hemorrhagic fever, Congo-Crimean hemorrhagic fever, dengue hemorrhagic fever, and Kyasanur forest disease.

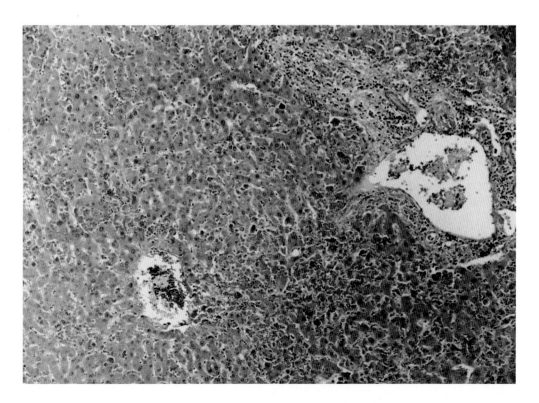

FIGURE 4-11. Liver from a fatal case of Lassa fever shows multifocal necrosis that is randomly distributed throughout the lobule and lacks the midzonal predominance found in yellow fever. A portal triad contains underlying nonspecific mononuclear inflammation (hematoxylin and eosin stain; original magnification, ×25).

FIGURE 4-12. Higher magnification of Lassa hepatitis shows contiguous foci of dead hepatocytes, some of which are contracted eosinophilic Councilman-like bodies; others resemble coagulative necrosis (hematoxylin and eosin stain; original magnification, ×100).

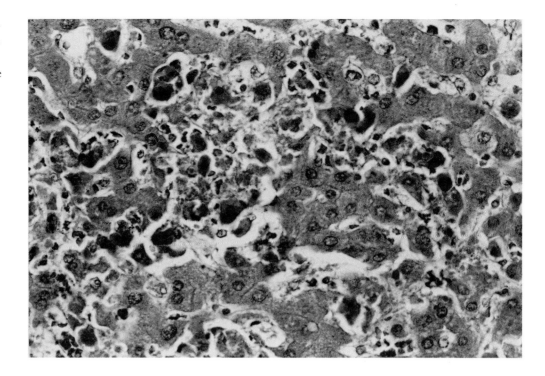

Microbiology

Thick and thin smears of peripheral blood contained no detected malarial parasites, and all blood cultures showed no growth. A sample of blood and postmortem liver was shipped to a reference laboratory with biosafety level 4 containment facilities for highly hazardous agents. Lassa virus was recovered in cell culture from the blood and liver. Indirect immunofluorescent antibody assay demonstrated IgM antibodies to Lassa virus at a titer of 1:16.

Comment

The incubation period of most exotic diseases is much longer than the air transport time from developing regions to developed regions. This is illustrated by a fatal case of Lassa fever reported from a hospital in middle America. The patient had returned from the funeral of his mother in West Africa. Although most pathologists think of viral hepatitis in immunocompetent patients and certain opportunistic pathogens in immunocompromised patients with febrile hepatic injury, they are generally unfamiliar with the pathologic lesions of arenaviral and filoviral infections, such as Lassa fever, the South American arenaviral hemorrhagic fevers, Ebola and Marburg disease, bunyaviral hemorrhagic fevers, and even yellow fever. Lassa fever and other arenaviral infections can be treated successfully with ribavirin given early in the course.

Lassa virus is maintained in an enzootic cycle involving *Mastomys natalensis*, an African rodent that when infected persistently sheds the virus in its urine asymptomatically. Humans are infected in West African villages, where approximately 300,000 cases occur each year. In endemic areas, most infections do not result in hospitalization, but Lassa fever is a major cause of adult febrile hospitalization and accounts for 30% of adult hospital deaths. Person-to-person transmission occurs, but universal precautions suffice to prevent nosocomial transmission to health care workers and others.

Diagnosis

Lassa viral hepatitis.

FULMINANT HEPATIC FAILURE

Clinical History

A 12-year-old girl, along with the rest of her family, developed flulike symptoms. Although the other family members recovered, she became jaundiced and 2 days later had markedly increased serum hepatic enzyme concentrations (AST, 2,160 IU/liter; ALT, 2,050 IU/liter). After 7 days of malaise and anorexia, she developed nausea, abdominal pain, and vomiting. Abnormal laboratory test results included a markedly prolonged prothrombin time and activated partial thromboplastin time, blood urea nitrogen less than 2 mg/dl, falling serum transaminase levels, and elevated serum ammonium concentration. She developed hepatic encephalopathy and died on the 21st day of illness.

Pathologic Findings

Autopsy revealed massive hepatic necrosis. The liver capsule was wrinkled, representing loss of hepatic mass, and weighed only 75% of the expected weight. The cut surface was nearly all red, congested sinusoids. Microscopically, hepatocytes were almost totally absent, and the lobules contained only sinusoids with Kupffer cells and blood (Figure 4-13). A few residual Councilman-like bodies were present. Regenerative activity was limited to marked proliferation of portal bile ducts and periportal

bile ductules and focal lobular islands or rosettes of 2–10 hepatocytes with canalicular cholestasis (Figure 4-14). Portal inflammation comprised more lymphocytes and macrophages than neutrophils (Figure 4-15). Many of the latter were seen in bile ducts. Kupffer cells and portal macrophages were laden with lipofuscin pigment that presumably originated from dead hepatocytes.

Differential Diagnoses

The differential diagnoses include the hepatic viruses; enteroviruses, particularly in the neonatal period; HSV during pregnancy; exposure to toxic chemicals; and treatment with medications that can have either idiosyncratic or dose-related hepatic toxicity, including massive hepatic necrosis.

Microbiology

Serologic investigation revealed negative assays for all of the following: IgM anti-HAV antibodies; HB_sAg; hepatitis B e antigen; antibodies to HB_c, surface, and e antigens; HCV; HEV; and dengue virus. The presence of only immunoglobulin G (IgG) to HAV established immunity to that agent and excluded it as a possible diagnosis. A toxicology screen was negative.

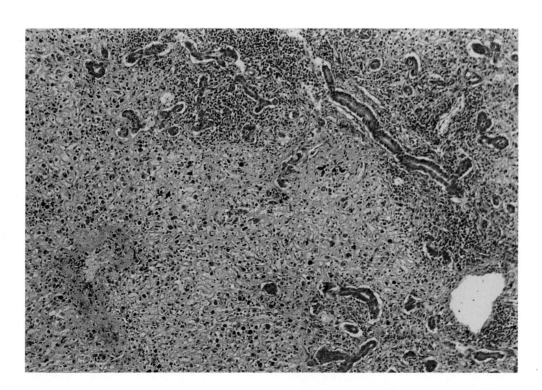

FIGURE 4-13. Photomicrograph of liver from a case of fulminant hepatitis shows massive hepatic necrosis. There is lobular collapse owing to near-total loss of hepatocytes. The remaining tissue consists of sinusoids, terminal hepatic vein, and portal triads containing ductular proliferation and a mononuclear cell infiltrate (hematoxylin and eosin stain; original magnification, ×25).

Figure 4-14. Photomicrograph of liver from a case of fulminant hepatitis shows a few rosettes of regenerating hepatocytes and many sinusoids with pigment-containing macrophages (hematoxylin and eosin stain; original magnification, ×100).

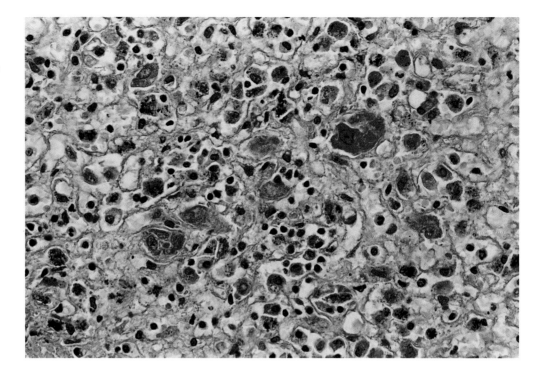

Comment

Fulminant viral hepatitis can be caused by HBV alone; HBV in conjunction with hepatitis delta virus; hepatitis E virus, which has been documented in Mexico; and, less frequently, HAV and HCV. In newborn infants, enteroviruses, especially echoviruses, also must be considered in the differential diagnosis, and cultures of blood, throat, and rectum (or involved tissue in fatal cases) should be submitted for viral culture. The serologic studies in this patient do not support any of these diagnoses. Although there is no evidence for toxic exposure, the possibility cannot be ruled out. It is important to bear in mind that acute hepatocellular injury accompanied by fever may be caused by occupational and accidental exposure to toxic agents, such as carbon tetrachloride, and that various medical treatments often induce hepatocellular injury. Acetaminophen and isoniazid are well-known examples among a myriad of drugs associated with hepatic damage. Suspicion of an infectious etiology based on clinical and pathologic grounds should not eliminate consideration of other exogenous diagnoses. Confluent hepatic necrosis resulting in fulminant hepatitis has a high mortality rate. With progressively longer duration of illness before death, the liver shrinks to 1,000 g or even 500 g. The prolonged prothrombin time reflects the severity of hepatocellular synthetic deficiency, and falling hepatic

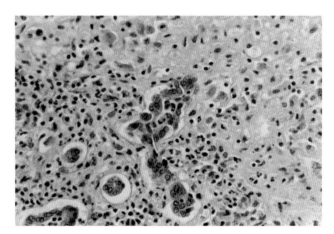

Figure 4-15. Photomicrograph of fulminant hepatitis shows ductular proliferation, portal triaditis, and absence of hepatocytes (hematoxylin and eosin stain; original magnification, ×100).

enzymes portend the gloomy prognosis of few remaining hepatocytes to release transaminases.

Diagnosis

Massive hepatic necrosis of unknown etiology.

GRANULOMATOUS HEPATITIS

Clinical History

A 48-year-old man who had a history of injection drug use came to an emergency department with complaints of productive cough and shortness of breath for 1 week and a 20-pound weight loss over the preceding 2 months. On physical examination, he was afebrile and had a pulse rate of 104 beats per minute, a respiratory rate of 23 breaths per minute, and blood pressure of 94/56 mm Hg. He had bilateral inguinal adenopathy and an enlarged lymph node (approximately 1.5 cm in diameter) in the left neck. His stool contained occult blood. A chest radiograph showed bilateral reticulonodular infiltrates. Pertinent laboratory test results included hemoglobin, 9.5 g/dl; white blood cell count 3,700 cells per μl (68% band forms); serum alkaline phosphatase, 244 IU/liter; serum lactate dehydrogenase, 1,517 IU/liter; and the presence of antibodies to human immunodeficiency virus. The differential diagnosis was disseminated tuberculosis or other bacterial infection or lymphoma. Sputum and blood specimens were submitted for bacterial, mycobacterial, and fungal stains and cultures. The patient was admitted, and empiric broad-spectrum antimicrobial treatment was begun.

The following day, a computed tomographic scan of the abdomen showed punctate lesions in the liver and spleen. Two days later, he developed bleeding from the upper gastrointestinal tract and respiratory distress, requiring intubation and mechanical ventilation. Despite aggressive supportive care, he died 6 days after admission.

Pathologic Findings

Autopsy revealed multiple, well-formed epithelioid granulomas, some with central caseation necrosis, involving the lungs, liver (Figure 4-16), spleen, kidneys, and abdominal and thoracic lymph nodes. A section of liver stained by the Ziehl-Neelsen method showed a few acid-fast bacilli (AFB).

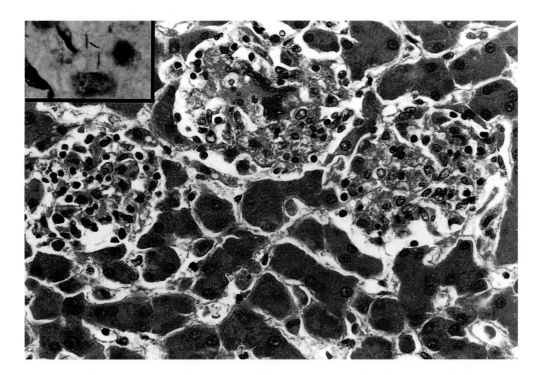

FIGURE 4-16. Section of a liver nodule from a patient with disseminated tuberculosis shows three mature granulomas composed of compact aggregates of lymphocytes and epithelioid histiocytes. One granuloma also has a giant cell (hematoxylin and eosin stain; original magnification, ×50). *Inset*: One granuloma contains a few acid-fast bacilli (Ziehl-Neelsen stain; original magnification, ×250). Postmortem culture of the tissue grew *Mycobacterium tuberculosis*.

Differential Diagnoses

The differential diagnoses of granulomas in the liver include noninfectious causes (Table 4-1) and a variety of infectious agents. The infectious causes correlate to a degree with the morphology of the granulomas, which in this case are noncaseating, mature granulomas. Organisms associated with mature granulomas include *Mycobacterium tuberculosis*, some nontuberculous mycobacteria, *Histoplasma capsulatum*, *Coccidioides immitis*, *Brucella* species, *Coxiella burnetii*, *Ehrlichia chaffeensis*, cytomegalovirus, and (rarely) *Toxoplasma gondii*. *Schistosoma* species also are associated with mature granulomas, but in most cases eosinophils and egg fragments also are present (Figure 4-17); these features were not observed in this patient. Based on this differential diagnosis, special stains for AFB and fungi should be performed.

Microbiology

Premortem mycobacterial cultures of sputum and postmortem cultures of granulomas in the lung and liver grew *M. tuberculosis*.

Comment

The finding of granulomas in the liver often is a diagnostic challenge for surgical pathologists. The granulomas may have a noninfectious or an infectious cause; because special stains for organisms often are negative, even in cases of an infectious etiology, arriving at a specific diagnosis may be difficult. Of the noninfectious etiologies (see Table 4-1), sarcoidosis is the single most common diagnosis. The sarcoid granuloma is the prototype of noncaseating granulomas (i.e., discrete, round, well-demarcated aggregates of epithelioid macrophages often intermingled with giant cells and surrounded by a rim of lymphocytes). The center may contain a focus of eosinophilic necrosis and nuclear debris, but caseation does not occur. The diagnosis is based on clinical and laboratory findings, the presence of typical granulomas in the liver and elsewhere, and the exclusion of an infectious cause. Controversy continues to surround the hypothesis that sarcoidosis is a reaction to mycobacterial antigens.

The investigation of infectious causes of mature granulomas of the liver should include special stains for AFB and fungi and mycobacterial and fungal cultures of liver tissue or other relevant specimens (e.g., sputum if the patient has pulmonary symptoms and an abnormal chest radiograph). If these tests fail to identify the etiology, serologic tests (e.g., assays for antibodies to *C. burnetii* or IgM antibodies to cytomegalovirus or *T. gondii*) should be performed. In this case, the Ziehl-Neelsen–stained section of the liver showed AFB.

Of the infectious causes of mature granulomas, *M. tuberculosis* is the most common etiology. A positive AFB

TABLE 4-1. Noninfectious Causes of Hepatic Granulomas

Sarcoidosis

Primary liver disease
    Cirrhosis (primary biliary, postnecrotic, alcoholic, nutritional)
    Biliary obstruction
    Acute and chronic pericholangitis
    Fatty infiltration
    Toxic or drug-induced hepatitis
    Chronic active hepatitis
    Acute hepatitis A viral infection

Hypersensitivity reactions
    Berylliosis
    Reactions to the following drugs
        Sulfonamides
        Penicillin
        Allopurinol
        Halothane
        β-Methyldopa
        Procainamide
        Quinidine
        Hydrochlorothiazide
        Phenytoin
        Sulfonylurea derivatives
        Phenylbutazone
        Oxyphenbutazone
        Clofibrate
        p-Aminosalicylic acid
        Cromolyn sodium
        Diazepam
        Progesterone-estrogen contraceptive
        Ethiocholanolone
        Copper (vineyard sprayers' lung)
        Other (extrinsic allergic alveolitis)

Allergic granulomatosis/granulomatous-vasculitis syndromes
    Wegener's granulomatosis
    Temporal arteritis
    Polymyalgia rheumatica
    Allergic granulomatosis
    Benign lymphocytic angiitis and granulomatosis
    Bronchocentric granulomatosis
    Hyalinizing granuloma

Host defense deficiency diseases
    Chronic granulomatous disease of childhood
    Hypogammaglobulinemia (various)

Malignancies
    Lymphomas, Hodgkin's disease
    Hepatocellular carcinoma
    Lung carcinoma (small cell)
    Thymoma
    Renal cell carcinoma
    Lymphomatoid granulomatosis

Other diseases
    Crohn's disease
    Ulcerative colitis
    Eosinophilic granuloma of the lung
    Post-ileal bypass surgery
    Celiac disease

Foreign bodies (starch, talc, silica)

Idiopathic granulomas

Source: Modified from PT Harrington, JJ Gutiérrez, CH Ramirez-Ronda, et al. Granulomatous hepatitis. Rev Infect Dis 1982;4:638.

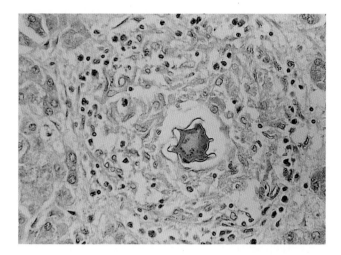

FIGURE 4-17. Section of liver shows a well-formed granuloma, in the center of which is a cross-section of an ovum of *Schistosoma mansoni* (hematoxylin and eosin stain; original magnification, ×100).

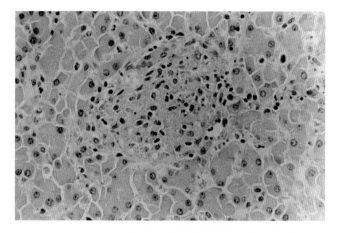

FIGURE 4-18. Section of liver from a patient with the acquired immunodeficiency syndrome and disseminated tuberculosis shows a poorly circumscribed aggregate of histiocytes with focal necrosis and a few degenerating neutrophils (hematoxylin and eosin stain; original magnification, ×100).

stain, however, is not sufficient for a diagnosis of tuberculosis. Certain nontuberculous mycobacteria may be associated with mature granulomas in the liver—for example, *Mycobacterium szulgai*, *Mycobacterium kansasii*, and *Mycobacterium avium* complex (MAC) in patients not infected with human immunodeficiency virus. Therefore, mycobacterial culture is necessary to identify the specific agent; in this case, *M. tuberculosis* was recovered. Culture should be done even if the patient has died, because a contact investigation must be performed if the patient had tuberculosis to prevent further spread of the disease.

The histopathology of disseminated tuberculosis varies. In addition to mature, well-formed epithelioid granulomas illustrated in this case, granulomas may show central caseation, or there may be focal areas of tissue necrosis with or without an infiltrate of neutrophils (Figure 4-18). The latter is particularly common in persons infected with human immunodeficiency virus.

Diagnosis

Disseminated tuberculosis.

AGGREGATES OF FOAMY MACROPHAGES

Clinical History

A 33-year-old man, diagnosed 3 years earlier with acquired immunodeficiency syndrome (AIDS), was admitted for evaluation of fever, diarrhea, and lethargy of 1 week's duration. History included *Pneumocystis carinii* pneumonia (the AIDS-defining illness), cytomegalovirus retinitis 1 year later, and a scrotal abscess with secondary bacteremia caused by *Staphylococcus aureus* 2 months before the current illness. On physical examination, his temperature was 38°C, his pulse rate was 110 beats per minute, his respiratory rate was 18 breaths per minute, and his blood pressure was 88/48 mm Hg. His abdomen was distended, and his liver was enlarged. The remainder of the examination was noncontributory. Pertinent abnormal laboratory test results included a hemoglobin concentration of 8.4 g/dl and an elevated serum alkaline phosphatase level. The differential diagnoses were bacteremia and disseminated infection with MAC or *H. capsulatum*. Blood cultures for aerobic and anaerobic bacteria, mycobacteria, and fungi were collected, and broad-spectrum antimicrobial therapy was initiated. Despite antibiotics and aggressive supportive care, however, his condition deteriorated. He died 6 days after admission.

Pathologic Findings

At autopsy, the liver and spleen were both enlarged, weighing 3,800 g (normal, 1,400–1,900 g) and 560 g (normal, 125–195 g), respectively; scattered throughout the parenchyma of both were several firm, white-to-tan nodules measuring 2 cm in greatest diameter. Similar-appearing lesions were found in the abdominal lymph nodes and adrenal glands. H and E–stained sections of the lesions in the liver, spleen, adrenal glands, and lymph nodes showed poorly formed granulomas characterized by well-circumscribed aggregates of foamy histiocytes (Figure 4-19), a few neutrophils, and small foci of necrosis. In sections stained by the Ziehl-Neelsen method, the histiocytes were filled with AFB (Figure 4-20).

Microbiology

Mycobacterial cultures of the antemortem blood culture and the enlarged lymph nodes observed at autopsy grew MAC.

Comment

Infectious agents that may be associated with aggregates of foamy histiocytes include (in addition to MAC) *Mycobacterium genavense*, the Whipple's bacterium (*Trophermyma whippleii*), *Encephalitozoon* (formerly *Septata*) *intestinalis*, *H. capsulatum* (which may also be associated with marked proliferation of Kupffer cells, as illustrated in Figures 4-21, 4-22, and 4-23, rather than actual histiocyte aggregates, in which case the infection must be differentiated from visceral leishmaniasis [Figure 4-24]), *Penicillium marneffii*, and *Ehrlichia chaffeensis*. Thus, stains for AFB and fungi should be

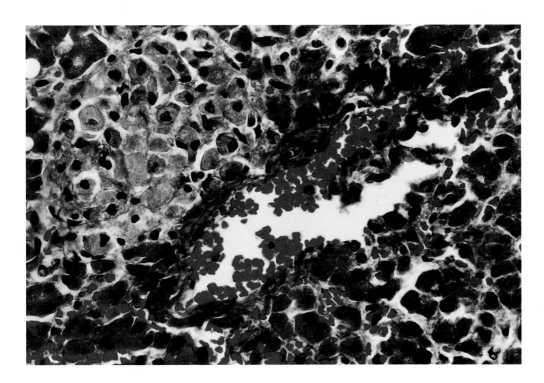

FIGURE 4-19. Section of a liver nodule from a patient with disseminated *Mycobacterium avium* complex disease shows aggregates of pale-staining histiocytes adjacent to a central vein (Masson trichrome stain; original magnification, ×100).

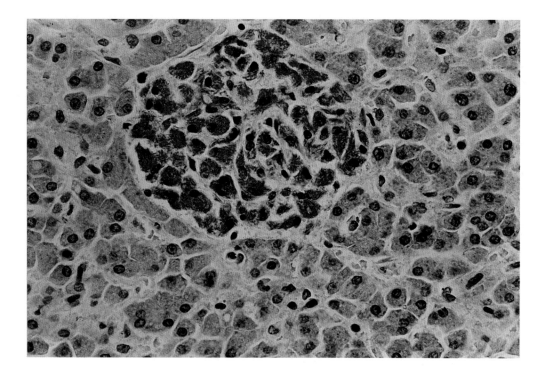

FIGURE 4-20. Section from a liver nodule stained by the Ziehl-Neelsen method from the case illustrated in Figure 4-19 demonstrates that the histiocytes are filled with numerous intracytoplasmic acid-fast bacilli (Ziehl-Neelsen stain; original magnification, ×100).

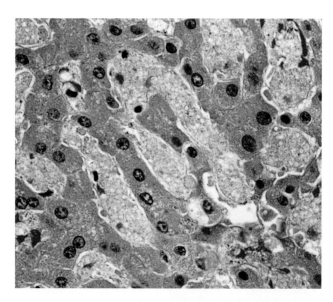

FIGURE 4-21. Section of liver from a patient with the acquired immunodeficiency syndrome who died from disseminated histoplasmosis shows dilatation of the sinusoids caused by marked hypertrophy of Kupffer cells, which have vacuolated cytoplasm (hematoxylin and eosin stain; original magnification, ×100).

performed to help identify the responsible pathogen in tissue sections, although yeast cells of *H. capsulatum* or *P. marneffii* often can be visualized in sections stained with H and E. If these stains are negative, a tissue Gram stain, which allows visualization of spores of *E. intestinalis*, or electron microscopy should be performed. In this case, the Ziehl-Neelsen stain revealed numerous AFB within the histiocytes' cytoplasm. The presence of AFB, however, does not allow a definitive diagnosis; mycobacterial culture is required to identify the specific mycobacterium.

The most likely pathogen in this patient is MAC. Disseminated MAC disease is the most common bacterial infection in persons with advanced AIDS; nearly 25% of all patients with AIDS are estimated to develop this infection during their lifetimes. Moreover, this patient demonstrated several of the typical characteristics of MAC disease, including fever, anemia, and elevated serum alkaline phosphatase. *M. genavense*, however, can cause similar symptoms and abnormal laboratory test results (discussed in more detail in Chapter 8); therefore, mycobacterial culture is essential. MAC grows well in mycobacterial culture in broth and on solid media, and the

FIGURE 4-22. Higher-power magnification of the section illustrated in Figure 4-21 shows that the cytoplasm of the Kupffer cells contains numerous small yeast cells surrounded by a clear halo (hematoxylin and eosin stain; original magnification, ×250).

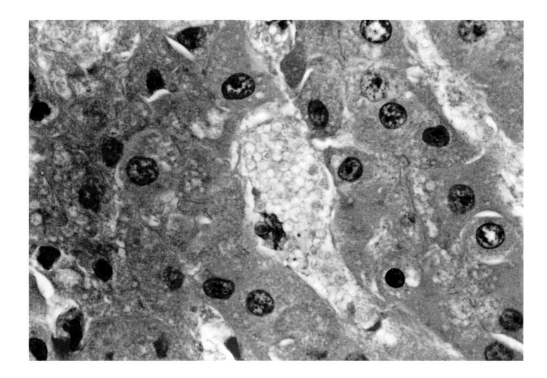

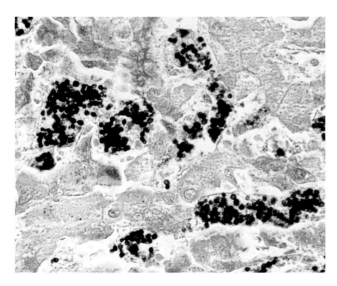

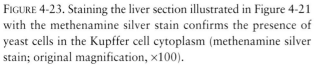

FIGURE 4-23. Staining the liver section illustrated in Figure 4-21 with the methenamine silver stain confirms the presence of yeast cells in the Kupffer cell cytoplasm (methenamine silver stain; original magnification, ×100).

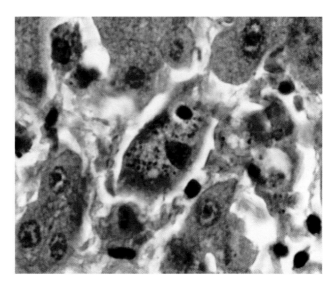

FIGURE 4-24. Section of liver from a patient with visceral leishmaniasis shows enlargement of Kupffer cells, a few of which have amastigotes of *Leishmania donovani* in their cytoplasm (hematoxylin and eosin stain; original magnification, ×250). In contrast to *Histoplasma capsulatum*, amastigotes do not stain by the methenamine silver method.

necessary tests for identification (e.g., nucleic acid probes and latex agglutination) are commercially available. In contrast, *M. genavense* grows very slowly in liquid media, requires a special supplement called *mycobactin J* (which most microbiology laboratories do not use routinely) to grow on solid media, and can be identified only by com-

plex molecular techniques generally performed only in reference or research laboratories.

Diagnosis

Disseminated MAC disease.

FEVER AND HEPATITIS WITH RING GRANULOMAS

Clinical History

A 45-year-old man developed fever, severe headache, myalgia, and malaise, followed 1 week later by a dull ache in the right upper quadrant of his abdomen, anorexia, and a mild, nonproductive cough. On the eleventh day of illness, he sought medical attention. Physical examination revealed fever (103°F) and hepatomegaly. A chest radiograph showed small nodular infiltrates in both lung fields. Clinical laboratory data included hematocrit of 38%, white blood cell count of 6,300 cells per µl, mildly elevated serum hepatic enzyme concentrations (AST, 81 IU/liter; ALT, 95 IU/liter; and alkaline phosphatase, 150 U/liter), serum bilirubin of 1.9 mg/dl, and serum albumin of 3.5 g/dl. Serologic evaluation for HAV, HBV, and HCV viruses was not diagnostic. A liver biopsy was performed on the thirteenth day of illness to determine the cause of the hepatitis and hepatic enlargement.

Pathologic Findings

Numerous discrete, well-formed granulomas were observed randomly distributed within the hepatic lobules. In the periphery of the granulomas were multinucleated giant cells, epithelioid macrophages, and lymphocytes. Some of the granulomas contained neutrophils scattered through the clusters of macrophages. Nearly half of the cut sections of profiles of granulomas revealed a large clear central vacuole (Figure 4-25). Phosphotungstic acid–hematoxylin stain demonstrated that

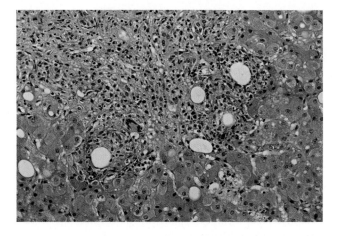

FIGURE 4-25. Section of liver shows several fibrin-ring granulomas and moderate steatosis in a case of Q fever (hematoxylin and eosin stain; medium-power magnification).

this clear space was surrounded by a ring of fibrin. Stains for bacteria, AFB, and fungi revealed no organisms.

Microbiology

Serologic data on the fifteenth day of illness included indirect immunofluorescent antibody (IFA) titers against phase II *Coxiella burnetii* of 1:64 for IgM and 1:128 for IgG. During convalescence 2 weeks later, the IFA IgG titer to *C. burnetii* phase II was 1:512. No antibodies were detected to phase I *C. burnetii*.

Comment

The general category of granulomatous hepatitis has a long list of infectious etiologies, including *Mycobacterium* species, *Brucella* species, *Listeria monocytogenes*, *Salmonella typhi*, *Bartonella* species, *H. capsulatum*, *C. immitis*, *Schistosoma mansoni*, and Q fever. Noninfectious causes include sarcoidosis, primary biliary cirrhosis, berylliosis, chronic granulomatous disease of childhood, Hodgkin's disease, and some cases of drug-associated hepatitis and toxic hepatitis (see Table 4-1). Tuberculosis and sarcoidosis are the leading causes in most case series.

Fibrin-ring granulomas (Figure 4-26), or so-called doughnut granulomas (as were observed in this case), are the characteristic lesion in Q fever hepatitis. However, ring granulomas have also been observed in association with cytomegaloviral and Epstein-Barr viral infection of the liver, viral hepatitis A, *M. avium* infection of the liver, Hodgkin's disease, and allopurinol-associated hepatic injury and thus are not pathognomonic of Q fever.

The spectrum of lesions observed in Q fever hepatitis likely reflects the temporal sequence of events of the hepatic involvement. Human volunteers infected by inhalation of aerosols containing *C. burnetii* developed focal hepatic lesions with death of hepatocytes and infiltration by lymphocytes, macrophages, and polymorphonuclear phagocytes during the incubation period. Granulomatous lesions were observed a short time later in the course and are much more highly associated with acute rather than chronic Q fever. Although Q fever granulomatous hepatitis is likely to follow infection by inhalation of organisms (usually from birth products of sheep, cattle, or goats or even cats, rabbits, or dogs, or by ingestion of *C. burnetii* in contaminated, unpasteurized milk or cheese), the source of infection is often not apparent. Q fever, a disease that is prevalent throughout the world, has received very little attention in the United States and is seldom diagnosed.

The serologic diagnosis of acute Q fever is established by demonstrating seroconversion to phase II *C. burnetii* (IFA titers of ≥1:200 for IgG or ≥1:50 for IgM). IFA titers of 1:200 or higher against phase I *C. burnetii* are indicative of chronic rather than acute Q fever.

Diagnosis

Q fever granulomatous hepatitis.

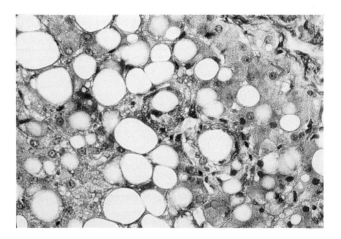

FIGURE 4-26. A fibrin-ring granuloma in this patient with acquired immunodeficiency syndrome and hepatic steatosis was documented by culture to have been caused by *Mycobacterium marinum* (Masson trichrome stain). (Courtesy of Dr. William K. Gourley.)

MULTIPLE ABSCESSES OF THE LIVER

Clinical History

A 62-year-old woman was seen in an emergency room for abdominal pain, anorexia, and nausea of 4 days' duration. The presumptive diagnosis was acute chole-cystitis. Her serum hepatic enzymes were elevated, and multiple hypodense lesions in an enlarged liver were demonstrated with a computed tomographic scan of the abdomen. The inferior vena cava was compressed. An isolated mass lesion in the apex of the right upper lobe of the lung was visualized on a chest radiograph. A clinical diagnosis of probable carcinoma of the lung with metastasis to the liver was made. Blood was collected for bacterial culture. She was started on empiric antimicrobial therapy, but she died within 24 hours of admission.

Pathologic Findings

The most striking abnormality at autopsy was in the liver, which weighed 2,500 g and contained multiple abscesses, the largest of which measured 11 cm in greatest diameter. Forty percent of the liver was estimated to have been replaced by necrotic tissue. Several of the abscesses communicated with the surface of the liver, and 700 ml of purulent fluid were present in the peritoneal cavity. Microscopically, the liver abscesses consisted of necrotic hepatocytes and masses of polymorphonuclear

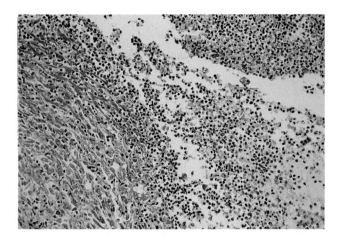

FIGURE 4-27. At the edge of the abscess, necrotic liver tissue and innumerable inflammatory cells, mostly polymorphonuclear leukocytes, are present. Bacteria are the most likely cause of such an abscess, but many etiologic agents are possible. Mixed infections with bacteria from the gastrointestinal tract are common in this clinical setting (hematoxylin and eosin stain; medium-power magnification).

neutrophils (Figure 4-27). Microabscesses were demonstrated in the lungs, heart, and brain.

Differential Diagnoses

Space-occupying lesions of the liver fall into two general categories: infectious and neoplastic. The most common infectious causes are bacterial and parasitic. During the first half of the twentieth century, amebic abscesses were common, and pyogenic abscesses often followed pylephlebitis of the portal vein after appendiceal disease. The amebiasis occurred predominantly in men during the third and fourth decades of life. Cultures for bacteria were often sterile because of amebic etiology and inadequate bacterial culture techniques. Amebic abscesses must still be considered when the patient comes from an area of the world in which *Entamoeba histolytica* is prevalent. In Western countries, however, bacterial etiologies now predominate. The most common underlying conditions are biliary tract disease, pancreatic disease, and disease of the gastrointestinal tract. Direct extension from adjacent infections are another major source for hepatic disease. Abscesses may follow trauma to the abdomen, and neoplasms of the biliary system, pancreas, and colon are frequent predisposing factors. Bacteremia and fungemia may result in hepatic abscesses, which are usually microscopic. Occasionally, no source is evident for the abscesses, which are termed *cryptogenic*.

Microbiology

The antemortem blood culture grew an alpha hemolytic streptococcus identified by biochemical tests as *Streptococcus anginosus* (*"milleri"*). A Gram stain of a smear of purulent material obtained from a liver abscess at autopsy contained gram-positive cocci in pairs and chains. A Brown-Hopps stain did not reveal any bacteria in tissue sections, but gram-positive bacteria were demonstrated with the Brown-Brenn stain (Figure 4-28). The liver abscesses were not cultured.

Comment

Reflecting the source of the infecting bacteria, mixed infections with biliary and fecal flora are common. Members of the *Enterobacteriaceae*, especially *Escherichia coli*, are the most frequently recovered bacteria. A variety of anaerobic bacteria may be isolated if adequate microbiologic techniques are used. *Candida* species are the most common fungal pathogens in disseminated infections. *S. aureus* is a common pathogen in primary bacteremic infection of the liver in children. Streptococci are frequent components of a mixed bacterial infection, but they also may produce abscesses in many organs as a single pathogen. The abscess-forming species of streptococci are termed *Streptococcus "milleri"* by British microbiologists. The species name is placed in quotation marks because it is not formally recognized as a valid taxonomic entity. In American identification systems, the most common identifications are *Streptococcus anginosus*, *Streptococcus constellatus*, and *Streptococcus MG-intermedius*; the currently preferred nomenclature is *Streptococcus anginosus*. As suggested by the confusion over bacterial taxonomy, the identification of alpha and gamma hemolytic streptococci is extremely difficult, because the biochemical reactions produced by these bacteria are variable, and considerable overlap exists among the species. If specific identification is attempted, determining whether the purported species fits the clinical situation must be done carefully.

Abscesses may be single or multiple. Single abscesses are most often found in the right lobe, perhaps because the greatest proportion of the portal blood supply goes to that lobe. The differentiation of hepatic abscesses from other abnormal conditions has been made increasingly easier as radiographic techniques have improved. Computed tomography and magnetic resonance imaging have replaced earlier diagnostic tools. The ultimate differentiation of the nature of the lesions, however, is made by aspiration of a lesion under radiographic guidance, or histologic examination of tissue sections. The therapy of amebic and bacterial abscesses is different; thus, the distinction is clinically important.

In cases of bacterial abscesses, the Brown-Brenn and Brown-Hopps stains, both of which are modifications of the Gram stain for histologic sections, are useful for preliminary classification of the responsible pathogen. In general, the Brown-Brenn stain colors gram-positive bacteria better than the Brown-Hopps

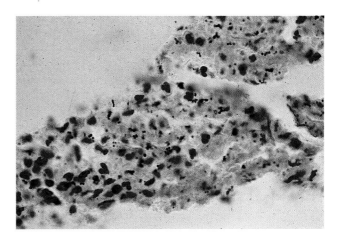

FIGURE 4-28. Gram-positive cocci in pairs and short chains are present in the inflammatory exudate, both within phagocytes and extracellularly (Brown-Brenn stain; oil immersion magnification).

stain, and the reverse is true with gram-negative bacteria. The dramatic difference in the performance of the two techniques that was seen in this case is a distinctly unusual occurrence for gram-positive bacteria. The case does illustrate, however, the importance of making smears of pathologic material for staining with a traditional Gram stain. Not only is this the reference method, but the morphology of the bacteria is also easier to study in cytologic preparations than in histologic sections. In addition, the results are available within minutes; Gram stain is the cheapest rapid test available, although its interpretation requires considerable experience in difficult cases.

Diagnosis

Bacterial liver abscesses caused by *Streptococcus "milleri."*

SPACE-OCCUPYING NECROTIZING LESION

Clinical History

A 45-year-old man was admitted to a hospital in the western United States with a chief complaint of abdominal pain. Clinical and radiographic evaluation of the patient disclosed a large, space-occupying lesion of the liver. An exploratory laparotomy was performed, and the mass was resected.

Pathologic Findings

The surgical material consisted of necrotic debris and stroma without recognizable hepatic tissue. Most of the necrotic matter was devoid of identifying structures (Figure 4-29); in better preserved areas, however, infiltrating trophozoites of *E. histolytica*, which appeared as oval to round structures in clear lacunae amid the necrotic debris (Figure 4-30), were visualized in the H and E–stained section. The characteristic ameboid forms could be seen in some cells as relatively pale-staining pseudopods extended from the darker-staining cell mass. The cytoplasm was vacuolar and relatively clear with little phagocytized debris. Erythrophagocytosis was demonstrated in some amebae (Figure 4-31), a characteristic feature that virtually assures the identification of the protozoa as *E. histolytica*. The typical nuclear structure, so important to parasitologists examining smears with the trichrome stain, is more difficult to visualize in histologic sections. In some cells, however, the fine peripheral chromatin and small karyosome (nucleolus) of *E. histolytica* could be appreciated.

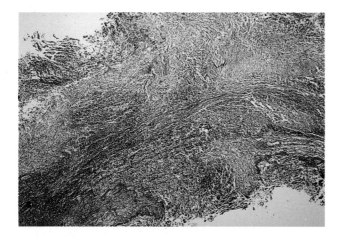

FIGURE 4-29. At low power, no discernible hepatic tissue remains; hepatocytes and stroma have undergone necrosis (hematoxylin and eosin stain, low-power magnification).

Comment

E. histolytica is a protozoan parasite that is widely distributed in the tropical and subtropical world. Most infected patients are asymptomatic, and the parasite is limited to the lower gastrointestinal tract. The stools of these patients contain the cyst form of the parasite (10–20 μm in diameter), which is either present as the only parasitic form or the predominant form. In active infection, the motile trophozoite form (12–50 μm in diameter) is present. Cysts that are passed in the stool are the infective form for individuals who ingest them. Infection most often is spread by the fecal-oral route, by means of contaminated water. Spread by colonic irrigation in a chiropractic clinic has been described, and sexual transmission may occur in populations in which oral-anal sex is practiced.

E. histolytica must be differentiated from the commensal intestinal amoeba, *Entamoeba coli*, and from artifacts and fecal leukocytes. It is now recognized that pathogenic strains and nonpathogenic strains exist that have the morphologic characteristics of *E. histolytica*. These biological variants are known as *zymodemes* (defined by different electrophoretic patterns of cellular enzymes); it has been proposed that the nonpathogenic strains be transferred to the genus *Entamoeba dispar*.

Amebic disease may be intestinal or extraintestinal. Invasive gastroenteritis is characterized by the gradual onset of abdominal pain and bloody diarrhea (amebic dysentery). The classic colonic lesion is an undermining ulcer with necrosis of the bowel wall. Chronic intestinal amebiasis may be less severe and mimic ulcerative colitis. Extension beyond the bowel most commonly involves the liver, but amebic lesions may occur in the lung, brain, genitourinary tract, and skin. Most patients with hepatic amebiasis do not have active gastrointestinal disease at the time. Amebic liver abscess has classically been described as a single large lesion in the right lobe of the liver (Figure 4-32), but modern radiographic techniques have documented the presence of multiple small lesions throughout the liver. Almost all patients with extraintestinal amebiasis have detectable antibodies by indirect hemagglutination or enzyme immunoassay. Although the presence of antibodies does not establish the diagnosis of active amebic infection, the absence of antibodies makes amebic abscess very unlikely.

Although monoclonal antibodies specific for *E. histolytica* have been described, the diagnosis of intestinal or extraintestinal disease is made by morphologic demonstration of the parasites in H and E–stained sections. The amebae also are well demonstrated by the period acid–Schiff (PAS) reaction (Figure 4-33), a useful

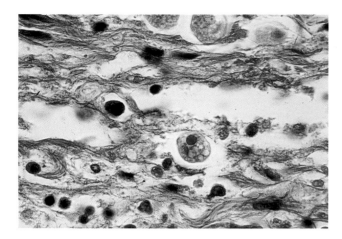

FIGURE 4-30. At high-power magnification, amebae can be seen within lacunae in the necrotic tissue. In histologic sections, the characteristic nucleus is not as easy to visualize as in cytologic preparations, such as are performed in the parasitology laboratory. The nucleus can be differentiated from nuclei of macrophages, however, by the pattern of the nuclear chromatin. The cytoplasm is vacuolated from phagocytic activity (hematoxylin and eosin stain; high-power magnification).

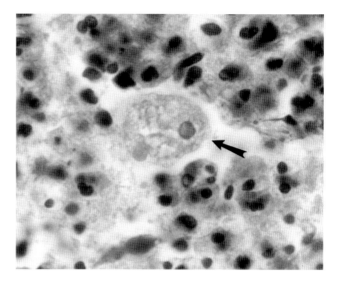

FIGURE 4-31. Section of tissue from a resected amebic abscess shows an *Entamoeba histolytica* trophozoite that has phagocytized an erythrocyte (*arrow*; hematoxylin and eosin stain; original magnification, ×250).

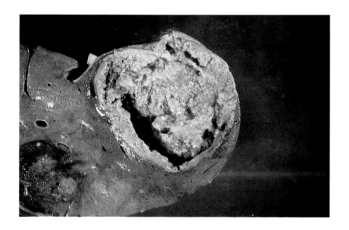

FIGURE 4-32. Liver from another patient with an amebic abscess. The solitary lesion is typically located in the right lobe and is filled with amorphous brown necrotic tissue sometimes called *anchovy paste*.

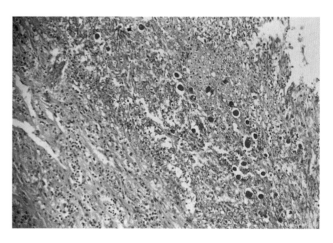

FIGURE 4-33. Even at low power, the amebae stand out sharply against the necrotic background when the section is stained by the periodic acid-Schiff with diastase method (periodic acid-Schiff stain; low-power magnification).

stain if this diagnosis is suspected and the protozoa are not detected in the H and E stain. The diagnostic morphology of the amebae is obscured, however, by the PAS reaction, and the cytologic detail should be evaluated with the H and E stain. Size (emphasizing the importance of using a micrometer) and the characteristics of the cytoplasm and nucleus must be evaluated to make the correct identification. The small ratio of nucleus to cytoplasm and the peripheral distribution of the nuclear chromatin distinguish amebae from macrophages. *E. histolytica* and *E. coli* are phagocytic, but only the former phagocytizes erythrocytes.

Diagnosis

Amebic abscess of the liver.

SPACE-OCCUPYING DISEASE OF THE LIVER CHARACTERIZED BY MULTIPLE THIN-WALLED CYSTS

Clinical History

A 72-year-old retired man noted a slowly enlarging abdomen for approximately 20 years and an increasingly bulging mass in his right flank for 6 months. Otherwise, he was asymptomatic. He was born on Cyprus and lived there until he was 22 years old, at which time he emigrated to the United States. Subsequently, he returned to Cyprus for periodic visits.

Physical examination was notable for a markedly enlarged abdomen. The liver edge extended below the pelvic margin. The edge was rounded, smooth, and nontender. The spleen was not palpable. Prominent abdominal veins, a small umbilical hernia, and a nodular prostate were present. The patient consumed alcohol, up to one bottle of whiskey per month or three glasses of wine per day.

Abnormal laboratory results included serum alkaline phosphatase, 276 U/μl; GGT, 95 U/μl; and hemoglobin that varied between 9.9 and 11.5 g/dl. The stool contained occult blood. A liver-spleen scan demonstrated little activity in the liver, which was replaced by a nonfunctioning mass. An ultrasound of the abdomen showed a large cystic mass in the right upper quadrant extending across the midline and inferiorly to 11 cm below the umbilicus. Multiple sonolucent areas ranged from 2 to 6 cm. The mass was not purely cystic but contained mul-

tiple internal echoes that suggested necrotic debris. Computed tomography of the abdomen revealed a large, low-density mass in the right upper quadrant with displacement of the left lobe of the liver and the aorta (Figure 4-34). Focal density in the mass compatible with calcification and a suggestion of nodularity were present. The spleen was intact. An aortogram documented avascularity of the mass with an absence of tumor blush.

In the operating room, the liver appeared pale and nodular. A cystic structure approximately 45 cm in diameter obliterated the right lobe of the liver, and the left lobe had hypertrophied to the approximate size of a normal liver. The cyst wall was approximately 8 mm thick and was adherent to the omentum, cystic duct, vena cava, and hepatic veins. Several small biliary and vascular radicles crossed through the cyst wall. The gallbladder was enlarged but contained no calculi. The spleen was minimally enlarged. An unsuccessful attempt was made to aspirate the cyst contents and inject a 20% saline solution. The cyst contents were removed as completely as possible without disrupting vital structures. The patient recovered uneventfully and returned to his local community.

Pathologic Findings

The surgical specimen consisted of a liver biopsy, resected gallbladder, and eight liters of cyst contents. Many cysts had thickened walls and gelatinous contents; others contained clear fluid with particulate matter visible in the fluid (hydatid sand). In an aspirate of fluid from the cysts were daughter cysts that contained multiple protoscolices of E. granulosus (Figures 4-35 and 4-36). The inverted hooklets were clearly visible. Sections of the liver, including the periphery of the cyst, demonstrated compression of the parenchyma and fibrosis and fragments of laminated membranes (Figure 4-37). The laminations of the chitin in the cyst walls were demonstrated with Gomori's methenamine silver stain.

Microbiology

Postoperatively, an indirect hemagglutination test performed in a reference laboratory was reported as positive for antibodies to Echinococcus granulosus.

Comment

Cystic hydatid disease of the liver is caused by E. granulosus, the dog tapeworm. Echinococcus multilocularis produces alveolar hydatid disease, characterized by mul-

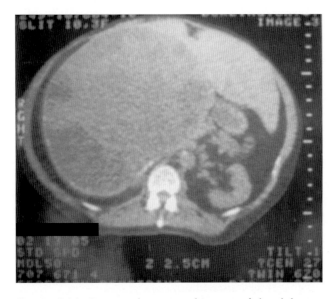

FIGURE 4-34. Computed tomographic scan of the abdomen demonstrates a hypodense lesion that fills and expands the entire left lobe of the liver.

FIGURE 4-35. Cell block section of material aspirated from an hydatid cyst shows three inverted scolices with hooklets and a few detached hooklets (*arrow*) in a background of necrotic debris (hematoxylin and eosin stain; original magnification, ×100). (Slide preparation courtesy of Dr. Assad J. Saad.)

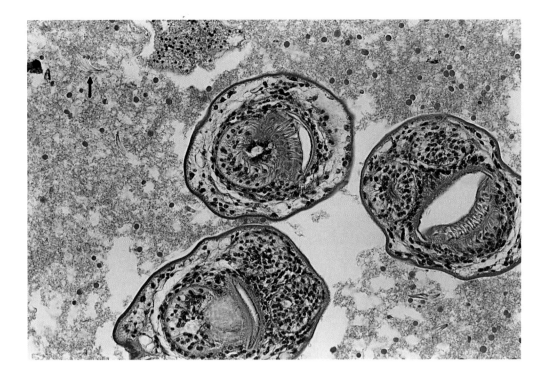

FIGURE 4-36. Smear of material aspirated from an hydatid cyst shows an everted scolex with an armed rostellum (*arrow*) and a cluster of detached hooklets (*arrowhead*; hematoxylin and eosin stain; original magnification, ×100). (Slide preparation courtesy of Dr. Assad J. Saad.)

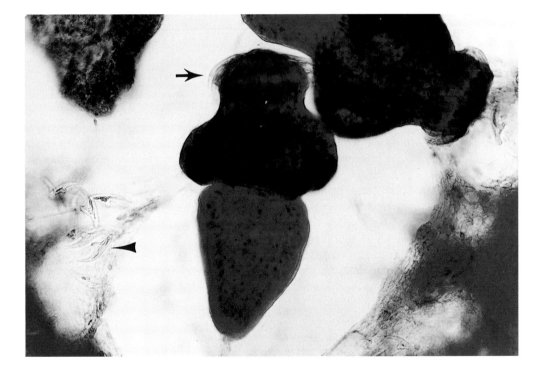

tilocular cysts that have an invasive tendency and may be mistaken for carcinoma of the liver. A third species, *Echinococcus vogeli*, may rarely produce human infection in South America. Other species have been identified in animals, but have not caused well documented human infection.

E. granulosus is widely distributed throughout the world, particularly where sheep are raised: the Middle East, the Mediterranean region, the Baltic states, Russia,

South Africa, India, and Australia. Echinococcal disease was described in the eastern United States by Osler, but most indigenous cases occur in sheep-raising areas of the southwest and California. The incidence of hydatid disease has been decreased by changes in animal husbandry as the life cycle of the parasite has been elucidated, but it has not been eliminated even in the United States.

The life cycle of *E. granulosus* includes a definitive host, in which the sexual phases of the cycle occur, and

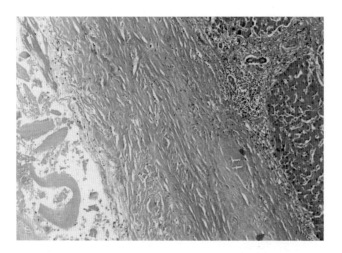

FIGURE 4-37. Section of liver taken to include the periphery of the cystic lesion shows a dense, fibrotic wall at the border between the liver and the larva. On the left are fragments of laminated larval cuticle (hematoxylin and eosin stain; original magnification, ×50).

an intermediate host, in which abortive infection results in the parasitic cyst. The definitive hosts are a variety of carnivores, primarily dogs, but occasionally coyotes and jackals. When the definitive host eats the infected organs of an herbivore, the protoscolices in the cysts are released in the gastrointestinal tract. There they develop into mature worms, which release eggs into the environment. The eggs of *E. granulosus* are indistinguishable from those of the pork and beef tapeworms *Taenia solium* and *Taenia saginata*. The eggs are ingested by herbivores, such as sheep, when they graze on contaminated vegetation. In the small intestine, the eggs hatch and the embryos migrate through the portal circulation, producing cysts most commonly in the liver, less often in the lung, and in virtually any organ on occasion. Certain traditional practices of shepherds, such as allowing herding dogs to eat the carcasses of dead sheep, foster maintenance of the cycle in nature. Humans are infected incidentally and are often termed *dead-end hosts*. This incidental role is a direct result of the organization of most societies. In parts of Africa, humans have functioned as active participants in the life cycle of the parasite (intermediate hosts); human corpses buried in shallow graves were preyed on by carnivores, such as dogs and jackals. A sylvatic form of cystic hydatid disease caused by *E. granulosus* has been reported in

Alaska, Canada, and the northern Plains states of the United States. The definitive host is the wolf, and large herbivores, such as moose, caribou, and large deer, serve as intermediate hosts. The clinical presentation of this variant is benign in comparison to classical infection, and conservative management is indicated.

E. multilocularis is found in Central Europe, Russia, and Japan, and cases have been reported in the northern portion of the Western Hemisphere. This species is primarily sylvatic and causes human disease infrequently. The life cycle includes rodents as intermediate hosts and foxes or dogs as definitive hosts.

In the infected organ, *E. granulosus* produces a unilocular cyst with a laminated acellular membrane and an internal germinative membrane (the mother cyst). From the germinative membrane, protoscolices develop in brood capsules that protrude into the cyst lumen. As the brood capsules break away from the wall, multiple generations of daughter cysts may be formed. Eventually the parasites die, producing amorphous debris including hooklets, which is termed *hydatid sand*. Portions of the cysts may calcify.

The most important complication of hydatid cysts is rupture, after which cysts may develop throughout the abdomen or in distant organs if protoscolices enter the vascular system. Bile peritonitis may result if a hepatic cyst ruptures. Pleural effusions result from rupture of lung cysts. Secondary bacterial infection converts the cysts into pyogenic abscesses in the liver, whereas empyema may develop in the pleural cavity. A potentially fatal complication of massive rupture is an acute anaphylactic reaction when large amounts of antigenic cyst fluid are released into the peritoneal cavity or the circulation. Slow leakage of cyst fluid may produce nonfatal anaphylaxis and eosinophilia, which is usually mild.

The diagnosis is usually made from the clinical history, epidemiology, and radiographic studies that demonstrate a cystic mass. Several serologic tests have been developed for detection of antibodies to *E. granulosus*. An enzyme-linked immunosorbent assay appears to have greater sensitivity and specificity than indirect immunofluorescence, indirect hemagglutination, and a classical intradermal skin test (Casoni test). A Western blot immunoassay is available for specific confirmation. The surgical treatment of hydatid disease depends on the extent of the cysts. Chemotherapy with scolicides, such as mebendazole or albendazole, is adjunctive to surgical therapy.

Diagnosis

Echinococcal cyst of the liver.

CHOLANGIOPATHY

Clinical History

A 28-year-old woman diagnosed with AIDS in 1992 presented with generalized pruritus, right upper quadrant pain, and weight loss of 10 pounds over the past 3 weeks. Her risk factor for AIDS was injection drug use. Pertinent medical history included two episodes of syphilis and cervical dysplasia. On physical examination, her temperature was 38°C, her heart rate was 82 beats per minute, and her respiratory rate was 18 breaths per minute. The abdomen was mildly distended, and moderate right upper quadrant tenderness was present. The remainder of the examination was unremarkable. Abnormal laboratory test results included a hemoglobin of 9.2 g/dl, white blood cell count of 3,400 cells per μl, and elevated liver enzymes. A stool specimen submitted to a microbiology laboratory for detection of microsporidia and cryptosporidia revealed microsporidial spores. An endoscopic retrograde cholescystopancreatogram revealed moderate dilatation of the midsection of the common bile duct and the intrahepatic bile ducts and narrowing of the distal common bile duct. A brush biopsy from the common bile duct mucosa and a needle biopsy of the liver were submitted for cytologic and histologic studies.

Pathologic Findings

The liver biopsy showed chronic cholangitis, cholangiolar hyperplasia with acute pericholangitis, and extensive portal fibrosis, consistent with obstructive sclerosing cholangitis. Formalin-fixed, paraffin-embedded sections of the common bile duct brush biopsy revealed a few degenerating bile duct epithelial cells and an inflammatory exudate consisting of histiocytes and neutrophils (Figure 4-38). Sections stained with a tissue Gram stain showed small, red-stained organisms (some of which had a prominent band in their center) within the histiocyte cytoplasm (Figure 4-39). Thick sections of the tissue processed for electron microscopic examination also showed multiple, oval organisms within histiocyte cytoplasm (Figure 4-40).

Comment

E. intestinalis is one of the species of microsporidia that infect humans and can disseminate. *E. intestinalis* infections of the intestine, kidneys, upper and lower respiratory tracts, and gallbladder, as occurred in this case, have been reported. In one review of five patients with AIDS who had chronic diarrhea due to *E. intestinalis*, four had right upper quadrant pain and ultrasound studies showing a dilated biliary tree, suggesting that the cholangiopathy in AIDS patients may occur commonly in *E. intestinalis* infection.

Histologically, in *E. intestinalis* infection of the small bowel, gallbladder, and bronchi, organisms are present in the cytoplasm of epithelial cells, as is true of infections with other species of microsporidia (see Chapter 3), and in macrophages in the lamina propria. *E. intestinalis* is believed to be able to reproduce in macrophages, thus facilitating its dissemination. In this case and a few other reports of *E. intestinalis* cholangitis, prominent clusters of foamy macrophages in the lamina propria were present, a potential clue to the diagnosis. Therefore, in patients with AIDS, *E. intestinalis* should be added to the list of pathogens that elicit an inflammatory response consisting of histiocytic aggregates, including MAC, *M. genavense*, and *H. capsulatum*. Based on this differential diagnosis, special stains for AFB and fungi should be obtained first. If neither mycobacteria nor fungi are identified, stains for microsporidia, such as the Brown-Brenn or Warthin-Starry stain or electron microscopy, or a combination of the two, should be performed.

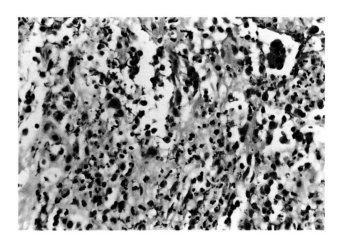

FIGURE 4-38. Formalin-fixed, paraffin-embedded section of material obtained by brush biopsy of the common bile duct reveals a few degenerating bile duct epithelial cells and an inflammatory exudate composed of histiocytes and neutrophils (hematoxylin and eosin stain; original magnification, ×100). (Courtesy of Dr. William Gourley.)

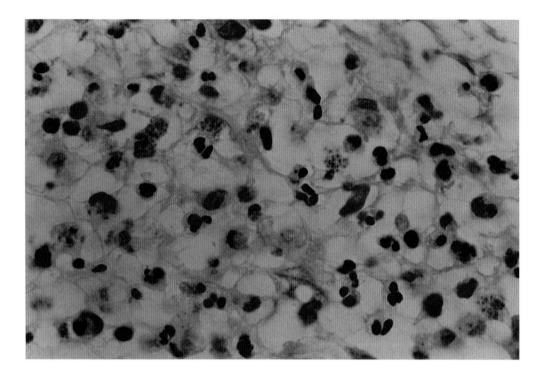

FIGURE 4-39. Section of the tissue illustrated in Figure 4-38 and stained with a tissue Gram stain shows clusters of red-staining microsporidia, some of which have a dark band near their centers (Brown-Brenn stain; original magnification, ×250). (Courtesy of Dr. William Gourley.)

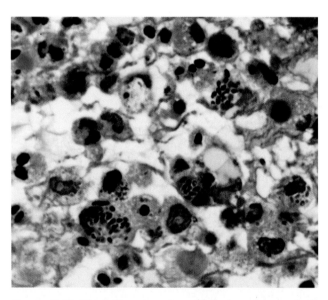

FIGURE 4-40. Thick (1 μm) section of bile duct tissue embedded in epoxy resin (Polybed) shows aggregates of histiocytes containing multiple small, oval microsporidia (toluidine blue stain; original magnification, ×250). (Courtesy of Dr. William Gourley.)

FIGURE 4-41. Electron photomicrograph shows a probable macrophage containing spores in spaces separated by thin septa. The epithelial location, host cell vacuoles, and septation are characteristic of *Encephalitozoon* (formerly *Septata*) *intestinalis* (original magnification, ×18,150).

Identification of microsporidia to the genus and, in some cases, species level requires electron microscopic analysis of tissue. Electron microscopy (Figure 4-41) demonstrates the presence of spores with a polar tube, a characteristic of all genera of microsporidia. Members of the genus *Encephalitozoon* are enclosed in a phagosome-like limiting vesicle produced by the host. In contrast, species of *Enterocytozoon* and *Nosema* develop in direct contact with host cell cytoplasm without a limiting vacuolar membrane. A distinguishing feature of *Nosema* species is the presence of paired, abutted nuclei.

Diagnosis

E. intestinalis cholangiopathy in a patient with AIDS.

RECOMMENDED READING

Viral Hepatitis

Abe H, Beninger PR, Ikejiri N, et al. Light microscopic findings of liver biopsy specimens from patients with hepatitis A and comparison with type B. Gastroenterology 1982;82:938.

Bach N, Thung SN, Schaffner F. The histological features of chronic hepatitis C and autoimmune hepatitis: a comparative analysis. Hepatology 1992;15:572.

DiBisceglie AM, Goodman ZD, Ishak KG, et al. Long-term clinical and histopathological follow-up of chronic post transfusion hepatitis. Hepatology 1991;14:969.

Esteban R. Epidemiology of hepatitis C virus infection. J Hepatol 1993;17:567.

Farci P, Alter HJ, Shimoda A, et al. Hepatitis C virus–associated fulminant hepatic failure. N Engl J Med 1996;335:631.

Kobayashi K, Hashimoto E, Ludwig J, et al. Liver biopsy features of acute hepatitis C compared with hepatitis A, B, and non-A, non-B, non-C. Liver 1993;13:69.

Krawczynski K. Hepatitis E. Hepatology 1993;17:932.

Lefkowitch JH, Schiff ER, Davis GL, et al. Pathological diagnosis of chronic hepatitis C: a multicenter comparative study with chronic hepatitis B. Gastroenterology 1993;104:595.

Scheuer PJ. Viral hepatitis. In RNM MacSween, PP Anthony, PJ Scheuer, et al. (eds), Pathology of the Liver. New York: Churchill Livingstone, 1994;816.

Scheuer PJ, Ashrafzadeh P, Sherlock S, et al. The pathology of hepatitis C. Hepatology 1992;15:567.

Teixeira MR Jr, Weller IVD, Murray A, et al. The pathology of hepatitis A in man. Liver 1982;2:53.

Lassa Fever

Holme GP, McCormick JB, Trock SC, et al. Lassa fever in the United States. Investigation of a case and new guidelines for management. N Engl J Med 1990; 323:1120.

McCormick JB, King IJ, Webb PA, et al. A case-control study of the clinical diagnosis and course of Lassa fever. J Infect Dis 1987;155:445.

McCormick JB, Walker DH, King IJ, et al. Lassa virus hepatitis: a study of fatal Lassa fever in humans. Am J Trop Med Hyg 1986;35:401.

Walker DH, McCormick JB, Johnson KM, et al. Pathologic and virologic study of fatal Lassa fever in man. Am J Pathol 1982;107:349.

Granulomatous Hepatitis

Albrecht H, Rusch-Gerdes S, Hans-Jurgen S, et al. Disseminated *Mycobacterium genavense* infection as a cause of pseudo–Whipple's disease and sclerosing cholangitis. Clin Infect Dis 1997;25:742.

Dupont HL, Hornick RB, Levin HS, et al. Q fever hepatitis. Ann Intern Med 1971;74:198.

Tissot Dupont H, Raoult D, Brouqui P, et al. Epidemiologic features and clinical presentation of acute Q fever in hospitalized patients: 323 French cases. Am J Med 1992;93:427.

Fishbein DB, Raoult D. A cluster of *Coxiella burnetii* infections associated with exposure to vaccinated goats and their unpasteurized dairy products. Am J Trop Med Hyg 1992;47:35.

Harrington PT, Gutiérrez JJ, Ramirez-Ronda CH, et al. Granulomatous hepatitis. Rev Infect Dis 1982;4:638.

Hill AR, Premkumar S, Brustein S, et al. Disseminated tuberculosis in the acquired immunodeficiency syndrome era. Ann Rev Respir Dis 1991;144:1164.

Hunt AC, Bothwell PW. Histological findings in human brucellosis. J Clin Pathol 1967;20:267.

Lupatkin H, Brau N, Flomenberg P, Simberkoff MS. Tuberculous abscesses in patients with AIDS. Clin Infect Dis 1992;14:1040.

McCluggage WG, Sloan JM. Hepatic granulomas in Northern Ireland: a thirteen-year review. Histopathology 1994;25:219.

Raoult D. Host factors in the severity of Q fever. Ann NY Acad Sci 1990;590:33.

Raoult D, Marrie T. Q fever. Clin Infect Dis 1995;20:489.

Spink WW, Hoffbauer FW, Walker WW, Green RA. Histopathology of the liver in human brucellosis. J Lab Clin Med 1949;34:40.

Walker DH. Pathology of Q fever. In DH Walker (ed), Biology of Rickettsial Diseases (vol 2). Boca Raton, FL: CRC Press, 1988;17.

Young EJ. Human brucellosis. Rev Infect Dis 1983;5:821.

Bacterial Liver Abscess

Barbour GL, Juniper K Jr. A clinical comparison of amebic and pyogenic abscess of the liver in sixty-six patients. Am J Med 1972;53:323.

Barnes PF, DeCook KM, Reynolds TN, Ralls PW. A comparison of amebic and pyogenic abscess of the liver. Medicine (Baltimore) 1987;66:472.

Chua D, Reinhart HH, Sobel JD. Liver abscess caused by *Streptococcus milleri*. Rev Infect Dis 1989;11:197.

Dehner LP, Kissane JM. Pyogenic hepatic abscesses in infancy and childhood. J Pediatr 1969;74:763.

Rubin RH, Swartz MN, Malt R. Hepatic abscess: changes in clinical, bacteriologic and therapeutic aspects. Am J Med 1974;57:601.

Sabbaj J, Sutter VL, Finegold SM. Anaerobic pyogenic liver abscess. Ann Intern Med 1972;77:627.

Amebic Abscess

Adams EB, MacLeod IN. Invasive amebiasis—amebic liver abscess and its complications. Medicine 1977;56:325.

Anonymous. Misdiagnosis of amoebiasis. BMJ 1978; 6134:379.

Lesh FA. Massive development of amebas in the large intestine. Am J Trop Med Hyg 1975;24:383.

Phillips SC, Mildvan D, William DC, et al. Sexual transmission of enteric protozoa and helminths in a venereal-disease-clinic population. N Engl J Med 1981;305:603.

Rab SM, Alam N, Hoda AN, Yee A. Amoebic liver abscess. Some unique presentations. Am J Med 1967;43:811.

Sorvillo FJ, Strassburg MA, Seidel J, et al. Amebic infections in asymptomatic homosexual men, lack of evidence of invasive disease. Am J Publ Health 1986; 76:1137.

Yang J, Kennedy MT. Evaluation of enzyme-linked immunosorbent assay for the serodiagnosis of amebiasis. J Clin Microbiol 1979;10:778.

Echinococcosis

Araujo FP, Schwabe CW, Sawyer JC, Davis WG. Hydatid disease transmission in California. A study of the Basque connection. Am J Epidemiol 1975;102:291.

Didier D, Weiler S, Rohmer P, et al. Hepatic alveolar echinococcosis: correlative US and CT study. Radiology 1985;154:179.

Katz AM, Pan CT. Echinococcus disease in the United States. Am J Med 1958;25:759.

Pappaioanou M, Schwabe CW, Sard DM. An evolving pattern of human hydatid disease transmission in the United States. Am J Trop Med Hyg 1977; 26:732.

Pitt HA, Korzelius J, Tompkins RK. Management of hepatic echinococcosis in southern California. Am J Surg 1986;152:110.

Microsporidia

Liberman E, Bendict Yen TS. Foamy macrophages in acquired immunodeficiency syndrome cholangiopathy with *Encephalitozoon intestinalis*. Arch Pathol Lab Med 1997;121:985.

Infections of the Skin and Subcutaneous Tissue

The skin and subcutaneous tissue can be used to observe and diagnose not only localized or disseminated superficial infectious lesions but also pathologic processes that may involve the visceral organs. Diagnostic dermatopathology tends to emphasize neoplasia ranging from the repetitious pattern recognition of epidermal lesions to the complexity of adnexal tumors. Inflammatory cutaneous lesions pose a more urgent challenge. Often, timely identification of the etiology of acute and progressive chronic lesions allows the implementation of effective specific therapy that is sometimes lifesaving.

In this era of acquired immunodeficiency syndrome (AIDS) and other conditions of immunocompromise, physicians readily perform biopsies of recently appearing skin lesions associated with fever and other signs and symptoms. The pathologist, whose task is to provide a timely diagnosis, requires an organized approach based on the relevant differential diagnosis. Knowledgeable clinical colleagues should provide a clear macroscopic description of the lesions, a pertinent clinical history, and their important diagnostic considerations. Important macroscopic characteristics include the form of the lesions (i.e., macular, papular, plaque-like, nodular, vesicular, bullous, or pustular) and whether lesions are erythematous or hemorrhagic. The anatomic distribution, progression of spread, and time of onset, relative to other symptoms, of the skin lesions are also pertinent information. Relevant clinical history includes recent medications; exposure to animals, arthropods, febrile persons, or sexually transmitted diseases; travel; and immunologic status.

A rash might be the result of a drug reaction or infectious or other noninfectious diseases. Infection-associated rashes may be viral, fungal, or bacterial in origin. Maculopapular rash is often caused by viral infections (e.g., rubella; measles; parvovirus B19; enteroviruses; dengue;

and bacterial diseases, such as Rocky Mountain spotted fever, meningococcemia, and typhoid fever). Nodular rash is often caused by fungal infections (e.g., candidemia, histoplasmosis, sporotrichosis, blastomycosis, or coccidioidomycosis) and by mycobacteria and nocardia. Vesicles are usually viral in origin (e.g., varicella-zoster virus [VZV], herpes simplex virus [HSV], or enteroviruses). Pustules may evolve from vesicles or develop from other causes, such as gonococcemia. Variability in rashes with a particular disease may result from changes in an individual patient during the course of illness or striking differences among patients; secondary syphilis may be manifested as a macular, maculopapular, papulosquamous, or pustular rash.

Viral diseases cause a rash often by viral replication in the skin and direct cytopathic effects that may be evident as a typical pattern of necrosis with the presence of viral inclusions. Histopathology was the original laboratory method for diagnosis of viral diseases. The Scottish pathologist John Brown Buist described the elementary bodies that we now call *virions* in fluid from the skin lesions of smallpox in 1886. Guarnieri described nuclear and cytoplasmic inclusion bodies in smallpox lesions in 1892. The neuronal cytoplasmic inclusions (Negri bodies) of rabies and nuclear inclusions of varicella were reported in the first decade of the 20th century. Barring a catastrophic reintroduction via bioterrorism or biologic warfare, smallpox has been eradicated, and viral inclusions are useful diagnostic clues for only a small proportion of viral diseases (HSV types I and II, VZV, cytomegalovirus, disseminated adenovirus, measles giant cell pneumonia, subacute sclerosing panencephalitis, progressive multifocal leukoencephalopathy, and rabies). Each of these etiologic diagnoses can be achieved with greater sensitivity, specificity, timeliness, or clinical relevance by other available methods. Many viral agents leave no inclusion body as a calling card (e.g., Epstein-Barr virus; influenza viruses; rubella; rotavirus; poliovirus; Coxsackie viruses; echoviruses; rhinoviruses; hepatitis A, B, C, delta, and E viruses; arboviruses; arenaviruses; hantaviruses; mumps; and, in most cases, parainfluenza viruses and respiratory syncytial virus). Diagnosis of the virus at the time of presentation for medical care can be achieved in some cases by cytopathology, demonstration of viral antigens or nucleic acids, electron microscopy, or viral isolation from the lesions. For other viral agents, rash may result largely from host responses to viral antigens in the skin (e.g., measles).

Bacteria, fungi, and protozoa cause rashes by the effect of exotoxins, by growth of organisms damaging the blood vessels, or by stimulation of kinins, prostaglandins, leukotrienes, cytokines, coagulation, complement, and cell-mediated immune mechanisms. Diagnosis of these agents is usually achieved by a combination of visualization in tissue, microbiological cultivation, and serology.

AIDS has brought a greater volume of pathology cases with cutaneous manifestations of infectious diseases. The list of etiologic agents is long: human immunodeficiency virus (HIV; seroconversion disease), HSV, VZV, *Cryptococcus neoformans*, mycobacteria, *Histoplasma capsulatum*, *Sporothrix schenckii*, *Candida*, molluscum contagiosum, papillomaviruses, *Bartonella* organisms of bacillary angiomatosis, spirochetes, dermatophytes, and scabies. The clinical and pathologic manifestations often differ from the classic picture qualitatively and quantitatively, not only for these infections but also for drug eruptions, neoplasms (e.g., Kaposi's sarcoma, lymphomas, and skin cancers), and other diseases (e.g., psoriasis, seborrheic dermatitis, idiopathic thrombocytopenic purpura, and telangiectasia). The dermatopathology of AIDS is an evolving challenge that demands an etiologic answer as critically as does an immunocompetent febrile patient with meningococcemia versus Rocky Mountain spotted fever versus viral exanthem. Appropriate, timely, lifesaving treatment often hangs in the balance.

VESICULAR RASH IN AN IMMUNOSUPPRESSED PATIENT

Clinical History

A middle-aged male heart transplant recipient, who was immunosuppressed with cyclosporine and prednisone, developed cutaneous lesions on his face that subsequently disseminated over his body. The lesions began as erythematous macules and rapidly became vesicular and then pustular. One week later, a biopsy of one lesion was submitted for histopathologic evaluation.

Pathologic Findings

The section of skin showed a vesicle that was in part intraepithelial and in part subepithelial with a basal layer of epithelium at the margins and denuded epithelium in the center of the lesion (Figure 5-1). The vesicle contained multinucleate giant cells (Figure 5-2), some with intranuclear inclusions, and necrotic epithelial cells, some of which also contained intranuclear inclusions (Figure 5-3). Necrosis involving the superficial dermis was evident.

Differential Diagnosis

Based on the pathologic findings, the differential diagnosis is between VZV and HSV.

Microbiology

The diagnosis was suggested by the clinical observations; a Tzanck preparation from a lesion showed multinucleated giant cells (Figure 5-4). Intranuclear inclusions in

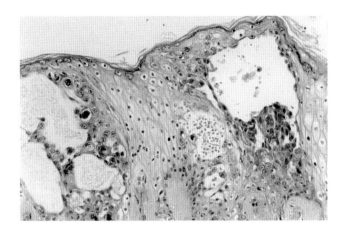

FIGURE 5-1. Photomicrograph of a skin lesion of disseminated varicella-zoster viral infection shows intraepidermal vesicles and inflammation and necrosis in the upper dermis (hematoxylin and eosin stain; original magnification, ×50).

suitably stained cytopathologic specimens, multinucleated giant cells, and intranuclear inclusions in a cutaneous punch biopsy (as in this case) do not distinguish VZV from HSV infection. Because VZV is labile and highly cell associated, viral culture is a relatively insensitive diagnostic method by which to detect VZV, but it is the most sensitive technique for detecting HSV. Detection of VZV antigens by immunofluorescence in a smear of cells from the vesicular fluid, or scraped from the base of a lesion, and tissue specimens is considerably more sensitive and

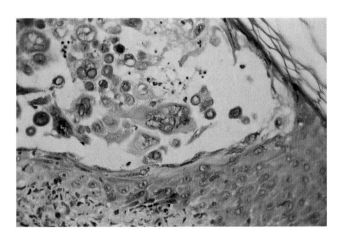

FIGURE 5-2. Photomicrograph of an intraepidermal vesicle of a varicella-zoster viral lesion that contains multinucleate giant cells and nuclear changes characteristic of herpesvirus group cytopathic effect (hematoxylin and eosin stain; high-power magnification).

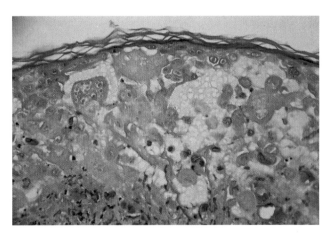

FIGURE 5-3. Photomicrograph of a cutaneous lesion of disseminated varicella-zoster viral infection shows an intraepidermal vesicle containing necrotic epithelial cells, some of which have prominent pink intranuclear inclusions (hematoxylin and eosin stain; high-power magnification).

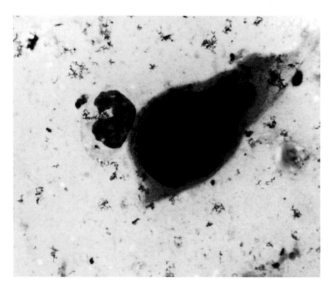

FIGURE 5-4. Tzanck preparation of a smear fluid collected from a vesicle of a patient with varicella-zoster virus infection shows a multinucleate epithelial cell characteristic of the cytopathic effect induced by this virus (Giemsa stain; original magnification, ×250).

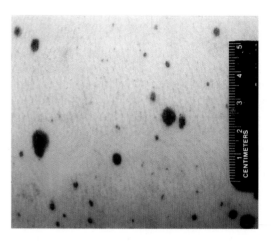

FIGURE 5-5. Skin of a severely immunocompromised teenager with disseminated varicella. Numerous macular and pustular lesions manifest striking hemorrhage.

was positive in this case. The specificity of these antigen tests is excellent in determining which patients have VZV and which have HSV infection. Serology is used virtually only to determine immune status.

Comment

VZV causes two distinct clinical syndromes: chickenpox (primary infection) and shingles or zoster (reactivation). VZV is a DNA virus of the herpesvirus group ultrastructurally similar to HSV-1, HSV-2, Epstein-Barr virus, and cytomegalovirus. After chickenpox (usually occurring in childhood), VZV remains latent in the neurons of the sensory ganglion supplying a dermatome that had been heavily involved in chickenpox. The virus intermittently reactivates when the host's cell-mediated immunity to the virus is low, viral proteins are synthesized, and viral replication occurs. Many persons undergo this reactivation

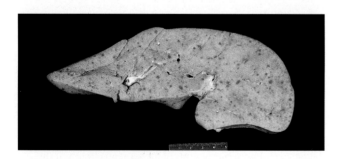

FIGURE 5-6. Cross section of gross liver from a patient with disseminated varicella-zoster viral infection shows numerous foci of hemorrhagic hepatic necrosis.

with only an asymptomatic boost in anti-VZV antibody titer. Some patients develop only neuralgia of the involved dermatome, and others also have centrifugal spread of the virus down the infected neurons to the skin where the vesicular eruption occurs. The histopathologies of chickenpox and zoster are similar, although greater dermal involvement in zoster more often leads to scarring, particularly in immunosuppressed patients. Nearly half of immunosuppressed cases, as in this patient, have cutaneous dissemination with 20–50 lesions outside the primary dermatome. Although visceral dissemination may have a fatal outcome, disseminated cutaneous VZV is seldom more serious than zoster itself. Other infectious diseases that cause a disseminated vesicular rash include rickettsialpox, enteroviral exanthem, HSV infection, cytomegalovirus infection, *Mycoplasma pneumoniae* infection, and *Vibrio vulnificus* infection.

The rash of disseminated VZV in immunosuppressed patients is not always vesicular. For example, it may be manifested as disseminated purpuric cutaneous lesions (as observed in the 19-year-old man with aplastic anemia who was exposed to a child with chickenpox, illustrated in Figure 5-5). A frozen section of a lesion showed multinucleate giant cells. The patient developed disseminated visceral lesions and disseminated intravascular coagulation; he died one week after onset of illness. Miliary foci of hemorrhagic necrosis were observed in the liver (Figure 5-6), lungs, skin, spleen, and esophagus.

Diagnosis

VZV infection.

FEVER AND MACULOPAPULAR RASH

Clinical History

A 70-year-old man experienced chills, fever, and severe headache. He subsequently developed myalgia, nausea, vomiting, and a nonproductive cough, consulted a physician, and was treated with erythromycin. On the sixth day of his illness, his wife noted a few red macules in his axilla, followed over the next two days by a maculopapular rash involving the trunk and, the next day, on the arms and legs. On the ninth day of illness, he went to an emergency room, where examination revealed bilateral rales, confusion, stupor, ataxia, and a petechial maculopapular rash. Laboratory data included a normal white blood cell count, thrombocytopenia (platelets, 35,000 per μl), elevated serum hepatic transaminases, and azotemia. Blood, cerebrospinal fluid (CSF), and urine were collected for bacterial and viral cultures. A biopsy of the skin rash was submitted for histopathologic studies.

Pathologic Findings

Sections of the punch biopsy of skin revealed dermal arteries, veins, and capillaries with markedly swollen endothelial cells, a lymphohistiocytic perivascular infiltrate, and focal hemorrhage (Figure 5-7). Immunohistologic staining for typhus group rickettsiae revealed that the swollen endothelial cells were distended by large quantities of cytoplasmic rickettsiae.

Differential Diagnosis

The differential diagnosis of febrile maculopapular exanthem with systemic flulike symptoms includes rickettsioses (Rocky Mountain spotted fever, boutonneuse fever, other geographic spotted fever rickettsioses, murine typhus, classic typhus, and scrub typhus), enteroviral infection, rubeola, rubella, dengue, meningococcemia, typhoid fever, toxic shock syndrome, secondary syphilis, disseminated gonococcal infection, leptospirosis, and Kawasaki syndrome. In the absence of a rash, which is recognized in only 54% of patients and often appears late, the cough and pulmonary infiltrates may suggest

pneumonia or bronchitis, central nervous system signs and symptoms and CSF pleocytosis may suggest viral or bacterial meningitis or encephalitis, and abdominal signs and symptoms may suggest gastroenteritis.

Microbiology

Cultures of blood, CSF, skin lesions, and urine revealed no pathogenic organisms. The anti-*Rickettsia typhi* indirect immunofluorescence antibody titers of sera collected on the tenth day of illness and 2 weeks later were 1:128 and 1:2,048, respectively. No antibodies against *R. rickettsii* were detected.

Comment

The diagnosis of murine typhus is difficult to establish during the acute stage of illness. Although immunohistologic identification of typhus group rickettsiae (Figure 5-8) and analysis of blood by the polymerase chain reaction

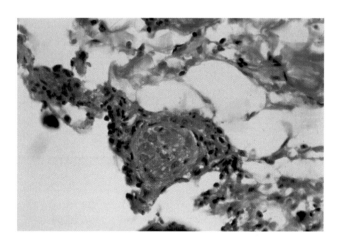

FIGURE 5-7. Photomicrograph of a classic typhus rickettsial lesion in the skin of a patient with murine typhus. Vascular injury is manifested as severe endothelial swelling, and the host immune response consists of a prominent perivascular lymphohistiocytic infiltrate (hematoxylin and eosin stain; high-power magnification).

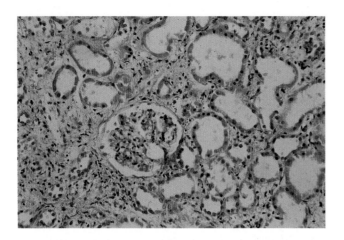

FIGURE 5-8. Photomicrograph of kidney from a fatal case of murine typhus shows a glomerulus with focal endothelial cells distended by numerous *Rickettsia typhi* organisms (anti–typhus group rickettsial monoclonal antibody-based immunohisto-chemistry; medium-power magnification).

can establish a diagnosis, serologic assays are usually the only tests that are available. Commercially available methods for detecting antibodies against *R. typhi* include indirect immunofluorescence assay (IFA), dot–enzyme-linked immunosorbent assay (ELISA), and *Proteus* OX-19 agglutination. IFA and dot-ELISA are substantially more sensitive and specific than the Weil-Felix test. Even with the sensitive and specific IFA, a diagnostic titer is present in only half of murine typhus patients during the first week of illness, when therapeutic decisions are critical.

The discovery of a novel rickettsia, *Rickettsia felis*, in cat fleas (which are also a vector of *R. typhi*) suggests that rickettsial infections should be a diagnostic consideration more often than they are.

Diagnosis

Murine typhus.

CENTRIFUGALLY EXPANDING RASH AND SYSTEMIC SYMPTOMS

Clinical History

A 28-year-old woman noted the presence of a red papule on her left thigh 1 week after she had attended a picnic in late June. She did not recall a tick bite at that site or elsewhere, but she did remove a very small tick approximately the size of a poppy seed from the scalp of her son while bathing him after the outing. The red papule expanded to a diameter of 11 cm over the next nine days and developed a bright red outer border with partial clearing within the outer erythematous ring (Figure 5-9). During this period, she was tired and had a headache for a few days that was followed by fever and myalgia, for which she sought medical attention. Physical examination revealed fever (38.2°C), a classic erythema migrans lesion on her thigh, and enlarged left inguinal lymph nodes. The patient gave informed consent for a cutaneous biopsy to be performed for research purposes. She was treated with oral doxycycline, and the rash and systemic symptoms resolved.

Pathologic Findings

The biopsy of the outer erythematous portion of the skin lesion showed dermal perivascular infiltrates of lymphocytes and plasma cells (Figure 5-10). Examination of four sections stained by the Warthin-Starry method revealed only one borrelial organism.

Differential Diagnoses

The differential diagnoses of the rash include erythema migrans (Lyme borreliosis), cellulitis, tinea, granuloma annulare, allergic reactions to an arthropod bite, erythema multiforme, urticaria, contact dermatitis, and fixed drug reaction.

Microbiology

Culture of an aspirate of the leading edge of the erythema migrans rash lesion in Barbour-Stoenner-Kelly medium yielded a borrelial isolate after 3 weeks of incubation. Polymerase chain reaction of DNA of a portion of the skin biopsy detected DNA of the plasmid gene encoding the surface protein OspA of *Borrelia burgdorferi*. The initial serologic test at the time of presentation, an enzyme immunoassay, did not detect any antibodies against *B. burgdorferi*. A second serum sample collected four weeks later contained immunoglobulin M (IgM) and immunoglobulin G (IgG) antibodies by screening enzyme immunoassay that were confirmed by immunoblotting. Immunoblot

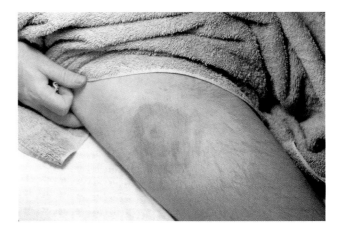

FIGURE 5-9. A typical lesion of erythema migrans on the right anterolateral thigh of a patient with Lyme borreliosis. Borreliae are more abundant in the outer margin of erythema. Note the inner area of partial clearing. (Courtesy of Dr. Justin D. Radolf.)

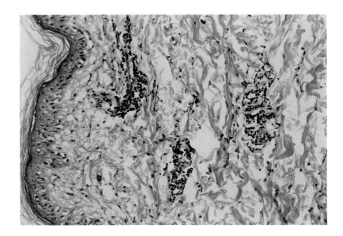

FIGURE 5-10. Photomicrograph of skin from an erythema migrans lesion of Lyme borreliosis shows an abundant lymphocyte-rich perivascular infiltrate in the dermis (hematoxylin and eosin stain; medium-power magnification).

bands of 24, 39, and 41 kd reacted with IgM antibodies; five of the 10 critical bands reacted with IgG antibodies in the patient's serum.

Comment

If the skin lesion disappears within 48 hours, erythema migrans is an unlikely diagnosis. A similar lesion occurs in southern states that is not associated with *B. burgdorferi* but is suspected to represent another unidentified tick-transmitted agent. Not all patients with Lyme borreliosis have erythema migrans, and those who do often have no other signs or symptoms. Transmitted by *Ixodes* species tick bite at the site of the erythema migrans, the illness manifests other similar hematogenously disseminated skin lesions in 25–50% of cases. Carditis with heart block (5%), arthritis (60%), and neuroborreliosis (15%) evolve later and may cause chronic illness.

The two-tiered approach to serologic diagnosis, screening EIA or IFA followed by Western immunoblotting of positive and equivocal sera, is the recommended method of laboratory testing, although testing patients with classic symptoms is not necessary. Performing serologic tests on patients without the established syndromes (e.g., erythema migrans or arthritis) results in numerous problems owing to false-positive results.

Diagnosis

Lyme borreliosis.

DERMAL HISTIOCYTIC AGGREGATES

Clinical History

A 17-year-old boy from eastern Texas presented to a clinic with the chief complaint of disseminated skin lesions. The lesions began approximately 4 months earlier as nontender, erythematous macules on his lower legs. During the next several weeks, the lesions enlarged, darkened, and became nodular, and new lesions appeared on the upper legs, arms, and ears. The patient had not traveled outside of Texas, and neither family members nor friends had similar lesions. The only pertinent findings on physical examination were the skin lesions, which had decreased sensation to pin-prick. Biopsies of a leg lesion were submitted for mycobacterial and fungal cultures and for histopathologic studies; a nasal swab specimen was submitted for mycobacterial culture. An auramine O–stained smear prepared from the submitted tissue and from the nasal swab showed numerous acid-fast bacilli (AFB).

Pathologic Findings

Histologic examination of the skin biopsy specimen showed findings consistent with lepromatous leprosy. Under low-power magnification, there was a diffuse infiltrate of vacuolated histiocytes in the dermis (Figure 5-11). High-power magnification of the infiltrate illustrated globi, consisting of aggregates of degenerating bacilli within intrahistiocytic vacuoles, and a few intradermal nerves surrounded by Virchow cells (Figures 5-12 and

5-13). Sections stained by Fite's method, which is essential for demonstration of bacilli of *Mycobacterium leprae*, showed numerous AFB in clumps and globi within the histiocytes (Figure 5-14).

Differential Diagnoses

Based on the history of the skin lesion and the positive AFB stain, the differential diagnosis is that of mycobacterial infections of the skin. The most likely diagnosis in this case, based on the clinical manifestations and histopathology of the lesions, is lepromatous leprosy. Other mycobacteria that may elicit a similar inflammatory response, especially in immunocompromised persons, include *Mycobacterium tuberculosis*, *Mycobacterium kansasii*, *Mycobacterium avium* complex, and *Mycobacterium fortuitum-chelonae* complex. If stains for AFB are negative in immunocompromised patients (particularly patients infected with HIV), other organisms, such as microsporidia, *H. capsulatum*, *Penicillium marneffei*, and *Leishmania* must be considered, and additional stains (i.e., tissue gram [for microsporidia], and silver [for fungi]) should be performed.

Microbiology

An auramine O–stained smear prepared from the leg lesion and from the nasal swab showed numerous AFB. Mycobacterial and fungal cultures were negative.

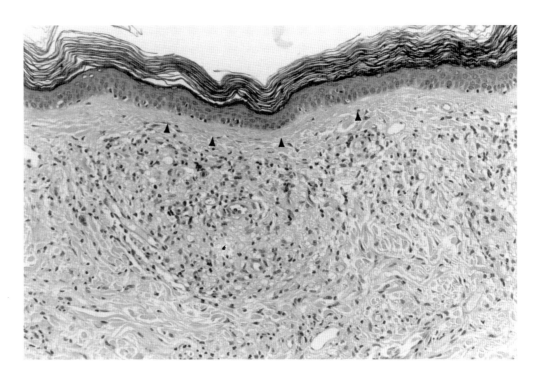

FIGURE 5-11. Section of a skin lesion from a patient with lepromatous leprosy shows a diffuse infiltrate of vacuolated histiocytes in the dermis, separated from the epidermis by a narrow rim of normal connective tissue, the Grenz zone (*arrowheads*) (hematoxylin and eosin stain; original magnification, ×50).

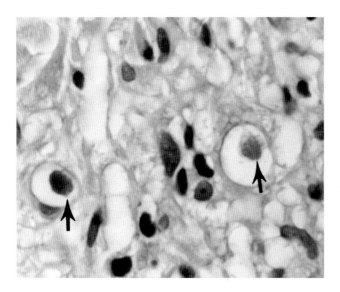

FIGURE 5-12. Higher-power magnification of the section illustrated in Figure 5-11 shows numerous vacuolated histiocytes (called *Virchow cells*) and two globi (*arrows*) consisting of aggregates of degenerating bacilli within intrahistiocytic vacuoles (hematoxylin and eosin stain; original magnification, ×250).

Comment

Between 10 and 15 million people in the world are estimated to have leprosy; approximately 62% are in Asia, and approximately 34% are in Africa. Approximately 6,000 persons in the United States have leprosy; most are immigrants, but some are natives of the Gulf Coast states, California, and Hawaii. The mechanism of transmission of *Mycobacterium leprae* is unknown, but the favored theory

is person-to-person aerosol spread of organisms from the nose of a person who has active lepromatous disease to the nasal mucosa of another individual. Transmission also may occur through skin, through penetrating wounds (e.g., a thorn stick or bite of an arthropod), and possibly from mother to infant in breast milk. The presence of naturally occurring *M. leprae* infections of armadillos of the Gulf Coast region and association of some cases with armadillo contact suggests that they may also serve as a reservoir for human infection. The lesions of leprosy develop after a 2- to 5-year incubation period and vary in appearance depending on the immune response of the host. The three cardinal signs of leprosy are skin lesions, areas of cutaneous anesthesia, and enlarged peripheral nerves.

The polar types of leprosy—lepromatous and tuberculoid—are generally clinically stable. Lepromatous leprosy, the disseminated anergic form of the disease, is characterized by cutaneous lesions that range from diffuse, generalized skin involvement to widespread, symmetrically distributed nodules typically involving the cooler parts of the body surface. In advanced disease, lesions are accompanied by sensory loss secondary to involvement of dermal nerve fibers. Histologically, lesions show foamy histiocytes containing numerous AFB, few or no lymphocytes, no significant intraneural inflammation, and many AFB in the Schwann cells of nerves, the perineurium, blood vessel walls, and arrector muscles. Tuberculoid leprosy, the localized form of the disease, is characterized by one or several well-circumscribed anesthetic macules or plaques often accompanied by an enlarged peripheral nerve near the skin lesions. Histologically, lesions demonstrate granulomas composed of epithelioid histiocytes, lymphocytes, and often Langhans' giant cells in the nerves

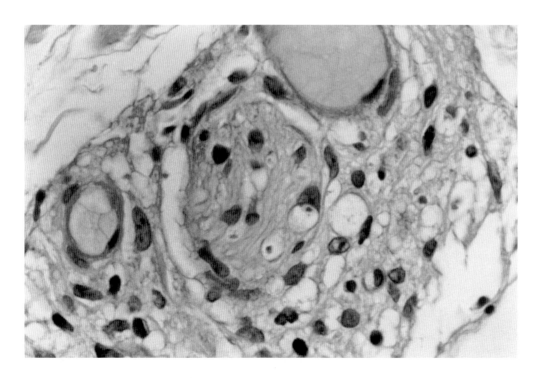

FIGURE 5-13. Higher-power magnification of the section illustrated in Figure 5-11 shows a dermal nerve surrounded by Virchow cells and two intravacuolar structures resembling globi within the nerve (hematoxylin and eosin stain; original magnification, ×250).

and the dermis, extending to involve the basal layer of the epidermis (Figure 5-15), and few (if any) AFB.

Borderline leprosy is a clinically unstable condition that may slowly develop features that more closely resemble either tuberculoid or lepromatous disease. Borderline tuberculoid leprosy resembles tuberculoid disease, with the following exceptions: Lesions are larger, more numerous, and have less distinct borders; damage to peripheral nerves is more widespread and more severe; and, histologically, granulomas do not involve the basal layer of the epidermis, and AFB often are found in nerves. Borderline lepromatous leprosy is similar to polar lepromatous leprosy except that some skin lesions are selectively anesthetic and have more distinct borders; peripheral nerve trunk involvement is more extensive; mucous membranes are less often involved; and, microscopically, lesions contain more lymphocytes and fewer AFB.

The diagnosis of leprosy is based on clinical manifestations, histopathologic findings on a skin biopsy, and failure to recover mycobacteria on culture of the lesion.

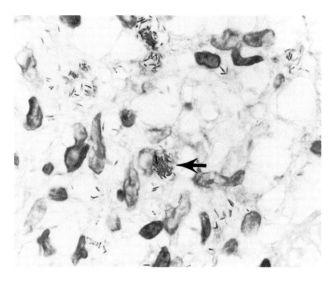

FIGURE 5-14. Staining the section illustrated in Figure 5-11 with Fite's method shows numerous acid-fast bacilli in clumps and a few globi (*arrow*; Fite's method; original magnification, ×250).

Diagnosis

Lepromatous leprosy.

FIGURE 5-15. Section of a skin lesion from a patient with tuberculoid leprosy shows several non-caseating granulomas in the dermis, some of which are close to the dermal-epidermal junction (hematoxylin and eosin stain; original magnification, ×50).

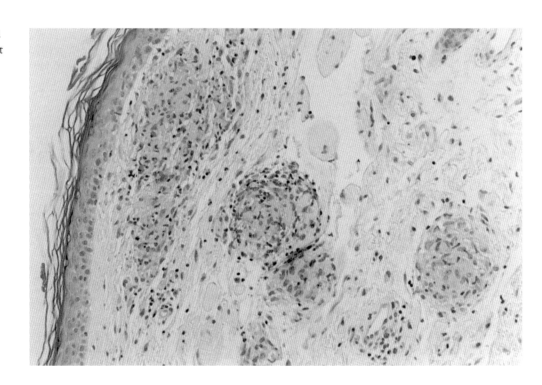

DISSEMINATED ULCERONODULAR "RASH"

Clinical History

A 59-year-old man diagnosed with systemic lupus erythematosus 3 years earlier was admitted for evaluation of skin "rash" that appeared on his buttocks and lower extremities while he was visiting Mexico 6 weeks earlier and acute onset of chills, diffuse arthralgias, and myalgia. His medications included high-dose corticosteroids, which he had taken for the past 3 years, and azathioprine (Imuran), which was added to the immunosuppressive regimen 3 months earlier. On physical examination, he was afebrile, his pulse was 98 beats per minute, his respiratory rate was 16 breaths per minute, and his blood pressure was 133/93 mm Hg. On the lower extremities and the buttocks, several red nodules 1–2 cm in diameter were present (Figure 5-16), some of which were centrally ulcerated and contained purulent material (Figure 5-17). The joints of the hands were mildly swollen but showed no evidence of an infectious process. The remainder of the examination was noncontributory. The differential diagnoses of the skin lesions included infection caused by a fungus or nontuberculous mycobacteria or a drug reaction. Biopsies of skin lesions on the buttocks and right lower leg were performed. Tissue was submitted for histologic studies, and separate samples were sent to the microbiology laboratory for fungal and mycobacterial stains and cultures.

Pathologic Findings

Sections of both lesions showed extensive acute necrotizing inflammation of the dermis and a mixed granulomatous and acute inflammatory infiltrate in the deep dermis and subcutaneous tissue (Figure 5-18). Staining with the Ziehl-Neelsen method demonstrated aggregates of AFB in the area of granulomatous inflammation (Figure 5-19). No organisms were seen in sections stained by the methenamine silver technique.

Differential Diagnoses

Infectious agents that may elicit a mixed suppurative and granulomatous response include certain nontuberculous mycobacteria (e.g., the rapidly growing mycobacteria), *Blastomyces dermatitidis, S. schenckii, Paracoccidioides brasiliensis,* and fungi associated with chromoblastomycosis and systemic phaeohyphomycosis. Based on the

presence of AFB and absence of fungi in tissue sections in this case, a diagnosis of a mycobacterial infection caused by a mycobacterium other than *M. tuberculosis* can be made. Mycobacterial cultures, however, are necessary for identification of the specific pathogen.

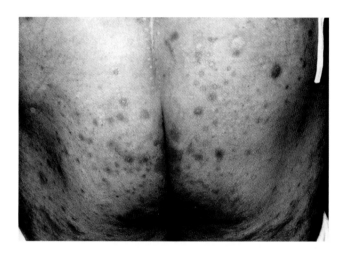

FIGURE 5-16. Photograph of the skin lesions on the buttocks of a patient with disseminated cutaneous *Mycobacterium chelonae* infection. (Courtesy of Dr. Saher Shebib.)

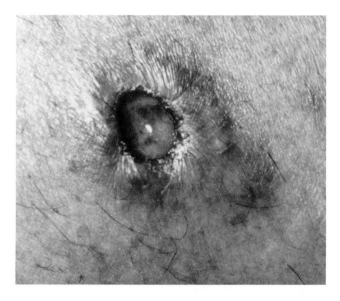

FIGURE 5-17. Closer examination of the lesions illustrated in Figure 5-16 shows a central area of ulceration containing purulent material. (Courtesy of Dr. Saher Shebib.)

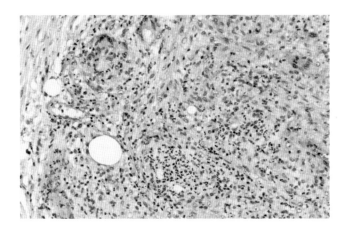

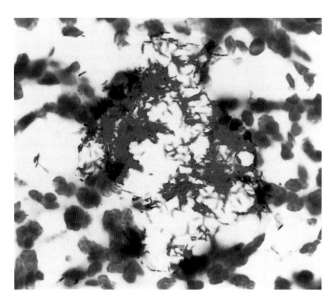

FIGURE 5-18. Section of a biopsy of one of the skin lesions shows a mixed granulomatous and suppurative inflammatory response in the dermis and subcutaneous tissue, characterized by aggregates of polymorphonuclear neutrophils, epithelioid histiocytes, and giant cells (hematoxylin and eosin stain; original magnification, ×100).

FIGURE 5-19. A section of the lesion illustrated in Figure 5-18 stained by Kinyoun carbol fuchsin demonstrates a cluster of acid-fast bacilli (Kinyoun carbol fuchsin stain; original magnification, ×250). The mycobacterial culture of tissue from the lesion grew *Mycobacterium chelonae*.

Microbiology

Mycobacterial cultures of the skin lesion grew *Mycobacterium chelonae*.

Comment

Several mycobacteria, including *M. tuberculosis*, can cause cutaneous disease, but those most commonly associated with skin lesions are *M. fortuitum-chelonae* complex (*Mycobacterium fortuitum*, *Mycobacterium chelonae*, and *Mycobacterium abscessus*), *Mycobacterium marinum*, *Mycobacterium haemophilum*, and *Mycobacterium ulcerans*. Primary cutaneous disease caused by *M. fortuitum-chelonae* complex may be manifested as localized cellulitis, draining abscesses, or minimally tender nodules occurring 3 weeks to 1 year (but usually 4–6 weeks) after a penetrating injury in persons with an intact immune system. Postoperative *M. fortuitum-chelonae* complex infections, which generally are manifested 3 weeks to 3 months after the procedure, are characterized by breakdown of a healed wound with serous drainage or a nonhealing wound. Disseminated disease, which most commonly affects immunocompromised adults, is manifested by multiple, recurrent skin and soft tissue abscesses with no apparent primary source of infection. Histologically, cutaneous lesions caused by *M. fortuitum-chelonae* complex are characterized by necrosis with minimal or no caseation and a mixed inflammatory infiltrate composed of neutrophils and granulomas with foreign body or Langhans' giant cells. Clumps of extracellular AFB, usually within aggregates of neutrophils, are found in less than one-third of cases. These findings, however, are not specific; identification of the species responsible for the infection requires mycobacterial culture. Species identification is important, because different species are treated with different antimicrobial agents.

Infection with *M. marinum* most often is acquired by trauma to the skin during contact with either nonchlorinated fresh or salt water, although infection may be acquired during trauma unassociated with water contact or contact with water in the absence of trauma. The most common presentation is a single papulonodular lesion on the elbow, knee, foot, toe, or finger 2–3 weeks after inoculation that often becomes verrucous or ulcerated. Occasionally, secondary nodules occur along the lymphatics, resembling sporotrichosis; rarely, in immunocompromised persons, cutaneous lesions become disseminated. The histopathologic changes vary based on the age of the lesion. In early lesions, neutrophil aggregates are surrounded by histiocytes; in later lesions, lymphocytes, epithelioid histiocytes, occasional giant cells, and fibrinoid necrosis are seen. In lesions present for more than 6 months, aggregates of lymphocytes are found in the dermis. Stains for AFB usually are negative, but occasionally, AFB are present within histiocytes.

Most persons with *M. haemophilum* infection have an underlying immunodeficiency, particularly infection with HIV. Disease most commonly is manifested by multiple cutaneous nodules, ulcers, or painful swellings involving the extremities. The lesions increase in size and occasionally become abscesses and open fistulas draining purulent material. Histologically, lesions show focal areas of necrosis without caseation surrounded by a polymorphous inflammatory infiltrate with occasional Langhans' giant cells in the lower dermis. Single or clusters of AFB often are seen, frequently within histiocytes.

M. ulcerans infection is endemic in parts of Africa, Malaysia, New Guinea, Guyana, Mexico, India, and Australia that lie between latitudes 25° north and 38° south. The infection begins as one (occasionally multiple) painless boil or subcutaneous lump on an exposed area, most often the leg. After several weeks, the lump ulcerates and satellite ulcers and nodules may develop. Acute infection is characterized by necrosis and edema, especially of adipose tissue, and an infiltrate of lymphocytes, plasma cells, histiocytes, and occasional giant cells. Neutrophils are present only if secondary bacterial infection is present. Clusters of AFB are found in areas of necrosis.

Diagnosis

Disseminated cutaneous *M. chelonae* infection.

ULCERATIVE NODULES

Clinical History

A 29-year-old man was admitted for evaluation of diffuse skin lesions (Figure 5-20), weight loss of approximately 90 pounds over the previous 6 months, and cough occasionally productive of blood-tinged sputum for the past 2 months. He had been in good health until 6 months before admission, when a nontender lump appeared on the left side of his abdomen. A few days later, several lumps developed on his upper and lower extremities, face, trunk, back, and head. These lumps began as pink, spherical soft masses approximately 1 cm in diameter. They gradually enlarged, became fluctuant, drained yellow-green pus, and then ulcerated and became crusted. He had a twelve-pack-year history of smoking cigarettes and had worked for 3 years in a gravel pit in south Texas.

On physical examination, he was afebrile, his pulse rate was 104 beats per minute, his respiratory rate was 22 breaths per minute, and his blood pressure was 142/84 mm Hg. Ulcerated skin lesions covered much of his body as described. The remainder of the examination was noncontributory. Results of his chest radiograph were normal. Abnormal laboratory test results included a hemoglobin concentration of 9.8 mg/dl and a serum alkaline phosphatase level of 323 IU per liter. A serologic test for antibodies to HIV was negative. Disseminated fungal infection was believed to be the most likely diagnosis. Biopsies of the skin lesions were submitted for histologic examination and fungal culture. The next day, he had an episode of hemoptysis. Because he was unable to produce a sputum specimen, bronchoscopy was performed. Biopsy specimens of the trachea and carina were submitted for histologic studies and fungal and mycobacterial cultures.

Pathologic Findings

Microscopic examination of hematoxylin and eosin (H and E)–stained sections of both the skin and transbronchial biopsies showed a mixed suppurative and granulomatous inflammatory infiltrate within the dermis (Figures 5-21 and 5-22) and bronchial mucosa. Staining these skin sections by the methenamine silver method revealed budding yeast cells, some with spherical buds but others with cigar-shaped buds (Figure 5-23), characteristic of *Sporothrix schenckii*.

FIGURE 5-20. Photograph of an ulcerative skin lesion of a man with disseminated *Sporothrix schenckii* infection.

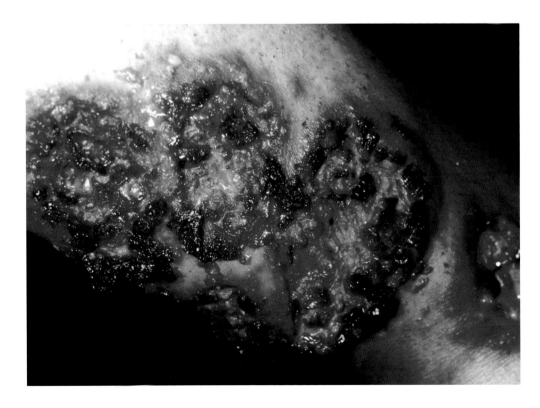

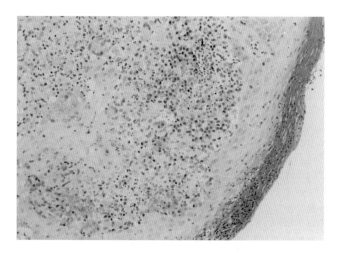

FIGURE 5-21. Section of a skin biopsy shows a mixed suppurative and granulomatous inflammatory infiltrate within the dermis (hematoxylin and eosin stain; original magnification, ×50).

Differential Diagnoses

Common infectious causes of skin lesions that histologically show a mixed suppurative and granulomatous inflammatory response are certain nontuberculous mycobacteria, especially members of the *M. fortuitum-chelonae* complex and *M. marinum*, and several fungi, including *S. schenckii* (illustrated in this case), *B. dermatitidis*, *Coccidioides immitis*, *P. brasiliensis*, and fungi associated with chromoblastomycosis, most often *Fonsecaea pedrosoi* and *Cladosporium carrionii*.

Microbiology

Fungal cultures of skin and transtracheal biopsy tissue grew *S. schenckii* after incubation for 5 days.

Comment

The etiology of skin lesions caused by infectious agents may be determined by examination of sections of the lesion stained by H and E. For example, yeast cells of *B. dermatitidis* (Figures 5-24 and 5-25), *C. immitis*, and fungi causing chromoblastomycosis (Figures 5-26 and 5-27) often are visible in H and E–stained sections. However, if organisms cannot be found in tissue sections stained by H and E, stains for AFB and fungi (including the Fontana-Masson stain, which is useful for visualization of sclerotic bodies associated with chromoblastomycosis) should be performed to help identify the pathogen. In addition to tissue pathology, clinical history is useful in making a diagnosis (Table 5-1), and a portion of the tissue specimen always should be cultured for fungi and mycobacteria.

Sporotrichosis is a chronic infection that occurs worldwide in temperate and tropical climates. It is caused by the dimorphic fungus *S. schenckii*, which is found in the soil and on plants, trees, timber, moss, and other organic materials. Infection most often is acquired by accidental percutaneous inoculation of the organism growing on plant materials like thorns, but rarely is acquired by inhalation of fungal conidia. The classic form of sporotrichosis (i.e., lymphocutaneous) consists of a primary nodular-ulcerative skin lesion, usually on the hand, arm, neck or less often,

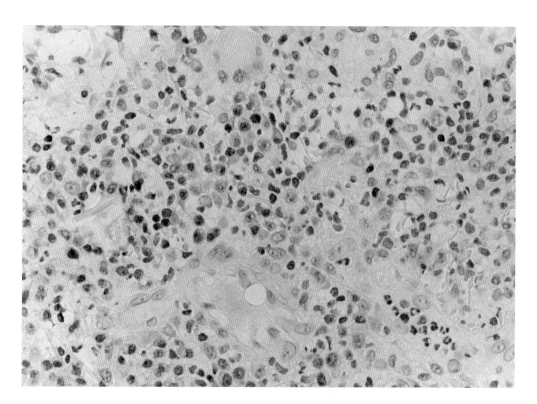

FIGURE 5-22. Higher-power magnification of the section illustrated in Figure 5-21 reveals aggregates of epithelioid histiocytes admixed with lymphocytes, plasma cells, and focal collections of neutrophils (hematoxylin and eosin stain; original magnification, ×100).

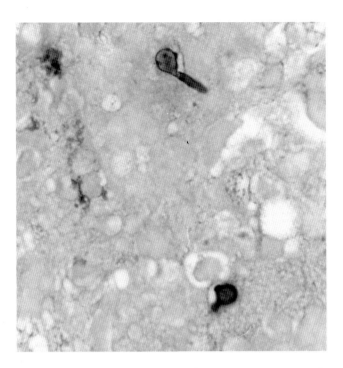

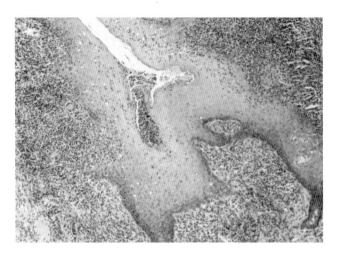

FIGURE 5-23. Staining the section shown in Figure 5-22 with methenamine silver demonstrates yeast cells, some with cigar-shaped buds typical of *Sporothrix schenckii* (fungal culture grew *S. schenckii*; Gomori's methenamine silver stain; original magnification, ×250).

FIGURE 5-24. Section of a skin biopsy shows prominent pseudoepitheliomatous hyperplasia, infiltration of the epidermis by neutrophils, and a mixed suppurative and granulomatous inflammatory infiltrate in the dermis (hematoxylin and eosin stain; original magnification, ×25).

FIGURE 5-25. Higher-power magnification of the section illustrated in Figure 5-24 shows a collection of neutrophils admixed with few multinucleated giant cells and rare yeast cells with broad-based buds (*arrow*) characteristic of *Blastomyces dermatitidis*, a diagnosis confirmed by culture (hematoxylin and eosin stain; original magnification, ×100).

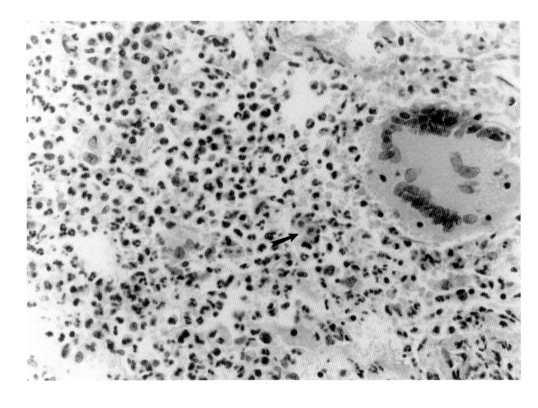

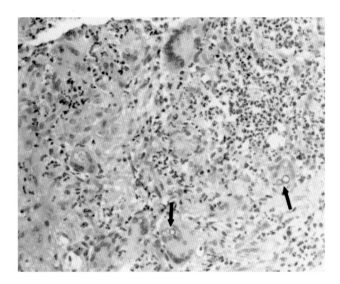

FIGURE 5-26. Section of skin shows a mixed suppurative and granulomatous inflammatory infiltrate composed of epithelioid histiocytes, giant cells, some with thick-walled spherical structures in the cytoplasm (*arrows*), and neutrophils within the dermis (hematoxylin and eosin stain; original magnification, ×50).

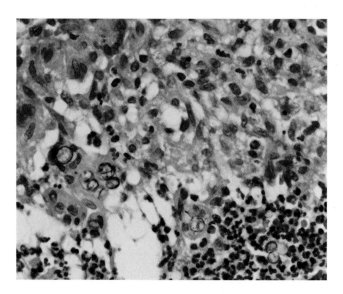

FIGURE 5-27. Higher-power magnification of the section illustrated in Figure 5-26 reveals thick-walled, brown sclerotic bodies, fungal cells (with cross septations in more than one plane), characteristic of the dematiaceous fungi that cause chromoblastomycosis (hematoxylin and eosin stain; original magnification, ×100). To identify the specific organism involved, fungal culture must be performed.

TABLE 5-1. Diagnosis of Skin Infections Characterized Histologically by a Mixed Suppurative and Granulomatous Inflammatory Response

Organism	Clinical Information
Mycobacterium fortuitum	History of trauma, including intramuscular injection and surgical procedures
Mycobacterium chelonae	History of trauma; chronic corticosteroid use with disseminated cutaneous lesions
Mycobacterium marinum	History of trauma associated with water contact ("swimming-pool granuloma")
Sporothrix schenckii	History of trauma associated with gardening (e.g., puncture from a thorn); lymphocutaneous disease (i.e., primary lesion followed by new lesions proximally along the lymphatics draining the area of the primary lesion)
Blastomyces dermatitidis	Patient lives in or has history of travel to endemic area (Mississippi River Basin and southeastern and south-central areas in the United States); often occurs in the absence of apparent active pulmonary disease
Coccidioides immitis	Patient lives in or has history of travel to endemic area (southwestern United States and bordering regions of northern Mexico)
Paracoccidioides brasiliensis	Patient lives in or has history of travel to endemic area (tropical and subtropical forests of Central America and South America from Mexico to Argentina [not in Caribbean Islands and Chile])

the foot or leg, and a linear chain of secondary subcutaneous nodules along the course of the lymphatics draining from the primary site. Other forms of sporotrichosis include primary verrucous skin lesions without lymphatic involvement and disseminated disease characterized by widespread cutaneous lesions and involvement of the

bones, joints, and lungs in a patient who is immunocompromised or has a serious underlying condition. The case presented here is unusual because no immune suppression or underlying disease could be found.

The characteristic histopathologic findings of cutaneous sporotrichosis are a mixed suppurative and granulomatous inflammatory reaction in the dermis, ulceration of the overlying epidermis, and pseudoepitheliomatous hyperplasia of the adjacent epidermis. Yeast cells generally are not seen in H and E–stained sections; in sections stained by methenamine silver or periodic acid-Schiff, preferably with diastase digestion, they appear as round, oval, or classic elongated ("cigar-shaped") single or budding cells 2–6 μm in diameter. The asteroid body, which consists of a yeast cell surrounded by a stellate, radial crown of eosinophilic Splendore-Hoeppli material, is found in microabscesses or necrotic centers of granulomas but is not present in all cases, nor is it specific for sporotrichosis. Lesions of systemic sporotrichosis resemble those of tuberculosis (i.e., caseating granulomas with organisms in the area of central necrosis).

Diagnosis

Disseminated sporotrichosis.

GRANULOMATOUS INFLAMMATION OF THE SKIN

Clinical History

A 50-year-old, previously healthy man participated in a tour of Peruvian archeological sites. While in remote areas, the group slept in tents equipped with mosquito netting. Several weeks after returning home, he noticed two papules on his arm. The moderately painful lesions slowly enlarged and underwent central ulceration (Figure 5-28). He was referred to a plastic surgeon, who débrided the ulcers, submitted tissue for histologic examination, and attempted skin grafting of the sites. Histologic examination of the tissue showed acute and chronic inflammation; no etiology of the process was provided. Meanwhile, the ulceration recurred, and the skin grafts were unsuccessful. Shortly before Christmas, he received a letter from another member of the tour, who related the appearance of a similar chronically ulcerated lesion on her leg that was diagnosed as leishmaniasis and resolved only after specific therapy. The patient consulted another physician, who requested that the original slides be reviewed. After a corrected diagnosis of leishmaniasis was rendered, the patient was treated appropriately and the lesions healed.

Pathologic Findings

The initial biopsy of the lesion showed extensive chronic inflammation in the dermis (Figure 5-29) and pseudoepitheliomatous hyperplasia of the overlying epidermis. The infiltrate consisted of lymphocytes and macrophages with focal aggregation of the macrophages into poorly defined granulomas. Polymorphonuclear neutrophils were also present in some areas. At low power, the process could be interpreted as nonspecific chronic inflammation; if stains for AFB and fungi were performed, they would have produced negative results. Under high power, numerous oval structures, located primarily within the cytoplasm of macrophages, are seen (Figure 5-30). The distinguishing feature of *Leishmania* amastigotes is the kinetoplast (a micronucleus containing the DNA of the mitochondrion), which is not always easily visualized in tissue sections, owing to its small size and frequent absence in a particular plane of section. If the lesion is aspirated, the morphology of the parasites is much more easily seen in Giemsa-stained smears (Figure 5-31).

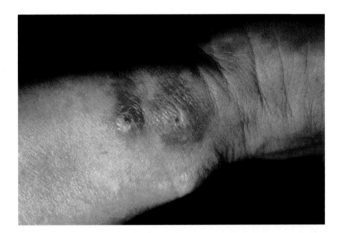

FIGURE 5-28. Two leishmanial ulcers on the arm of a patient who acquired the infection while traveling, probably by *Leishmania tropica*. A central ulcer is surrounded by a thickened rim and erythema. Injection of a small amount of sterile saline into the edge of the ulcer, followed by aspiration of tissue fluid, is the diagnostic approach of choice.

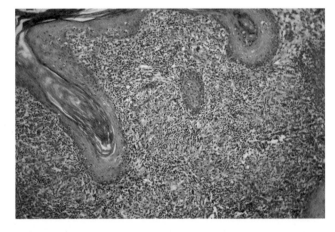

FIGURE 5-29. Section of a skin lesion from a patient with cutaneous leishmaniasis shows hyperplasia of the overlying squamous epithelium and an extensive dermal infiltrate, primarily of mononuclear cells. The presence of poorly formed granulomas is suggested by eosinophilic aggregates of macrophages (hematoxylin and eosin stain; low-power magnification).

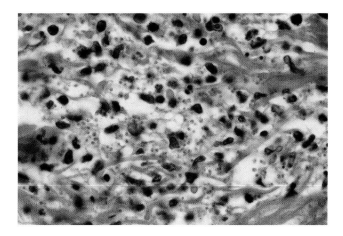

FIGURE 5-30. At high-power magnification, numerous amastigotes surrounded by a clear space (i.e., a pseudocapsule) are visible within the cytoplasm of macrophages (hematoxylin and eosin stain; high-power magnification).

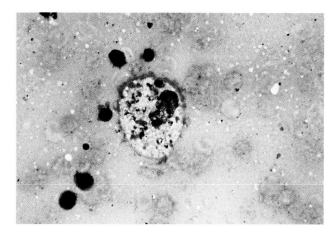

FIGURE 5-31. Aspirate from an ulcer shows lymphocytes and a single degenerating, infected macrophage. The presence of both a nuclear mass and an elongated, bar-shaped kinetoplast is clearly demonstrated in some of the organisms (Giemsa stain; high-power magnification).

Differential Diagnoses

The differential diagnoses of leishmaniasis includes histoplasmosis, penicilliosis (due to *P. marneffei*), and the rare localized cutaneous form of American trypanosomiasis (Chagas' disease). When Darling first observed the lesions of histoplasmosis in tissue, he believed he was dealing with an organism that was related to *Leishmania*, hence the genus name suggesting a tissue parasite and the species name referring to the appearance of a clear space around the organisms in section. *H. capsulatum* can be differentiated from *Leishmania* species by the absence of a kinetoplast in the organism and positive staining with Gomori's silver methenamine stain. In smears of solitary cutaneous lesions of Chagas' disease, amastigotes may be seen.

Comment

Leishmaniasis occurs throughout the tropical and subtropical areas of the world. The vector is one of several species of biting flies (*Phlebotomus* in the Old World and *Lutzomyia* in the New World). The different clinical manifestations of infection have been recognized for many decades, and specific clinical presentations have been associated with defined geographic areas and genetic groups of parasites (Table 5-2). The immunologic responsiveness of the host is an additional determinant of clinical disease. The most severe form of disease is disseminated (visceral) leishmaniasis, also known as *kala-azar*, *Dumdum fever*, or *Assam fever*. Kala-azar occurs worldwide, with the most important foci being in China, the Indian subcontinent, and East Africa.

Mucocutaneous leishmaniasis has intermediate severity. In addition to skin lesions, patients experience infection of the mouth and nose that may lead to disfiguring ulceration. Mucocutaneous disease, which is also known as *espundia*, is most commonly found in northern South America. The most benign form of leishmaniasis is cutaneous disease, as exemplified by this case. The lesions may be multiple and may cause chronic morbidity with cosmetic damage, but the process is not life-threatening. Cutaneous disease occurs in the Middle East and Central America. In the Middle East, it has been called *Baghdad boil*, *Oriental sore*, or *Aleppo evil*. A localized lesion on the ear in Mexico, known as *chiclero ulcer*, is explained by the predilection for the vector to inhabit vegetation that is 5–6 feet off the ground.

Diagnosis is made most easily by examination of smears of material aspirated from the affected tissue. Aspiration provides better material for study of morphology in thin smears and avoids the scarring that may result from biopsy. Amastigotes are more numerous in localized cutaneous disease than in mucocutaneous disease. The rolled edge of a cutaneous ulcer is aspirated after infiltration with sterile saline. Smears are then stained with a Giemsa stain (or a similar Romanovsky stain). In kala-azar, splenic aspiration provides the highest diagnostic yield, but splenic rupture or leakage may occur. Bone marrow, liver, and, more rarely, buffy coat provide alternative specimens with a lower yield but fewer complications.

In culture, the amastigotes produce flagella and develop into the promastigote form, which is the stage found in infected sandflies. If media are available locally or through the Centers for Disease Control and Preven-

TABLE 5-2. Clinical Forms of Leishmaniasis and Their Associated Etiologic Agents, Geographic Locations, and Vectors

Clinical Disease	Most Common Agents	Less Common Agents	Geographic Locations	Vectors
Old World visceral (kala-azar) disease	*Leishmania donovani* *Leishmania infantum*	*Leishmania archibaldi* *Leishmania amazonensis* *Leishmania tropica*	Indian subcontinent, China, East Africa, Middle East, Mediterranean	*Phlebotomus* species
New World visceral (kala-azar) disease	—	*Leishmania chagasi*	South and Central America	*Lutzomyia* species
Old World cutaneous disease	*L. tropica* *Leishmania major* *Leishmania aethiopica*	*L. infantum* *L. archibaldi*	China, Middle East, Mediterranean, East Africa	*Phlebotomus* species
Old World disseminated cutaneous disease	*L. aethiopica*	—	East Africa	*Phlebotomus* species
New World cutaneous disease	*Leishmania mexicana* *L. amazonensis*	*Leishmania pifanoi* *Leishmania garnhami* *Leishmania venezuelensis* *Leishmania guyanensis* *Leishmania peruviana* *Leishmania panamensis* *L. chagasi*	Mexico, Central and South America	*Lutzomyia* species
New World diffuse cutaneous disease	*L. amazonensis*	*L. pifanoi* *L. mexicana*	Mexico, Central and South America	*Lutzomyia* species
Mucocutaneous disease	*Leishmania braziliensis*	Other species are rare	South America	*Lutzomyia* species

Source: Adapted from RD Pearson, A DeQueiroz Sousa. *Leishmania* spp. In GL Mandell, JE Bennett, RA Dolin (eds), Principles and Practice of Infectious Diseases (4th ed). New York: Churchill-Livingstone, 1995.

tion, culture can provide definitive characterization of the parasite. Molecular structure of the protozoa corresponds well to the geographic distribution of disease. Knowledge of the molecular structure, however, has given us a much stronger feeling of the diversity in the species-disease relationships. Particularly in geographic watershed areas, the knowledge that the *Leishmania* are of the cutaneous type is reassurance that destructive mucocutaneous lesions will not occur.

With time, most cutaneous lesions heal. Mucocutaneous disease and kala-azar are less likely to heal spontaneously. Appropriate therapy enhances the healing process in cutaneous disease and is essential for kala-azar and mucocutaneous infection. The mainstay of therapy is one of several antimony compounds, all of which have considerable toxicity and should be administered in consultation with an expert in tropical medicine. Pentamidine, also a toxic compound, has been used in recalcitrant cases, and ketoconazole has been used successfully in some cutaneous infections.

Diagnosis

Cutaneous leishmaniasis.

CHROMOBLASTOMYCOSIS

Clinical History

A 47-year-old man presented with a progressive skin lesion on his left hand and arm. Four years before admission, he noted the presence of pruritic vesicles and pustules on the posterior surfaces of the left hand and fingers. These lesions developed into elevated, scaling, verrucous nodules; the hand, wrist, and lower two-thirds of the forearm were gradually covered by a warty growth. The underlying soft tissues became progressively more swollen, and the size and weight of the arm eventually necessitated the use of a sling. Increased swelling and some pain were present when the arm was held in a dependent position, but the only other symptoms were local itching and burning. The skin of the lower two-thirds of the forearm and of the hand and fingers posteriorly was replaced by a nearly contiguous, hard, dry, rough, verrucous growth. The appearance suggested that adjacent lesions had coalesced, but nothing suggested an advancing border, and no erythema surrounded the lesions. A biopsy of the skin was performed, and scrapings from the involved areas were examined microscopically after digestion with KOH.

Pathologic Findings

The dermis contained a mixture of suppurative inflammation and granulomas with epithelioid macrophages, multinucleate giant cells, lymphocytes, plasma cells (many of which manifested Russell bodies), and extensive fibrosis. The epidermis showed pseudoepitheliomatous hyperplasia and an infiltrate of leukocytes and macrophages. Extracellularly within foci of suppuration and intracellularly in macrophages in the dermis and epidermis and at the dermal-epidermal junction, chestnut brown thick-walled yeast cells were present (5–12 μm in diameter) (Figures 5-32 and 5-33).

Differential Diagnoses

The inflammatory lesions suggested a differential diagnosis of cutaneous blastomycosis, paracoccidioidomycosis, chromoblastomycosis, phaeohyphomycosis, tuberculosis, leishmaniasis, lobomycosis, sarcoidosis, and squamous cell carcinoma. The observation of dematiaceous fungi narrowed the consideration to mainly chromoblastomycosis and phaeohyphomycosis.

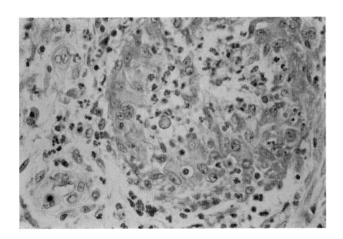

FIGURE 5-32. Polymorphonuclear leukocytes and mononuclear cells are present in the dermis and in the adjacent epidermis where a dematiaceous (melanin-containing) yeast is visible (hematoxylin and eosin stain; high-power magnification).

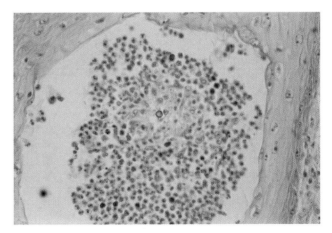

FIGURE 5-33. Transepithelial elimination of a dematiaceous yeast is observed with a suppurative inflammatory reaction surrounding an organism in transit to the surface of the skin in a patient with chromoblastomycosis (hematoxylin and eosin stain; medium-power magnification).

Microbiology

The KOH preparation revealed brown muriform cells (fungi with septa in the vertical and horizontal planes; see Figure 5-27). Fungal cultures yielded *F. pedrosoi*.

Comment

Chromoblastomycosis is a chronic, progressive, indolent infection that, despite vigorous host cellular and humoral immune reactions and inflammation, does not respond to treatment. It occurs mostly among tropical and subtropical farmers whose bare feet encounter these fungi that grow in the soil and on woody plants when they receive wounds from contaminated splinters. Chromoblastomycosis and phaeohyphomycosis represent a spectrum in which the predominant melanin-containing fungi are muriform cells or hyphae, respectively.

The observation of intraepithelial fungi in foci of inflammation represents the interesting process of transepithelial elimination, by which foci of fungal infection in the dermis are transported through the epidermis and are expelled on the epidermal surface.

Diagnosis

Cutaneous and subcutaneous chromoblastomycosis.

GRANULOMATOUS INFECTION OF SOFT TISSUE

Clinical History

A 17-year-old girl was evaluated for an erythematous, warm, indurated lesion (Figure 5-34) on the ulnar aspect of the distal palmar crease on her right hand. Nine months earlier, a thin-walled ganglion cyst was removed from that area. The cyst recurred and was aspirated 6 months previously, after which steroid injections of the area were given. Four months before admission, fibrotic tissue was removed from the site; histologic examination did not show inflammation or organisms. Several weeks before admission, the lesion became acutely inflamed and swollen. It was incised, and several milliliters of pus were drained from around the flexor tendon sheaths, after which necrotic tissue was débrided. She was treated with cephalexin, but the infectious process extended to the hypothenar region and along the little finger, requiring several additional surgical procedures. The inflammatory process was controlled completely by 5 months, at which time she had regained approximately half of the original function of the hand.

Pathologic Findings

The initial inflammatory mass contained fibrosis, lymphocytic infiltrates, and a necrotic mass that included large numbers of *Prototheca* organisms (Figure 5-35). Scattered collections of lipid consistent with the previously injected steroids were present. The morphology of the yeastlike cells, which stained well with H and E, was quite variable. Single-cell organisms had a thick wall and measured 8 μm to 20 μm in diameter. In the absence of asexual sporulation, these cells could be mistaken for systemic yeast, such as *B. dermatitidis*, but neither budding cells nor hyphae were present. Many of the organisms contained multiple endospores, each of which resembled the parent organism. When these endospores are arranged in a concentric form around a central spore, the cell is called a *morula form* (Figure 5-36). The morphology of *Prototheca* is distinctive and not likely to be mistaken for other pathogens if the observer is familiar with the agent. The algal forms stain well with the periodic acid-Schiff and methenamine silver techniques. Differentiation from fungi must be accomplished, and the endosporulating cells may be mistaken in H and E–stained sections for bizarre, multinucleated tissue cells.

Subsequent biopsies from this patient demonstrated a prominent granulomatous reaction with central necrosis and multinucleated giant cells. Algal cells were present in smaller numbers, usually within the cytoplasm of macrophages or multinucleated giant cells. Although the differences among the biopsies could be related to sampling of tissue, the first biopsy with necrotic tissue and masses of algal cells is likely to have represented overwhelming infection, whereas the later granulomatous lesions resulted from a more effective host response after the mass of pathogens had been debulked surgically.

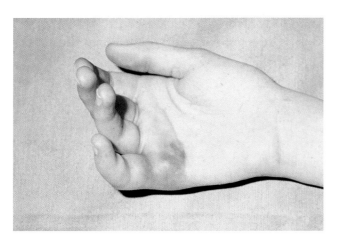

FIGURE 5-34. Intense erythema and swelling involves an extensive area of the palm. The initial lesion (not shown) was considered to be a ganglion cyst on the finger, which was injected with a steroid solution.

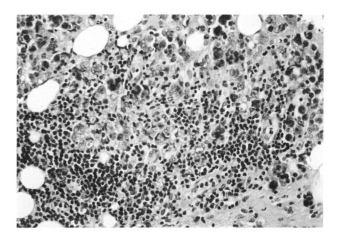

FIGURE 5-35. The initial biopsy contained mononuclear inflammatory cells and masses of *Prototheca* cells, which could be mistaken for tissue cells (hematoxylin and eosin stain; medium-power magnification).

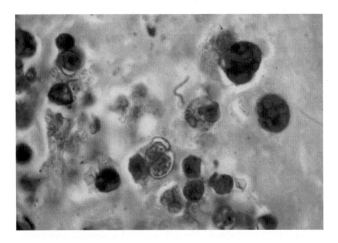

FIGURE 5-36. At high-power magnification, the morphology of distinctive algal cells is apparent. Some cells (sporangia) contain multiple sporangiospores, including cells in which the sporangiospores are arranged in a circle (morula cells). If the observer is familiar with *Prototheca*, the answer is obvious and immediate (hematoxylin and eosin stain; high-power magnification).

Microbiology

Cultures from each of the biopsies in which algal cells were demonstrated yielded a pure culture of *Prototheca wickerhamii*. On agar, the colonies were creamy and yeastlike. The isolated algae demonstrated a cellular morphology that was identical in range to the forms documented in tissue. The isolate was identified biochemically by assimilation tests, as performed in the mycology laboratory. A specific fluorescent antiserum to *P. wickerhamii* reacted with the isolate at the Centers for Disease Control and Prevention. In vitro susceptibility studies documented susceptibility to amphotericin B and resistance to 5-flucytosine.

Comment

Prototheca species are achlorophyllous algae that are ubiquitous in nature and are primarily associated with vegetation and contaminated waters. A number of species exist, but the most important human pathogens are *P. wickerhamii* and *Prototheca zopfii*, of which the former has caused the majority of reported infections. They were initially considered to be fungi, but the algal nature of the genus was deduced from reproductive mechanisms and ultrastructure.

Prototheca species must be differentiated from systemic fungi, including genera that reproduce by endosporulation (such as *Coccidioides* and *Rhinosporidium*). In addition to morphologic clues, the type of clinical disease and geographic location of the patient are useful data. They must also be distinguished from green algae, which may very rarely cause human infection. The green algae contain chloroplasts when studied ultrastructurally. They also have cytoplasmic glycogen bodies, which are demonstrable by a periodic acid-Schiff stain only before diastase digestion.

Despite the ubiquity of the algae, they only infrequently produce human infection. Cases have been described worldwide, with the greatest number coming from the southern United States. The most common infections have been localized lesions of the soft tissue, presumably after direct inoculation of environmental algae. Infection of synovial and bursal structures has figured prominently in some cases. Rare cases of deep tissue or disseminated infection have been described.

Therapy consists of aggressive surgical débridement, therapy with amphotericin B, or both.

Diagnosis

Prototheca infection of soft tissue.

SUBCUTANEOUS ABSCESSES

Clinical History

A 26-year-old man from the Rio Grande River Valley presented with the chief complaint of back pain. After further questioning, he also admitted to having a non-productive cough and night sweats for approximately 1 month. On physical examination, his temperature was 39.4°C, his blood pressure was 116/60 mm Hg, his pulse rate was 88 beats per minute, and his respiratory rate was 20 breaths per minute. The only additional relevant finding was a 4-cm, firm, tender, subcutaneous nodule on his back at approximately the T12 level just to the right of the midline. A radiograph of his chest showed diffuse, bilateral interstitial infiltrates. Pertinent laboratory test results were a hemoglobin of 10.1 g/dl, a white blood cell count of 19,600 per μl with 14% eosinophils, and negative serologic test results for antibodies to HIV. The differential diagnosis included an infectious process versus a spinal cord tumor. Blood and sputum specimens were submitted for bacterial, mycobacterial, and fungal cultures. A fine needle aspirate of the lesion was performed; material was submitted for cytologic and micro-biologic studies.

Pathologic Findings

Examination of smears of the aspirated material stained by the Papanicolaou method (Figure 5-37) showed inflammatory cells, necrotic debris, and spherules of *C. immitis*.

Differential Diagnoses

Organisms that may cause solitary or multiple subcutaneous abscesses include *C. immitis*; *B. dermatitidis*; *Cryptococcus neoformans*; *P. marneffei*; *Nocardia* species; *M. tuberculosis* and some of the nontuberculous mycobacteria (especially *M. kansasii*, *M. marinum*, *M. fortuitum-chelonae* complex, and *M. ulcerans*); and bacteria, such as *Staphylococcus aureus*. In this case, spherules were present in the material aspirated from the lesion, thus allowing the diagnosis of coccidioidomycosis.

Microbiology

Fungal cultures of the material aspirated from the subcutaneous nodule and the sputum specimen grew *C. immitis*.

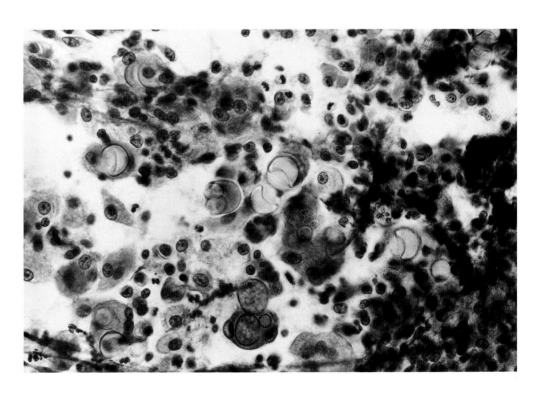

FIGURE 5-37A. Smear of material aspirated from a subcutaneous abscess of a patient with disseminated coccidioidomycosis shows an inflammatory infiltrate composed of histiocytes and a few neutrophils and several spherules of *Coccidioides immitis*, some of which are old and devoid of endospores and others that are mature and contain endospores (Papanicolaou stain; original magnification, ×100). Fungal culture of the material grew *C. immitis*.

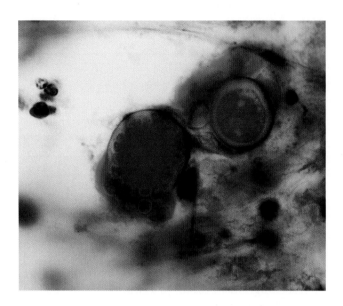

FIGURE 5-37B. High-power magnification of the aspirate illustrated in **A** shows intracellular mature spherules (Papanicolaou stain; original magnification, ×250).

Comment

Coccidioidomycosis is caused by the thermally dimorphic fungus *C. immitis,* which is endemic to the United States (in the area corresponding to the Lower Sonoran Life Zone of California, Arizona, Nevada, Utah, and New Mexico), Mexico, Guatemala, Honduras, Colombia, Venezuela, Bolivia, Paraguay, and Argentina. Infection is acquired by inhalation of *arthroconidia;* therefore, persons in endemic areas whose occupations involve exposure to soil dust are at greatest risk for contracting the disease. After primary infection, based on positive coccidioidin skin-test results, only approximately 40% of patients develop disease. Symptoms include fever, cough, and pleuritic or dull aching chest pain. A diffuse, erythematous skin rash may appear during the first few days of the illness. Other cutaneous manifestations of primary disease include erythema nodosum or erythema multiforme, which may appear at any time from several days to 3 weeks after the onset of respiratory symptoms.

Disseminated coccidioidomycosis usually is a complication of primary infection. It is more likely to occur in blacks, Filipinos, and immunosuppressed persons. Among the most common manifestations of hematogenous dissemination are lesions of the skin and subcutaneous tissues, including verrucous papules, which may resemble squamous cell carcinoma, ulcers, draining sinuses, or subcutaneous abscesses, as occurred in this patient. These lesions may involve virtually any site on the body and may persist for long periods. Other possible manifestations of disseminated disease are bone lesions, arthritis, miliary pulmonary disease, and meningitis.

Diagnosis

Disseminated coccidioidomycosis with subcutaneous abscesses.

MULTIPLE ERYTHEMATOUS CUTANEOUS PAPULES AND COUGH IN A FEBRILE PATIENT WITH ACQUIRED IMMUNODEFICIENCY SYNDROME

Clinical History

A 22-year-old woman with HIV-1 infection and a CD4 lymphocyte of 4 per µl 1 year earlier sought medical care for an illness of 3 weeks' duration characterized by fever, chills, headache, nonproductive cough, nausea, vomiting, diarrhea, abdominal pain, night sweats, and weight loss of 20 pounds. On admission, she was febrile (39.3°C) and had scattered 8-mm erythematous papules on her abdomen and legs. A chest radiograph showed bilateral diffuse interstitial infiltrates, patchy opacities, and enlarged paratracheal lymph nodes. She had been admitted three times during the previous year for disseminated histoplasmosis but had been noncompliant in her long-term antifungal therapy.

On the third hospital day, two skin lesions were biopsied with the clinical suspicion of disseminated involvement by histoplasmosis. Tissue was sent to the surgical pathology department for histopathologic examination and to the microbiology laboratory for fungal culture. On the next day, bronchoscopy was performed with biopsy of pedunculated endobronchial lesions. Serum was sent to a reference laboratory for detection of antibodies to *Bartonella* species.

Pathologic Findings

The cutaneous and bronchial lesions were located in the dermis and bronchial submucosa, respectively. Both contained lobular proliferations of spindle-shaped endothelial cells with admixed interstitial neutrophils, leukocytoclastic debris, and focal accumulations of extracellular amorphous granular material (Figure 5-38). The granular masses were demonstrated to be microcolonies of small, thin bacilli by a Warthin-Starry silver impregnation stain (Figure 5-39).

Differential Diagnoses

The vascular spindle-cell mass suggested a differential diagnosis of Kaposi's sarcoma, bacillary angiomatosis, pyogenic granuloma, granulation tissue, mycobacterial spindle cell pseudotumor, *verruga peruana*, and a variety of sarcomas.

Microbiology

Serologic testing revealed IFA antibody titers of 1:1,024 against *Bartonella* (formerly *Rochalimaea*) *henselae* and *Bartonella quintana*. Results of fungal cultures were negative.

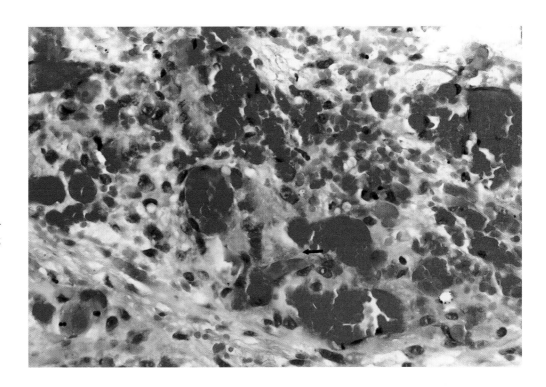

FIGURE 5-38. Photomicrograph of a lesion of bacillary angiomatosis contains an abundant proliferation of small, capillary-like blood vessels, some of which are lined by plump endothelial cells. The intervening edematous stroma contains extravasated erythrocytes and foci of hazy, bluish-purple material (*arrow*), representing microscopic colonies of extracellular bacteria (hematoxylin and eosin stain; original magnification, ×100).

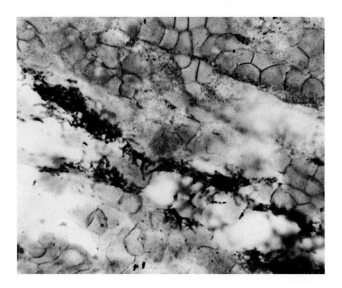

FIGURE 5-39. Numerous clusters of extracellular bacilli are distinctly demonstrated by silver impregnation staining in a perivascular location in the same lesion of bacillary angiomatosis (Warthin-Starry stain; original magnification, ×250).

Comment

The lesions of bacillary angiomatosis that have been recognized in the United States, mainly in immunocompromised patients and in particular those with AIDS, are caused by *B. henselae* and *B. quintana*. The lesions are virtually identical to *verruga peruana*, cutaneous lesions associated with the late stage of *Bartonella bacilliformis* infections in the Andes. A component of the *Bartonella* stimulates the proliferation of endothelial cells in vitro and angiogenesis in vivo. Bacillary angiomatosis can involve nearly any organ, including the spleen and liver (in which the lesion is termed *bacillary peliosis*), lymph node, bone, gastrointestinal tract, brain, mouth, nose, anus, and lung, as observed in this patient.

Owing to the slow growth of those fastidious organisms, the diagnosis of bacillary angiomatosis is usually established by histopathology and can be confirmed by specific polymerase chain reaction.

Diagnosis

Bacillary angiomatosis associated with *Bartonella* infection.

FEVER AND GANGRENE OF THE EXTREMITIES

Clinical History

A 39-year-old man presented to an emergency room with swelling and pain of both lower extremities. He reported that he had fallen and lost consciousness 2 days before. He had a history of ethanol abuse and had eaten raw oysters 2 days before admission. He was admitted to the hospital with a blood pressure of 66/44 mm Hg and a serum creatine kinase of 9,377 U/liter, which was attributed to striated muscle damage. Despite aggressive hydration and dopamine treatment, his condition rapidly worsened, with ecchymoses, bullous cutaneous lesions, increased swelling and pain of his lower extremities and arms (Figure 5-40), metabolic acidosis, renal insufficiency, and persistent hemodynamic instability. On the second hospital day, bilateral below-the-knee amputations were performed for apparent gangrene and submitted for pathologic evaluation.

Pathologic Findings

The microscopic appearance of the skin lesions in the amputated legs varied by lesion type and duration. The localized cellulitis-like lesions contained extravasated erythrocytes and many neutrophils in the dermis and subcutaneous tissue. The bullae were subepidermal with dermal perivascular infiltration by neutrophils and mononuclear cells (Figure 5-41). The gangrenous lesions showed dermal and epidermal necrosis with transmural necrosis of blood vessels, some of which contained thrombi. Gram-negative bacteria were present in the adventitia surrounding the injured blood vessels (Figure 5-42) and were vividly demonstrated by a Warthin-Starry silver impregnation strain (Figure 5-43).

Differential Diagnoses

Organisms that may cause peripheral gangrene include enteric gram-negative bacilli, *Vibrio* species (especially *Vibrio vulnificus*), *Pseudomonas aeruginosa*, *Aeromonas* species, meningococci, clostridia, *Rickettsia rickettsii*, and *Rickettsia prowazekii*. The perivascular distribution of gram-negative bacteria is observed in *V. vulnificus* septicemia and *Pseudomonas* ecthyma gangrenosa.

Microbiology

V. vulnificus was cultivated from soft tissues and bullous fluid from the legs and later in the course from the arms.

Comment

Among 11 *Vibrio* species known to cause human illness, *V. vulnificus* is the most important in the United States. *V. vulnificus* occurs naturally in warm coastal and estuarine salt water. In cold water, *V. vulnificus* enters a viable but nonculturable state. In warm water temperatures, quantities of *V. vulnificus* rise, with highest levels in the intestines of bottom-feeding coastal fin fish, substantial levels in molluscans and crustaceans such as oysters and crabs, and lower levels in the water itself. *V. vulnificus* multiplies in raw oysters, the principal source of human infection, after harvesting if they are not refrigerated.

Human infections with *V. vulnificus* occur in three forms: primary septicemia following ingestion of contaminated uncooked seafood (58%), wound infections (28%), and gastroenteritis (14%) in a series from Florida. Cases occur during seasons of warm water and predominantly

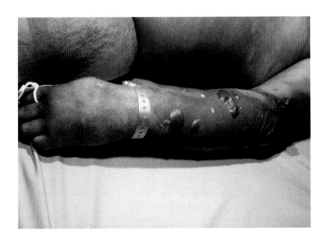

FIGURE 5-40. The arm of the patient showed the early lesions associated with *Vibrio vulnificus* sepsis, subepidermal bullae, and dermal ecchymoses.

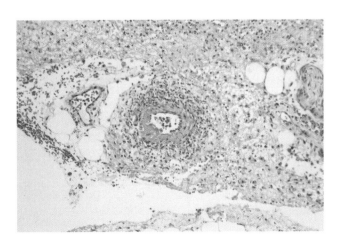

FIGURE 5-41. A dermal blood vessel demonstrates a perivascular leukocytic infiltrate and surrounding edema (hematoxylin and eosin stain; medium-power magnification).

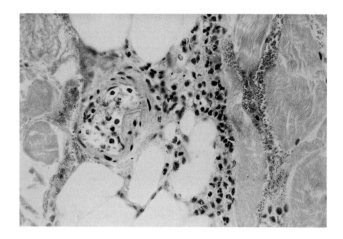

FIGURE 5-42. A myriad of gram-negative bacteria is present in the adventitia and adjacent spaces between skeletal muscle cells (Brown-Hopps stain; high-power magnification).

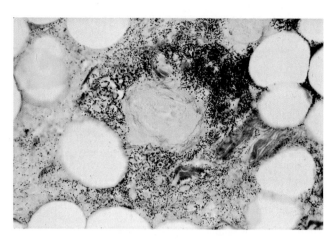

FIGURE 5-43. Silver impregnation staining demonstrates enormous quantities of perivascular bacteria (Warthin-Starry stain; high-power magnification).

affect men (71–96%). The case-fatality rate is slightly more than 50% for primary *V. vulnificus* septicemia, approximately 25% for wound infections, and essentially none for uncomplicated gastroenteritis. The risk of illness is 80 times higher for persons with liver disease who eat raw oysters than in persons without liver disease. Fatal septicemia is usually a result of eating contaminated raw oysters, and death is 200 times more likely to occur in patients with underlying liver disease, such as alcoholic cirrhosis or hemochromatosis, than in patients without liver disease. Immunosuppression is also a risk factor for disease caused by this organism, to which many immunocompetent persons are exposed without pathologic effects.

Diagnosis

V. vulnificus septicemia with bilateral lower extremity gangrene and extensive cutaneous necrosis.

RECOMMENDED READING

Varicella-Zoster Virus

Drew WL, Mintz L. Rapid diagnosis of varicella-zoster virus infection by direct immunofluorescence. Am J Clin Pathol 1980;73:699.

Hyman RW, Ecker JR, Tenser RB. Varicella-zoster virus RNA in human trigeminal ganglia. Lancet 1983; 2:814.

Oberg G, Svedmyr A. Varicelliform eruptions in herpes zoster—some clinical and serological observations. Scand J Infect Dis 1969;1:47.

Schmidt NJ, Gallo D, Devlin V, et al. Direct immuno-fluorescence staining for detection of herpes simplex and varicella-zoster virus antigens in vesicular lesions and certain tissue specimens. J Clin Microbiol 1980;12:651.

Ziegler T. Detection of varicella-zoster viral antigens in clinical specimens by solid-phase enzyme immunoassay. J Infect Dis 1984;150:149.

Murine Typhus

Dumler JS, Taylor JP, Walker DH. Clinical and laboratory features of murine typhus in South Texas, 1980 through 1987. JAMA 1991;266:1365.

Schriefer ME, Sacci JB Jr, Dumler JS, et al. Identification of a novel rickettsial infection in a patient diagnosed with murine typhus. J Clin Microbiol 1994;32:949.

Silpapojakul K, Chayakul P, Krisanapan S. Murine typhus in Thailand: clinical features, diagnosis and treatment. Q J Med 1993;86:43.

Silpapojakul K, Pradutkanchana J, Pradutkanchana S, Kelly DJ. Rapid, simple serodiagnosis of murine typhus. Trans R Soc Trop Med Hyg 1995;89:625.

Walker DH, Feng HM, Ladner S, et al. Immunohisto-chemical diagnosis of typhus rickettsioses using an anti-lipopolysaccharide monoclonal antibody. Mod Pathol 1997;10:1038.

Walker DH, Parks FM, Betz TG, et al. Histopathology and immunohistologic demonstration of the distribution of *Rickettsia typhi* in fatal murine typhus. Am J Clin Pathol 1989;91:720.

Lyme Disease

Bakken LL, Callister SM, Wang PJ, Schell RF. Interlaboratory comparison of test results for detection of Lyme disease by 516 participants in the Wisconsin State Laboratory of Hygiene/College of American Pathologists Proficiency Testing Program. J Clin Microbiol 1997;35:537.

Craven RB, Quan TJ, Bailey RE, et al. Improved serodiagnostic testing for Lyme disease: results of a multicenter serologic evaluation. Emerg Infect Dis 1996;2:136.

Nadelman RB, Nowakowski J, Forseter G, et al. The clinical spectrum of early Lyme borreliosis in patients with culture-confirmed erythema migrans. Am J Med 1996;100:502.

Schmidt BL. PCR in laboratory diagnosis of human *Borrelia burgdorferi* infections. Clin Microbiol Rev 1997;10:185.

Mycobacteria

Asnis DS, Bresciani AR. Cutaneous tuberculosis: a rare presentation of malignancy. Clin Infect Dis 1992; 15:158.

Beyt BE, Ortbals DW, Santa Cruz DJ, et al. Cutaneous mycobacteriosis: analysis of 34 cases with a new classification of the disease. Medicine (Baltimore) 1980;60:95.

Binford CH, Meyers WM. Leprosy. In CH Binford, DH Connor (eds), Pathology of Tropical and Extraordinary Diseases. Vol 1. Washington, DC: Armed Forces Institute of Pathology, 1976;205.

Blake LA, West BC, Lary CH, Todd JR IV. Environmental nonhuman sources of leprosy. Rev Infect Dis 1987;9:562.

Cruz DJS, Strayer DS. The histologic spectrum of the cutaneous mycobacterioses. Hum Pathol 1982; 13:485.

Gaylord H, Brennan PJ. Leprosy and the leprosy bacillus: recent developments in characterization of antigens and immunology of the disease. Ann Rev Microbiol 1987;41:645.

Hastings RC, Gillis TP, Krahenbuhl JL, Franzblau SG. Leprosy. Clin Microbiol Rev 1988;1:330.

Kester KE, Turiansky GW, McEvoy PL. Nodular cutaneous microsporidiosis in a patient with AIDS and successful treatment with long-term oral clindamycin therapy. Ann Intern Med 1998;128:911.

Lumpkin LR III, Cox GF, Wolf JE Jr. Leprosy in five armadillo handlers. J Am Acad Dermatol 1983;9:899.

Modlin RL, Melancon-Kaplan J, Young SM, et al. Learning from lesions: patterns of tissue inflammation in leprosy. Proc Natl Acad Sci USA 1988;85:1213.

Neil MA, Hightower AW, Broome CV. Leprosy in the United States, 1971–1981. J Infect Dis 1985;152: 1064.

Ridley DS, Jopling WH. Classification of leprosy according to immunity: A five group system. Int J Lepr 1964;34:255.

Rietbroek RC, Dahlmans RPM, Smedts F, et al. Tuberculosis cutis miliaris disseminata as a manifestation of miliary tuberculosis: literature review and report of a case of recurrent skin lesions. Rev Infect Dis 1991;13:265.

Wabitsch KR, Meyers WM. Histopathologic observations on the persistence of *Mycobacterium leprae* in the skin of multibacillary leprosy patients under chemotherapy. Lepr Rev 1988;59:341.

Sporothrix schenckii

Kauffman CA. Old and new therapies for sporotrichosis. Clin Infect Dis 1995;21:981.

Kwon-Chung KJ, Bennett JE. Sporothrichosis. In KJ Kwon-Chung, JE Bennett (eds), Medical mycology. Philadelphia: Lea and Febiger, 1992;707.

Lynch PJ, Voorhees JJ, Harrell ER. Systemic sporotrichosis. Ann Intern Med 1970;73:23.

Sanders E. Cutaneous sporotrichosis: beer, bricks, and bumps. Arch Intern Med 1971;127:482.

Wilson DE, Mann JJ, Bennett JE, Utz JP. Clinical features of extracutaneous sporotrichosis. Medicine (Baltimore) 1967;46:265.

Cutaneous Leishmaniasis

Desowitz RS. Kala-azar: the long anguish of the black sickness. Hosp Pract (Off Ed) 1992;27:201.

Fernandez-Guerrero ML, Aguado JM, Buzon L, et al. Visceral leishmaniasis in immunocompromised hosts. Am J Med 1987;83:1098.

Magill AJ, Grögl M, Gasser RA Jr, et al. Visceral infection caused by Leishmania tropica in veterans of operation desert storm. N Engl J Med 1993;328:1383.

Melby PC, Kreutzer RD, McMahon-Pratt D, et al. Cutaneous leishmaniasis: review of 59 cases seen at the National Institutes of Health. Clin Infect Dis 1992;15:924.

Chromoblastomycosis

Connor DH, Gibson DW. Association of splinters with chromomycosis and phaeomycosis cysts [Letter]. Arch Dermatol 1985;121:168.

Fader RC, McGinnis MR. Infections caused by dematiaceous fungi: chromoblastomycosis and phaeohyphomycosis. Infect Dis Clin N Am 1988;2:925.

Uribe JF, Zuluaga AI, Leon W, Restrepo A. Histopathology of chromoblastomycosis. Mycopathologia 1989;105:1.

Prototheca

Chandler FW, Kaplan W, Callaway CS. Differentiation between Prototheca and morphologically similar green algae in tissue. Arch Pathol Lab Med 1978;102:353.

Holcomb HS III, Behrens F, Winn WC Jr, et al. Prototheca wickerhamii—an alga infecting the hand. J Hand Surg [Am] 1981;6:595.

Nosanchuk JS, Greenberg RD. Protothecosis of the olecranon bursa caused by achloric algae. Am J Clin Pathol 1973;59:567.

Sudman MS. Protothecosis. A critical review. Am J Clin Pathol 1974;61:10.

Sudman MS, Kaplan W. Identification of the Prototheca species by immunofluorescence. Appl Microbiol 1973;25:981.

Tindall JP, Fetter BF. Infections caused by achloric algae (Protothecosis). Arch Dermatol 1971;104:490.

Coccidioides immitis

Raab SS, Silverman JF, Zimmerman KG. Fine-needle aspiration biopsy of pulmonary coccidioidomycosis. Am J Clin Pathol 1993;99:582.

Singh VR, Smith DK, Lawerence J, et al. Coccidioidomycosis in patients infected with human immunodeficiency virus: review of 91 cases at a single institution. Clin Infect Dis 1996;23:563.

Stevens DA. Coccidioidomycosis. N Engl J Med 1995;332:1077.

Bacillary Angiomatosis

Arias-Stella J, Lieberman PH, Erlandson RA. Histology, immunohistochemistry, and ultrastructure of the verruga in Carrion's disease. Am J Surg Pathol 1986;10:595.

Koehler JE, Quinn FD, Berger TG, et al. Isolation of Rochalimaea species from cutaneous and osseous lesions of bacillary angiomatosis. N Engl J Med 1992;327:1625.

LeBoit PE, Berger TG, Egbert BM, et al. Bacillary angiomatosis: the histopathology and differential diagnosis of a pseudoneoplastic infection in patients with human immunodeficiency virus disease. Am J Surg Pathol 1989;13:909.

Relman DA, Loutit JS, Schmidt TM, et al. The agent of bacillary angiomatosis. An approach to the identification of uncultured pathogens: the agent of bacillary angiomatosis. N Engl J Med 1990;323:1573.

Vibrio vulnificus

Ali A, Mehra MR, Stapleton DD, et al. Vibrio vulnificus sepsis in solid organ transplantation: a medical nemesis. J Heart Lung Transplant 1995;14:598.

Centers for Disease Control and Prevention. Vibrio vulnificus infections associated with raw oyster consumption—Florida, 1981–1992. MMWR Morb Mortal Wkly Rep 1993;42:405.

Chuang Y-C, Yuan C-Y, Liu C-Y, et al. Vibrio vulnificus infection in Taiwan: report of 28 cases and review of clinical manifestations and treatment. Clin Infect Dis 1992;15:271.

Kizer KW. Vibrio vulnificus hazard in patients with liver disease. Western J Med 1994;161:64.

Park SD, Shon HS, Joh NJ. Vibrio vulnificus septicemia in Korea: clinical and epidemiologic findings in seventy patients. J Am Acad Dermatol 1991;24:397.

Infections of the Central Nervous System

Infections of the central nervous system (CNS) represent potentially treatable conditions that generally have a more favorable prognosis (if diagnosed efficiently) than malignant neoplasms, demyelinating diseases, dementia, and other neurologic disorders. The etiologic agents of CNS infections include viruses, bacteria, fungi, protozoa, and helminths, which respond to distinctly different classes of pharmaceutical therapy. Patients may present for medical attention with an acute or chronic course, with a febrile or afebrile condition, and with or without focal neurologic signs. The two major categories of clinical problems are meningoencephalitis and space-occupying lesions; the status of the patient's immune system strongly influences the clinical differential diagnosis. Among patients with acquired immunodeficiency syndrome (AIDS), the list of diseases involving the CNS is extensive, including toxoplasmosis, progressive multifocal leukoencephalopathy, cryptococcal meningitis, tuberculous meningitis, *Mycobacterium avium-intracellulare* or *Mycobacterium fortuitum* meningitis, *Listeria monocytogenes* meningitis, disseminated candidiasis or histoplasmosis, primary CNS lymphoma (frequently associated with Epstein-Barr virus), nocardiosis, *Acanthamoeba* and *Balamuthia* meningoencephalitis, cytomegaloviral encephalitis, and human immunodeficiency virus (HIV) encephalopathy. In contrast, the differential diagnosis of acute meningoencephalitis of previously healthy persons comprises a rather different set of conditions, such as herpes simplex virus (HSV) encephalitis, arboviral encephalitides, Rocky Mountain spotted fever, murine typhus, human monocytotropic ehrlichiosis, and *Naegleria* meningoencephalitis.

Neuroimaging investigations, particularly computed tomographic (CT) scanning and magnetic resonance imaging, frequently assist greatly in the characterization and localization of the lesions within the CNS, such as brain abscess, toxoplasma encephalitis, neurocysticercosis, tuberculoma, and primary or metastatic tumor. For patients in whom increased intracranial pressure does not preclude its collection, cerebrospinal fluid (CSF) can often lead to a diagnosis by isolation of bacteria, fungi, or viruses or by detection of antigens or specific nucleic acid sequences. Biopsy of the brain is often a last resort; many patients are diagnosed by the neuropathologist at autopsy. These postmortem diagnoses have proved to be of public health importance for meningococcal infection, mosquito-borne encephalitis (e.g., St. Louis encephalitis), louse-borne typhus, hemorrhagic anthrax meningitis following inhalational exposure, and poliomyelitis, in which prophylactic antibiotics, arthropod vector control, preventive measures to avoid occupational or biologic warfare exposure, or vaccination may be appropriate measures. An etiologic diagnosis is key to the response to all of these situations.

ACUTE MENINGITIS

Clinical History

A 4-year-old girl was taken to an emergency department by her parents for evaluation of fever, vomiting, and headache for 1 day and a skin rash that had appeared the morning of evaluation and progressed over the next several hours. On physical examination, her temperature was 39.4°C, her pulse rate was 120 beats per minute, and her respiratory rate was 40 breaths per minute. She appeared lethargic and was unable to walk. Tenting of the skin was present on her forehead, her mucous membranes were dry, and numerous pinpoint, dark-red macules were scattered diffusely over her body. Pertinent abnormal laboratory test results included pancytopenia (hemoglobin concentration, 8.2 g/dl; white blood cell count, 3,200 cells per µl; platelet count, 27,000 U/µl), prolonged prothrombin and partial thromboplastin times, decreased fibrinogen concentration, and elevated fibrin degradation products. Meningococcemia was suspected. Blood cultures were obtained, and appropriate antimicrobial therapy was initiated immediately thereafter. Despite aggressive supportive care, her condition deteriorated, and she died approximately 24 hours after admission.

Pathologic Findings

At autopsy, the predominant findings were in the CNS. The brain was diffusely swollen (weight, 1,329 g; expected weight, 1,150 ± 150 g), and opacity of the leptomeninges overlying the convexities of the cerebral hemispheres and at the base of the brain was evident (Figure 6-1). A subarachnoid hemorrhage was present in the superior vermis of the cerebellum. Microscopic examination of the area of leptomeningeal opacity showed acute purulent meningitis, characterized by an extensive infiltrate of neutrophils (Figure 6-2). In one section stained by the Brown-Hopps method, rare intracellular gram-negative diplococci were seen.

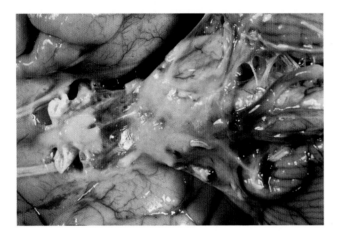

FIGURE 6-1. Brain from a patient with fatal meningococcal meningitis shows a purulent subarachnoid exudate.

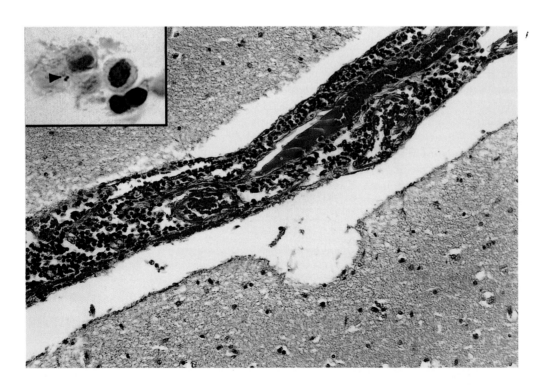

FIGURE 6-2A. Section of left frontal lobe of a child with meningococcal meningitis (based on blood cultures that grew *Neisseria meningitidis*) shows a perivascular infiltrate of neutrophils and a few histiocytes in a fissure (hematoxylin and eosin stain; original magnification, ×50). *Inset*: Rare intracellular gram-negative diplococci (*arrowhead*; Brown-Hopps stain; original magnification, ×250).

FIGURE 6-2B. Section of left frontal lobe of a child with meningococcal meningitis (based on blood cultures that grew *Neisseria meningitidis*) shows a perivascular infiltrate of neutrophils and a few histiocytes in the cerebrum (hematoxylin and eosin stain; original magnification, ×100).

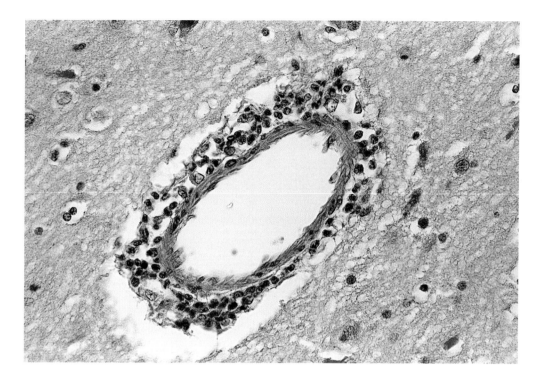

Differential Diagnosis

A meningeal infiltrate composed predominantly of neutrophils in conjunction with the clinical course in this case are characteristic of meningitis caused by one of the "pyogenic" bacteria, the most common of which are group B streptococcus, *Escherichia coli*, *Haemophilus influenzae* type b, *Neisseria meningitidis*, and *Streptococcus pneumoniae*.

Microbiology

In this case, premortem blood cultures grew *N. meningitidis*.

Comment

In a 4-year-old child, the bacteria most likely to cause meningitis are *N. meningitidis* and *S. pneumoniae*; of these two, *N. meningitidis* is most likely to be associated with a cutaneous rash (Figure 6-3). *H. influenzae* type b meningitis has become uncommon in the United States as a result of widespread use of the vaccine. Antemortem, the cause of bacterial meningitis is made by Gram stain and culture of CSF. However, if the diagnosis is not confirmed until autopsy, sections of the involved meninges should be stained with a tissue Gram stain to help determine the pathogen. Bacteria, however, cannot always be found, especially in cases of partially treated meningitis, such as this case. Therefore, culture

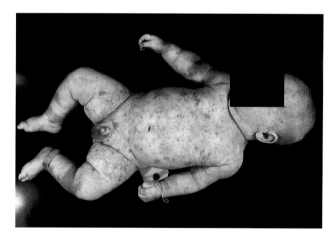

FIGURE 6-3. Photograph of an infant who died from meningococcemia shows the typical diffuse purpuric rash.

of blood, CSF, and meningeal tissue should be performed. Additionally, testing CSF for bacterial antigens (*H. influenzae*, *N. meningitidis*, and *S. pneumoniae*) may be useful, particularly in cases of partially treated meningitis.

Diagnosis

Meningococcal meningitis.

CHRONIC MENINGITIS

Clinical History

A 50-year-old man, with a history of injection drug use and alcohol abuse, was admitted for evaluation of disorientation, nausea, and vomiting for "several days." On physical examination, he was disoriented but had a normal response to painful stimuli. No localizing neurologic deficits were detected. His temperature was 38°C, his pulse rate was 105 beats per minute, his respiratory rate was 20 breaths per minute, and his blood pressure was 157/80 mm Hg. Abdominal examination revealed a fluid wave, and pitting edema of the lower extremities occurred bilaterally. The remainder of the examination was noncontributory. Pertinent abnormal laboratory test results included a white blood cell count of 17,300 cells per µl (78% segmented neutrophils, 12% band forms), bilirubin concentration of 4.4 mg/dl, slight elevation of the liver enzymes, and markedly prolonged prothrombin time and partial thromboplastin time. The differential diagnoses on admission were cirrhosis with hepatic encephalopathy, sepsis, and meningitis. After blood cultures were collected, CSF obtained by lumbar puncture was submitted for laboratory analysis, and empiric broad-spectrum antimicrobial therapy was initiated. Analysis of the CSF revealed a white blood cell count of 25 cells per µl (100% lymphocytes), protein concentration of 79 mg/dl, and a glucose concentration of 6 mg/dl; budding yeast cells were seen in the gram-stained smear. Based on this report, antifungal therapy was added to the antimicrobial regimen.

On hospital day 5, the patient had several seizures, all localized to the head and neck. An electroencephalogram showed epileptiform activity in the left frontal area. Anticonvulsant therapy was begun, but the seizure activity could not be controlled. A second electroencephalogram revealed diffuse slowing, reported as consistent with encephalopathy. He continued to deteriorate and died the following day.

Pathologic Findings

At autopsy, the most prominent findings were in the brain. The leptomeninges were fibrotic and firmly adherent to the pia, and a whitish-gray exudate was present in the leptomeningeal space (Figure 6-4), especially at the base of the brain. The brain was slightly swollen but showed no evidence of herniation. On cut section, the Virchow-Robin space around blood vessels penetrating the basal ganglia was distended, creating typical "soap bubble" lesions consisting of numerous perivascular yeasts (Figure 6-5). Microscopic examination of hematoxylin and eosin (H and E)–stained sections of the meninges and underlying brain parenchyma showed marked thickening of the subarachnoid space by predominantly yeast cells and very few inflammatory cells (Figures 6-6A and 6-6B). The mucinous capsule of these yeasts is illustrated in sections stained by the mucicarmine method (Figure 6-7), allowing a histologic diagnosis of cryptococcosis.

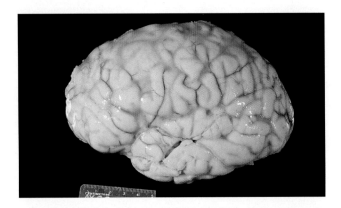

FIGURE 6-4. Brain from a patient with cryptococcal meningitis shows opacification of the leptomeninges overlying the cerebral hemispheres with milky white appearance of many sulci. The mucopolysaccharides of the fungal capsule made the surface of the brain very slippery to handle. (Courtesy of Dr. Gerald Campbell.)

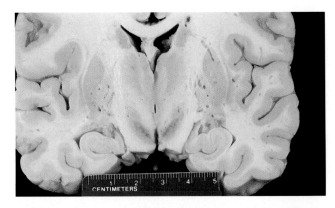

FIGURE 6-5. Section of brain from a patient with cryptococcal meningitis demonstrates distention of the Virchow-Robin space around blood vessels penetrating the basal ganglia. These "soap-bubble lesions" consist of large quantities of perivascular yeasts. (Courtesy of Dr. Gerald Campbell.)

Differential Diagnosis

The CSF Gram stain findings in this case (Figure 6-8) are very suggestive of cryptococcal meningitis. Yeast cells of *Blastomyces dermatitidis* can resemble those of *Cryptococcus neoformans*, but meningitis is an uncommon feature of blastomycosis. The gross features demonstrated by this case are consistent with chronic meningitis, and are caused by *C. neoformans*, *Histoplasma capsulatum*, *B. dermatitidis*, and *Mycobacterium tuberculosis*.

Microbiology

The day after antifungal therapy was initiated, the CSF cryptococcal antigen test was reported as positive (titer, 1:512). The CSF fungal culture grew *C. neoformans* after incubation for 4 days. The serologic test for antibodies to HIV was negative.

Comment

The histologic findings in the tissue sections stained by H and E and mucicarmine allow a diagnosis of cryptococcal meningitis. In this case, however, the diagnosis was made antemortem based on a positive result from CSF cryptococcal antigen test and the results of fungal culture.

C. neoformans, a saprophyte in nature, is found worldwide and is most commonly associated with excreta of pigeons. Infection most likely is acquired by inhalation of aerosolized conidia. Cryptococcal disease is most com-

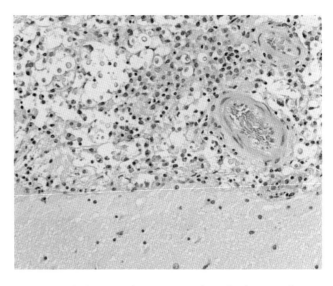

FIGURE 6-6A. Section of meninges and cerebral cortex shows a scanty lymphohistiocytic exudate and round yeast forms surrounded by a clear halo, an appearance highly suggestive of *Cryptococcus neoformans* (hematoxylin and eosin stain; original magnification, ×50).

mon in men (male to female ratio is 3 to1). Whites are affected more frequently than persons of other races. Factors associated with increased risk of cryptococcosis include infection with HIV, administration of corticosteroids, lymphoreticular malignancies (especially Hodgkin's disease),

FIGURE 6-6B. Higher-power magnification of the section illustrated in **A** shows the variably-sized yeast cells of *Cryptococcus neoformans* intermixed with an infiltrate of macrophages and lymphocytes (hematoxylin and eosin stain; original magnification, ×100).

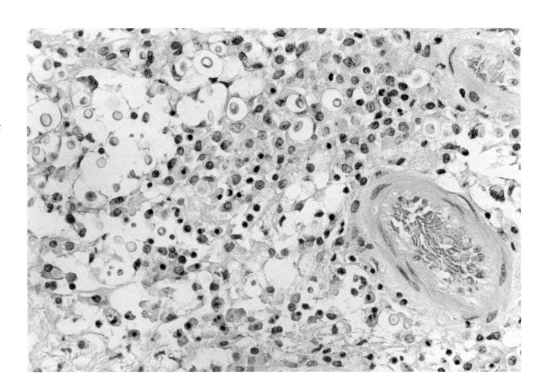

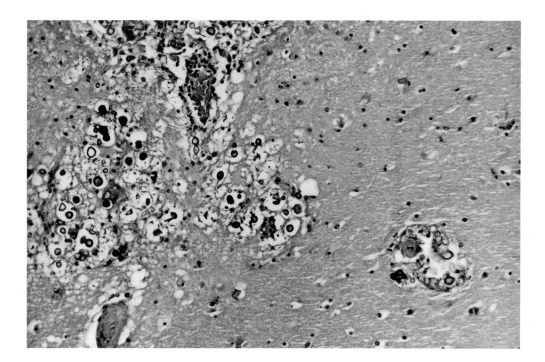

FIGURE 6-7. Section of brain from the case illustrated in Figure 6-6 shows cryptococcal yeast cells within the Virchow-Robin spaces and brain parenchyma. The intense coloring of the mucinous capsules of the yeasts provides a histologic diagnosis of cryptococcosis (Mayer's mucicarmine; original magnification, ×50).

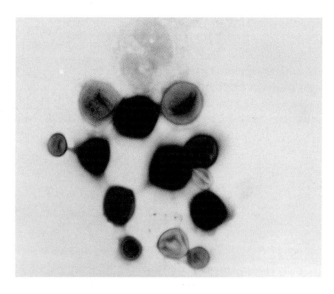

FIGURE 6-8. Smear of cerebrospinal fluid stained with Gram stain shows variably sized budding yeast cells (Gram stain; original magnification, ×250). The failure of the yeast cells to stain with crystal violet, and hence appear gram-negative, is typical of *Cryptococcus neoformans*.

and sarcoidosis; in more than 50% of cases, however, no predisposing condition is recognized.

The histopathologic findings associated with cryptococcal meningitis vary depending on the immune status of the host. In immunocompromised patients, such as persons infected with HIV, minimal (if any) inflammatory response occurs. In patients who have cryptococcal meningitis but who are not as severely immunocompromised as persons infected with HIV, the meningeal infection is associated with an inflammatory cell exudate comprised of histiocytes and lymphocytes (Figure 6-9). *C. neoformans* also can cause a fibrocaseous lesion, termed a *cryptococcoma* (Figure 6-10). For both of these manifestations, the gross features and histologic findings in H and E–stained tissue sections resemble those of tuberculosis (i.e., an inflammatory infiltrate composed of epithelioid histiocytes, lymphocytes, and fibroblasts; Figures 6-11 and 6-12). Capsule-deficient cryptococci stimulate a more vigorous granulomatous response. Although these capsule-deficient yeasts cannot be demonstrated with mucin stains, they are visualized very effectively by the Fontana-Masson stain. The presence of acid-fast bacilli

FIGURE 6-9. Section of cerebral cortex and meninges from a patient with a history of alcohol abuse shows a meningeal inflammatory cell infiltrate of macrophages and lymphocytes (hematoxylin and eosin; original magnification, ×100). *Inset*: Staining with Mayer's mucicarmine shows few encapsulated yeast forms, consistent with *Cryptococcus neoformans* (Mayer's mucicarmine; original magnification, ×250).

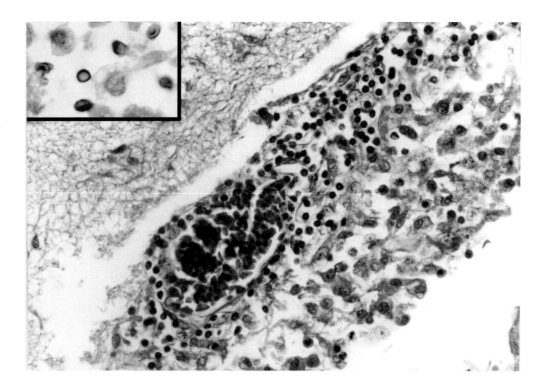

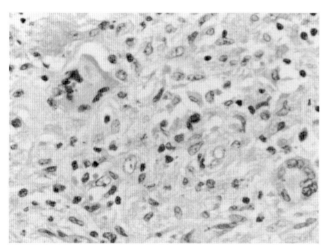

FIGURE 6-10. Section of a mass lesion removed by open brain biopsy from a patient with diabetes mellitus shows granulomatous inflammation including multinucleate giant cells (hematoxylin and eosin; original magnification, ×100). Sections stained by methenamine silver and mucicarmine methods (not illustrated) revealed rare yeast forms with mucinous capsules, allowing a diagnosis of cryptococcoma.

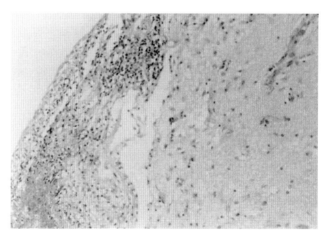

FIGURE 6-11. Section of cerebral cortex and meninges from a patient who died with a clinical diagnosis of chronic tuberculous meningitis shows thickening of the subarachnoid space with an inflammatory cell infiltrate composed of epithelioid histiocytes, lymphocytes, and fibroblasts (hematoxylin and eosin stain; original magnification, ×50).

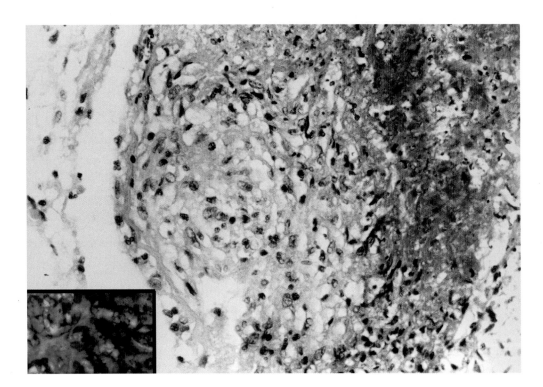

FIGURE 6-12. Higher-power magnification of the section illustrated in Figure 6-11 shows a granuloma and adjacent necrosis (hematoxylin and eosin stain; original magnification, ×100). *Inset*: Staining by the Ziehl-Neelsen method demonstrates a few acid-fast bacilli (Ziehl-Neelsen stain; original magnification, ×250). The mycobacterial culture of the cerebrospinal fluid collected antemortem grew *Mycobacterium tuberculosis*.

in tissue sections stained by the Ziehl-Neelsen method (see Figure 6-12) confirms a mycobacterial infection, but bacilli are not found in all cases of tuberculous meningitis or tuberculomas. *M. tuberculosis* is the most likely mycobacterial pathogen, but some of the nontuberculous mycobacteria (e.g., *M. fortuitum* and *Mycobacterium avium* complex) can cause meningitis. Therefore, culture is necessary to confirm the diagnosis.

Diagnosis

Cryptococcal meningitis.

ACUTE MENINGOENCEPHALITIS

Clinical History

A 62-year-old man from eastern Texas was admitted in late August for evaluation of fever and rapid neurologic deterioration. Before this illness, he had been in good health. On physical examination, he was somnolent, but arousable, and disoriented to person, place, and time. His temperature was 40°C, his pulse rate was 120 beats per minute, his respiratory rate was 40 breaths per minute, and his blood pressure was 120/70 mm Hg. Marked nuchal rigidity and a diffuse increase in muscle tone were present. The remainder of the examination was noncontributory. His white blood cell count was 11,600 cells per μl (84% neutrophils, 2% band forms, 5% lymphocytes, and 9% monocytes), and the erythrocyte sedimentation rate was 125 mm/hour. His serum electrolytes and liver enzyme values were within normal limits. A CT scan of the brain showed prominence of the cortical sulci and minimal enlargement of the ventricular system; no abnormal enhancement or mass effect was seen. A radionuclide brain scan demonstrated a diffusely abnormal increase in uptake of the radionuclide bilaterally in the temporal, occipital, and parietal lobes. Lumbar puncture was performed, and analysis of the CSF showed a white blood cell count of 125 cells per μl (23% neutrophils, 77% lymphocytes), a protein concentration of 124 mg/dl, and a glucose concentration of 74 mg/dl (the concomitant serum glucose concentration was 107 mg/dl). No organisms were visualized in smears of CSF stained by Gram stain or with auramine O.

Based on the patient's clinical presentation, the results of radiologic studies, and the CSF findings, a diagnosis of acute meningoencephalitis was made. Serologic studies for detection of antibodies to arthropod-borne viruses in CSF and serum were requested. Additional microbiologic tests included culture of CSF for viruses, mycobacteria, and fungi and examination of CSF by polymerase chain reaction (PCR) for HSV nucleic acids. Empiric broad-spectrum antimicrobial therapy, including an agent effective against HSV, and aggressive supportive care were initiated. His condition deteriorated, however, and he died 1 week after admission.

Pathologic Findings

At autopsy, the predominant findings were in the brain. On gross inspection, the brain appeared diffusely swollen, but no evidence of herniation was present. Sections of the cortex showed a perivascular inflammatory infiltrate composed of mononuclear cells and focal areas of necrosis with associated gliosis (Figures 6-13 and 6-14).

FIGURE 6-13. Section of brain tissue from a patient with St. Louis viral encephalitis shows a perivascular inflammatory infiltrate and a focus of necrosis associated with mononuclear cell infiltrate (hematoxylin and eosin stain; original magnification, ×50).

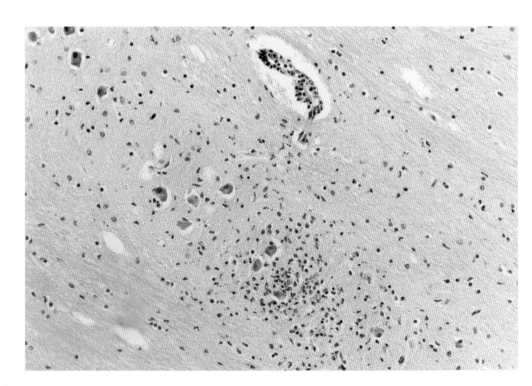

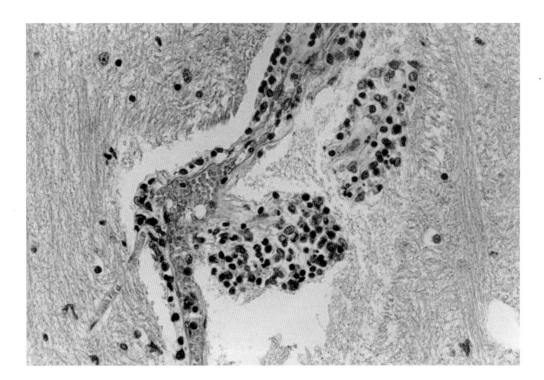

FIGURE 6-14. Examination of the section illustrated in Figure 6-13 under higher-power magnification shows that the perivascular inflammatory cell infiltrate is composed predominantly of lymphocytes and macrophages (hematoxylin and eosin stain; original magnification, ×100).

Differential Diagnoses

Among the potential pathogens, the arthropod-borne viruses, St. Louis encephalitis virus, western equine encephalitis virus, eastern equine encephalitis, and La Crosse and California encephalitis viruses are the agents most likely responsible for the illness. Less likely, but possible, causes are the enteroviruses and HSV.

Comment

The histopathologic findings are characteristic of viral encephalitis caused by any one of the arthropod-borne viruses included in the differential diagnosis or the enteroviruses. Based on the patient's age, geographic location (i.e., eastern Texas), absence of recent travel, season (i.e., summer), and recent weather conditions (i.e., heavy rains followed by a marked increase in the mosquito population), the etiologic agents most likely responsible are St. Louis encephalitis virus and eastern equine encephalitis virus. Encephalitis caused by the California encephalitis viruses (including La Crosse virus) or enteroviruses also occur during the summer season, but both are much more common in children than adults. Diagnosis requires detection of specific antibodies in CSF, serum, or both. Results of serologic studies performed premortem on CSF and serum confirmed a diagnosis of St. Louis encephalitis.

Diagnosis

St. Louis encephalitis.

HEMORRHAGIC ENCEPHALITIS

Clinical History

A 12-day-old female infant was admitted for evaluation of lethargy. The infant had been born at term, and had Apgar scores of 9 and 9 at 1 and 5 minutes, respectively. The day after admission, the infant became pale and limp. The differential diagnoses included meningitis and pneumonia. A CT scan of the head was normal, and lumbar puncture was performed. The CSF showed a white blood cell count of 23 cells per µl (92% lymphocytes, 8% neutrophils) and a protein concentration of 146 g/dl; no organisms were seen in the Gram-stained smear, and bacterial cultures were negative. Blood cultures were collected, and empiric antimicrobial therapy was initiated.

The next day, the baby had a right-sided seizure and developed severe respiratory distress requiring intubation and mechanical ventilation. Chest radiograph showed alveolar consolidation of the right lung with right-sided pleural effusion. A repeat CT scan of the head was reported as meningitis versus subarachnoid hemorrhage with diffuse cerebral edema. Pertinent abnormal laboratory test results included a hemoglobin concentration of 8.2 mg/dl and elevated prothrombin and partial thromboplastin times. HSV encephalitis was added to the differential diagnoses, and appropriate antiviral therapy was added to the therapeutic regimen. However, the baby's neurologic condition continued to deteriorate, and she died 2 weeks after admission.

Pathologic Findings

The predominant findings at autopsy were in the brain. There was widespread hemorrhagic necrosis of all lobes of the cerebrum, most marked in the temporal and inferior frontal lobes. This pattern of involvement suggested HSV encephalitis. Additional findings included a large hematoma in the left thalamus and focal areas of hemorrhagic necrosis in the cerebellum and brain stem. Tissue from the temporal lobes was submitted to the microbiology laboratory for viral culture. Histologic examination of areas of hemorrhagic necrosis in the temporal lobe showed extensive necrosis (Figure 6-15) and occasional cells showing intranuclear inclusions consistent with HSV (Figure 6-16).

Differential Diagnoses

Entities to consider in the differential diagnosis of focal lesions of HSV encephalitis, especially when viral inclusions are not recognizable, include toxoplasmosis, brain abscesses, and tumors.

Microbiology

After incubation of the culture for 1 week, HSV type 2 was recovered from the viral culture of brain tissue collected at autopsy.

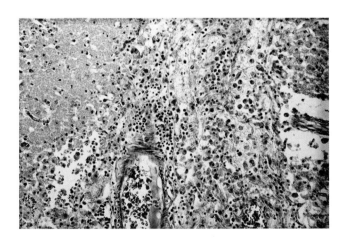

FIGURE 6-15. Necrosis with numerous lipid-laden macrophages and perivascular lymphocytic infiltration in a case of herpes viral encephalitis (hematoxylin and eosin stain; medium-power magnification).

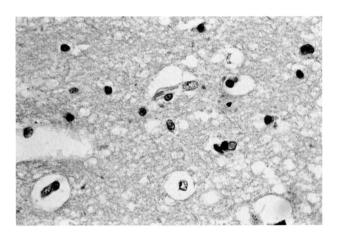

FIGURE 6-16. Herpes viral encephalitis with two neurons containing prominent eosinophilic intranuclear viral inclusions (hematoxylin and eosin stain; high-power magnification).

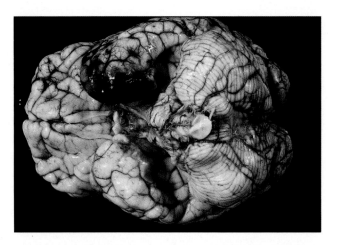

FIGURE 6-17. Photograph of the brain from a patient with fatal herpes simplex encephalitis shows the classic hemorrhagic necrosis of the temporal lobe.

Comment

HSV causes a broad spectrum of clinical manifestations. In neonates, 60–70% of cases are due to HSV type 2, which is acquired during delivery or via retrograde spread from the genital tract of the mother, who frequently has no symptoms of genital herpes. Neonatal disease becomes manifest before age 4 weeks, depending on the time of infection; it is categorized according to its extent as disseminated; CNS; or skin, eyes, and mouth. Localized CNS disease, as occurred in this case, is characterized by tremors, lethargy, irritability, paralysis, seizures, and coma. If untreated, the mortality rate is about 50%; of the babies who survive, fewer than 10% develop normally.

In adults, infection of the brain with HSV is the most common cause of fatal sporadic encephalitis in the United States. It occurs year-round, affects persons of all ages, and almost always is due to HSV type 1. HSV is believed to reach the brain by neural routes during primary or recurrent infection, localizing predominantly in the temporal lobes, where necrotizing, hemorrhagic encephalitis ensues (Figure 6-17). Clinical illness begins abruptly or after an influenzalike prodrome with fever, headache, stiff neck, behavior disorders, speech difficulties, focal seizures, and occasionally, olfactory hallucinations. Examination of the CSF frequently shows moderate pleocytosis with mononuclear cells and neutrophils, minimally elevated protein levels, and a normal glucose concentration, but these parameters may be completely normal. The mortality rate if untreated is 60–80%, and more than 90% of persons who survive have neurologic sequelae.

Diagnosis of HSV encephalitis often is not easy. Viral cultures of spinal fluid usually are negative, except in cases of congenital HSV. Nucleic acid amplification tests, such as the PCR, which allow detection of viral DNA in CSF, have become the diagnostic method of choice. However, PCR is available only in research and reference laboratories. In fatal cases or when brain biopsy is performed, the pathologist must make the diagnosis. Unfortunately, cells demonstrating classic cytopathic effects of HSV infection (i.e., intranuclear inclusions in oligodendroglia, astrocytes, or nerve cells) are not always visible, especially in areas of marked necrosis or when the patient has received antiviral therapy. When this occurs, the diagnosis requires viral culture of brain tissue or demonstration of HSV DNA by nucleic acid amplification or in situ hybridization.

Diagnosis

HSV type 2 encephalitis.

CONFUSION, ATAXIA, AND PULMONARY INFILTRATES IN A PREVIOUSLY HEALTHY MAN

Clinical History

A 74-year-old man was evaluated in an emergency department for chronic cough and paresthesia and weakness in his right arm. He was discharged but returned 4 days later with complaints of shortness of breath, confusion, vomiting, and right arm weakness and was admitted. On physical examination, he was afebrile. Pertinent physical findings included right arm weakness, bilateral ptosis, severe dysarthria, ataxia, and confusion. A chest radiograph showed bilateral pulmonary infiltrates. Lumbar puncture was performed, and analysis of the CSF revealed a white blood cell count of 1,000 cells per μl (predominantly lymphocytes) and a protein concentration of 174 mg/dl. The differential diagnoses included pneumonia and cerebrovascular accident.

During the first day of admission, the patient became progressively agitated, more confused, and ultimately unresponsive. He was intubated and placed on mechanical ventilatory support. Over the next 9 days, he remained unconscious and intermittently spiked a fever (as high as 39.3°C). He died 10 days after admission.

Pathologic Findings

At autopsy, the etiology of the patient's illness was found in the brain. H and E–stained sections of the cerebral cortex showed a perivascular mononuclear cell infiltrate (Figure 6-18). Examination of these tissue sections under higher-power magnification revealed neurons with intracytoplasmic inclusions (Figure 6-19) characteristic of rabies virus infection (i.e., Negri bodies). Rabies virus antigen was detected in paraffin-embedded sections of brain tissue by direct fluorescent antibody staining (performed at the Centers for Disease Control and Prevention). Nucleotide sequence analysis of the viral RNA present in the brain tissue identified the rabies virus variant associated with the silver-haired bat.

Differential Diagnoses

The diagnosis of rabies is not difficult in a patient who presents with hyperactivity, hydrophobia, or aerophobia, all of which are virtually pathognomonic of rabies, and is known to have been bitten by a potentially rabid animal.

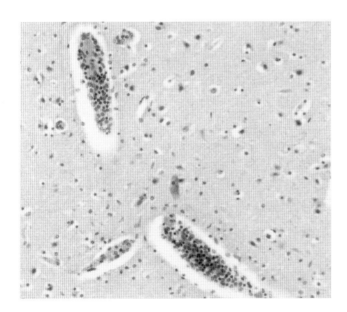

FIGURE 6-18. Section of cerebral cortex from a case of rabies shows a prominent perivascular mononuclear cell infiltrate (hematoxylin and eosin stain; original magnification, ×50).

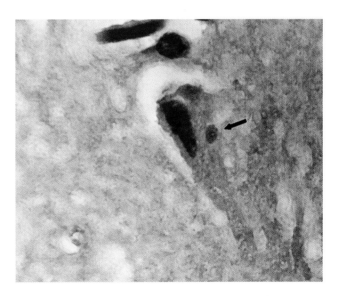

FIGURE 6-19. Higher-power magnification of the section illustrated in Figure 6-18 shows a neuron with an intracytoplasmic inclusion (*arrow*), characteristic of the Negri body associated with rabies virus infection (hematoxylin and eosin stain; original magnification, ×250).

However, not all patients with rabies give a history of possible rabies exposure, nor do all patients have hydrophobia and aerophobia. In this latter group of patients, rabies must be differentiated from other viral causes of encephalitis, such as HSV and the arboviruses, and paralytic rabies must be distinguished from poliomyelitis, Guillain-Barré syndrome, and transverse myelitis.

Comment

Rabies virus is an RNA virus classified in the family Rhabdoviridae. Rabies is predominantly a disease of wild and domestic animals. Most cases of human rabies result from direct or indirect exposure to a rabid animal. Where domestic rabies has not been well controlled, dogs account for at least 90% of cases; in countries where domestic rabies is well controlled, such as in the United States, Canada, and many western European countries, they account for fewer than 5% of cases. Domestic animals other than dogs (predominantly cats and cattle) are responsible for 5–10% of reported animal rabies worldwide. The principal wildlife vectors of rabies are the striped skunk, raccoon, and insectivorous bats in the United States; the fox in Europe, the Arctic, and sub-Arctic; the vampire bat in Latin America; the wolf in Western Asia; and the mongoose and jackal in Africa. Human-to-human transmission of rabies has been reported rarely in recipients of corneal transplants, and occasionally, no source of infection is recognized. In the United States, the proportion of cases of human rabies that have no known exposure to rabid animals has increased over the years. Between 1960 and 1979, no source was identified in 16%

of cases, and since 1980, no source could be identified in 60% of cases. Of the 20 rabies virus variants obtained from human rabies acquired in the United States from 1980 to 1996, 17 (85%) were associated with insectivorous bats, but unequivocal evidence of a bite was found in only one of the 17 cases.

Premortem, rabies is diagnosed most reproducibly by detection of rabies viral antigens using immunofluorescent antibody staining in a full-thickness punch skin biopsy specimen; the specimen should contain as many hair follicles as possible from the posterior neck above the hair line. Rabies virus may be recovered from saliva, brain tissue, CSF, urine, and tracheal secretions, and viral neutralizing antibodies may be detected in serum early in the second week after the onset of symptoms and in the CSF 4–7 days later.

Histopathologic examination of antemortem or postmortem brain tissue from patients with rabies shows perivascular mononuclear cell infiltrates in the gray matter in some but not all cases, neuronal degeneration, and (in 70–80% of the cases) one or more characteristic, sharply defined, eosinophilic intracytoplasmic inclusions called *Negri bodies*. The inclusions are round or oblong, 2–10 µm in diameter, and often contain basophilic spots. Negri bodies are most commonly found in the hippocampus, the horn of Ammon, and the Purkinje cells of the cerebellum; they are less often found in the motor area of the cerebral cortex or spinal ganglia.

Diagnosis

Rabies encephalitis.

FEVER AND COMA DURING TRAVEL IN THE TROPICS

Clinical History

The body of a 48-year-old man was delivered to a county medical examiner's office for postmortem evaluation of the brain (all abdominal organs had been previously removed and examined elsewhere). The only history provided to the medical examiner regarding the case indicated that the decedent had been a businessman on assignment in Brazil. Before leaving the United States, he had received the recommended immunizations, and while in Brazil, he supposedly had taken prescribed medication for malaria prophylaxis. The man developed fever and headache a few days before death but did not seek medical attention. He was found comatose and taken to a local hospital in Brazil, where he died a few hours thereafter.

Pathologic Findings

At autopsy in the medical examiner's office, the brain weighed 1,250 g. Gross findings included marked congestion of the cerebral vessels, diffuse flattening of the gyri and narrowing of the sulci, and grooving of the unci bilaterally. Sections of brain tissue showed marked engorgement of cerebral capillaries (Figure 6-20). Under high-power magnification, brown, granular pigmented material was visualized in several erythrocytes, predominantly those that were marginated along the endothelial lining of the blood vessel (Figure 6-21). Sections stained

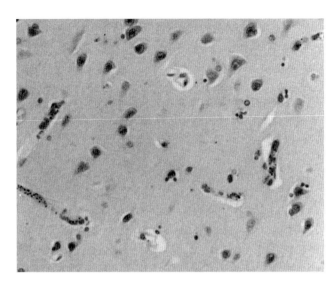

FIGURE 6-20. Section of cerebral cortex from a patient with cerebral malaria shows marked congestion of the capillaries, the lumens of which appear to contain many small, dark dots (hematoxylin and eosin stain; original magnification, ×50).

by Romanovsky's method demonstrated trophozoites, merozoites, and a rare gametocyte of *Plasmodium falciparum* (Figure 6-22).

FIGURE 6-21. Higher-power magnification of the section illustrated in Figure 6-20 reveals erythrocytes containing brown-pigmented granules, located predominantly along the endothelial lining of the vessel (hematoxylin and eosin stain; original magnification, ×250).

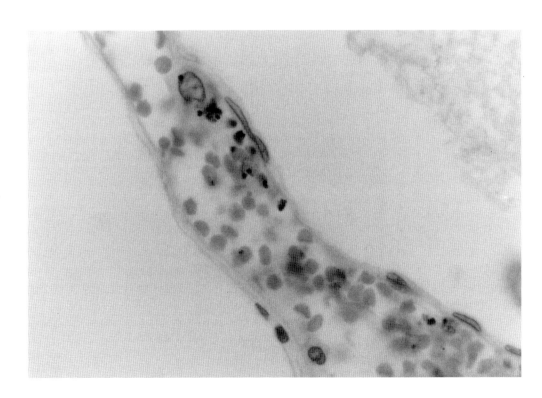

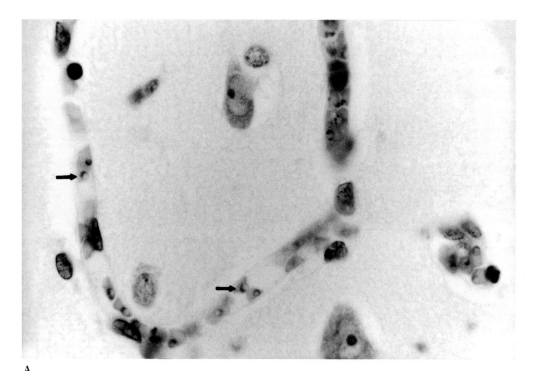

A

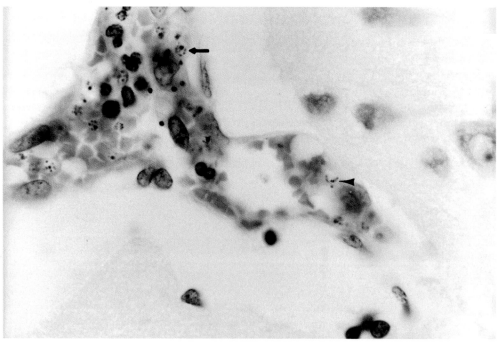

B

FIGURE 6-22. Section of cerebral cortex from the case illustrated in Figure 6-21 stained by Romanovsky's method demonstrates *Plasmodium falciparum* parasites, including (**A**) ring forms (*arrows*) and (**B**) schizont (*arrow*) and a gametocyte (*arrowhead*; azure-eosin stain; original magnification, ×250).

Comment

Malaria is caused by infection with any of the four species of *Plasmodium*: *Plasmodium falciparum*, *Plasmodium vivax*, *Plasmodium ovale*, and *Plasmodium malariae*. Of these, only infection with *P. falciparum* is potentially fatal. Infection is transmitted by the bite of an infective female *Anopheles* species mosquito. The signs and symptoms of malaria vary, but most patients have fever. Headache, back pain, chills, increased swelling, myalgia, nausea, vomiting, diarrhea, and cough also are common. The diagnosis of malaria should be considered for any person who has these symptoms and who has traveled to an area where malaria is transmitted, and for persons who have a fever of unknown origin, regardless of their travel history. In complicated malaria caused by *P. falciparum*, different signs and symptoms are present, depending on the predominant organ system involved. In cerebral malaria, as occurred in this case, drowsiness and headache followed by rapid development of coma and death are common; meningismus, paresis, mental changes, and seizures also may occur.

The histologic changes caused by infection with *P. falciparum* result from the development of the parasite within red blood cells attached to the endothelium of medium and small blood vessels and capillaries. In cerebral malaria, the cerebral gyri are usually flattened due to marked swelling. The blood vessels are congested, and the cut surface of the brain is pink with a cortex that is dark gray from the presence of pigment. Histopathologically, capillaries are distended by masses of red blood cells. In small blood vessels, erythrocytes containing parasites, which have darkly staining nuclei, are found attached to the endothelial surface by specific cytoadherence mechanisms. Malarial pigment, which is birefringent if viewed under polarized light, is present in parasitized red blood cells and macrophages and occasionally is free in the circulation. If cerebral malaria lasts more than 10 days, small areas of hemorrhage (called *ring hemorrhages*), owing to endothelial damage with thrombosis and leakage of blood into the tissue, develop around medium-sized blood vessels. In cases of nonfatal cerebral malaria, the hemorrhagic areas heal, forming areas of fibrosis called *Durck's granulomas*.

Diagnosis

Cerebral malaria caused by *P. falciparum*.

PROGRESSIVE NEUROLOGIC DISEASE WITH DEMYELINATING LESIONS

Clinical History

A 66-year-old man was admitted from another hospital for evaluation of right hemiparesis with sensory involvement, aphasia, and fever. The illness began approximately 3 months previously with mild right hemiparesis that involved the arm and leg and spared the face. Six weeks earlier, he lost all motor function in the right extremities and was admitted to another hospital. A CT scan at that time showed what was reported to be a stroke in the left parietal lobe with no evidence of hemorrhage. He was discharged to a rehabilitation center. One month before the current admission, he developed right facial weakness. His speech became garbled and slurred; over the next few weeks it was diminished to only yes and no responses. He was readmitted to the same hospital. Laboratory test results were normal, with the exception of a slightly elevated erythrocyte sedimentation rate (50 mm/hour). During this hospitalization, he became febrile with tachycardia and elevated blood pressure. Prednisone and empiric broad-spectrum antimicrobial agents were given; his con-

dition did not improve, however, and he was transferred to a tertiary-care medical center for further evaluation.

On physical examination at the tertiary-care center, the patient was confused and appeared chronically ill. His temperature was 38.6°C, his pulse rate was 100 beats per minute, his respiratory rate was 30 breaths per minute, and his blood pressure was 170/100 mm Hg. He responded to voice and light touch but remained mute and did not follow oral or demonstrated instructions. The right corneal reflex was diminished, and right-sided facial drop, right hemiparesis, and bilateral Babinski's signs were present. The remainder of the physical examination was within normal limits. Pertinent medical history included a questionable diagnosis of rheumatoid arthritis 4 years earlier, managed with prednisone.

Magnetic resonance imaging of the brain performed before and after gadolinium administration showed an extensive signal abnormality in the left parietal lobe and both frontal lobes that was confined to the white matter and crossed the genu of the corpus callosum. A focal area of increased signal also was present in the region of the junction of the left thalamus and the posterior limb of the internal capsule. No definite enhancement by gadolinium was evident. An electroencephalogram showed generalized, irregular slowing of delta activity without focal features. All hematologic and chemistry laboratory test results were normal. A serologic test for infection with HIV was negative. A test for antinuclear antibodies was positive at a titer of 1:1,024. Lumbar puncture was performed, and results of all hematologic, chemical, microbiologic, and cytologic studies performed on the CSF were normal. Based on the pattern of evolution of the patient's neurologic symptoms and the results of the neuroimaging and CSF studies, progressive multifocal leukoencephalopathy (PML) was considered to be the most likely diagnosis. Stereotactic brain biopsy was performed, and two samples of tissue from the left frontal lobe were submitted for histopathologic examination.

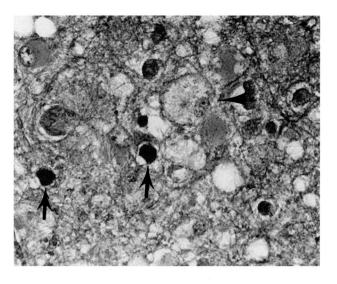

FIGURE 6-23. Autopsy section of cerebrum from a different patient with acquired immunodeficiency syndrome who died from progressive multifocal leukoencephalopathy shows extensive demyelinization, several smudgelike intranuclear inclusions in enlarged oligodendrogliocytes (*arrows*), reactive astrocytes, and one macrophage with phagocytized, degenerated myelin in its cytoplasm (*arrowhead*; Luxol fast blue stain; original magnification, ×100). These cytopathic changes are characteristic of infection with JC virus, which is responsible for the oligodendrogliocyte inclusions.

Pathologic Findings

The fragments of brain tissue measured 10 mm × 2mm × 1 mm and 8 mm × 2 mm × 1 mm. Microscopic examination of tissue sections stained with H and E showed lesions characteristic of PML, including giant astrocytes with large, irregular, hyperchromatic nuclei, oligodendrogliocytes with intranuclear inclusions, and lipid-laden macrophages. Special stains for myelin showed these same features and an absence of myelin (Figure 6-23). Electron microscopic examination showed that the oligodendroglial cell nuclei contained polyomavirus virions (Figure 6-24).

Comment

PML is caused by infection with JC virus, a nonenveloped, double-stranded DNA virus in the family Papovaviridae. Before the epidemic of infection with HIV, PML occurred predominantly in older patients with an underlying hematologic malignancy, although it occasionally was seen in patients with other causes for depression of cell-mediated immunity and rarely developed in persons with no identifiable immunodeficiency. It is estimated that more than 50% of deaths caused by PML are associated with HIV infection and that 1–4% of patients infected with HIV develop PML.

Patients with PML typically present with rapidly progressive focal neurologic deficits (most commonly hemiparesis, visual field deficits, and cognitive impairment) without signs of increased intracranial pressure. Manifestations that occur later include cortical blindness, quadriparesis, profound dementia, and coma. Most patients undergo rapid deterioration and die within 6 months of diagnosis.

Radiographic tests that are useful in the diagnosis of PML are the CT scan, which characteristically demonstrates hypodense, nonenhancing lesions of cerebral white matter, and magnetic resonance imaging, which reveals areas of increased signal intensity corresponding to the white matter lesions. CSF cell count and protein and glucose concentrations usually are normal. JC virus can be recovered from CSF or brain tissue, but this requires a special type of cell culture that generally is not available in clinical virology laboratories. Therefore, virus culture is not helpful diagnostically. A definitive diagnosis of PML requires histopathologic examination of brain tissue and visualization of findings characteristic of PML, as illustrated in this case. Typically, multiple asymmetric foci of demyelination are present at different stages of evolution in the cerebral white matter. Oligodendrogliocytes infected with JC virus demonstrate cytopathic effects that include nuclear enlargement, loss of the usual nuclear

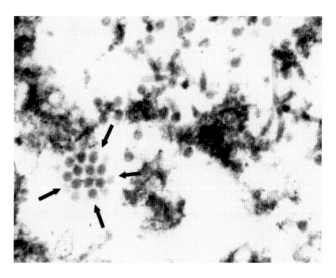

FIGURE 6-24. Electron photomicrograph of an oligodendroglial cell from a patient with progressive multifocal leukoencephalopathy demonstrates numerous (55 nm) papovaviruses, some of which are packed in clusters (*arrows*; uranyl acetate–lead citrate stain; magnification, ×90,000). (Courtesy of Dr. Benjamin Gelman and Julie Wen.)

chromatin pattern, and deeply basophilic intranuclear inclusions. Many lesions contain markedly enlarged astrocytes (some of which have hyperchromatic and irregularly shaped nuclei) and lipid-laden macrophages. JC virus nucleic acid may be detected in CSF by PCR, but this assay is available only in certain reference and research laboratories and is not necessary for diagnosis if the typical histopathologic findings are present in brain tissue.

Diagnosis

Progressive multifocal leukoencephalopathy.

INSIDIOUS NEUROLOGIC DISEASE IN A PATIENT WITH HUMAN IMMUNODEFICIENCY VIRUS INFECTION

Clinical History

A 46-year-old woman, diagnosed with HIV infection 6 months earlier, was admitted for frontal headache unrelieved by acetaminophen and dizziness of 1 week's duration. On physical examination, she was afebrile, her pulse rate was 85 beats per minute, her respiratory rate was 14 breaths per minute, and her blood pressure was 98/74 mm Hg. Neurologic examination revealed no abnormalities. The remainder of the examination was noncontributory. A CT scan of the head showed diffuse cerebral atrophy. By hospital day 3, the headache and dizziness appeared to have resolved, and the patient was discharged with instructions to begin antiretroviral therapy and prophylaxis against *Pneumocystis carinii* pneumonia.

One week later, she was readmitted for evaluation of severe frontal headache, lethargy, short-term memory loss, and disorientation. On physical examination, her temperature was 38.5°C. She was lethargic, disoriented to place and time, and able to follow only simple, one-step commands. The remainder of the results of the neurologic examination appeared to be normal, although thorough evaluation of cerebellar function was not possible because of poor cooperation by the patient. An enhanced magnetic resonance imaging study of the head demonstrated increased signal intensity in the periventricular region, reported as characteristic of ventriculitis; no mass lesion was evident. The CSF showed 116 white blood cells per µl (87% lymphocytes, 7% monocytes, 6% neutrophils), a protein concentration of 139 mg/dl, and a glucose concentration of 36 mg/dl (concomitant serum glucose concentration was 90 mg/dl). CSF was submitted to the clinical microbiology laboratory for bacterial, fungal, and mycobacterial stains and cultures and for viral culture, including shell vial centrifugation cell culture for detection of cytomegalovirus (CMV). Antiviral therapy directed against CMV was initiated, but her condition continued to deteriorate. Based on directives stated in the patient's living will, no further therapy was instituted. She died 3 weeks after admission.

Pathologic Findings

At autopsy, the predominant findings were in the brain. The cerebral ventricles were mildly enlarged, and the surface of the ventricular walls had a shaggy, granular appearance. On cut section, softening and congestion of the subependymal area was present throughout the entire ventricular system, including the fourth ventricle and cerebral aqueduct. The remainder of the gross examination of the cerebral hemispheres, brain stem, cerebellum, and spinal cord was unremarkable. Tissue sections from the right occipital lobe and lateral ventricle showed necrotic brain parenchyma and several enlarged cells in the area of necrosis (Figure 6-25). Examination of these enlarged cells under higher magnification revealed intranuclear inclusions and numerous, small intracytoplasmic inclusions (Figure 6-26) consistent with cytopathic changes caused by CMV.

Microbiology

No organisms were detected in CSF smears stained by Gram stain or with auramine O. The centrifugation cell culture stained with a CMV-specific fluorescent labeled antibody demonstrated characteristic intranuclear inclusions of CMV, and CMV was recovered in conventional tissue culture 2 weeks later.

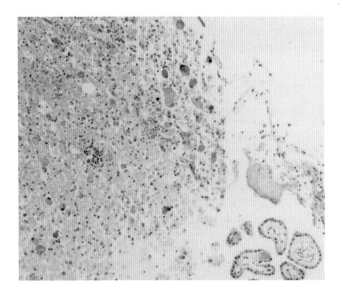

FIGURE 6-25. Section of right occipital lobe and lateral ventricle from an acquired immunodeficiency syndrome patient with cytomegalovirus ventriculoencephalitis shows choroid plexus (right) and necrotic brain parenchyma (left). Many enlarged cells are seen within the area of necrosis (hematoxylin and eosin stain; original magnification, ×25).

Comment

Gross findings often associated with CMV ventriculoencephalitis are ventricular dilation, necrosis, and hemorrhage or fibrinous exudates covering the ventricular system. Typical microscopic features include focal or diffuse destruction of the ependymal lining, necrosis of periventricular parenchymal tissue, and many cytomegalic cells in the ependymal and periependymal areas. In situ hybridization studies demonstrate diffuse and uniform infection of ependymal and subependymal lining cells by CMV.

Ventriculoencephalitis, demonstrated by this case, is only one of four pathologic lesions that have been associated with CMV encephalitis in patients with AIDS. The other three lesions are (1) isolated cytomegalic cells without associated microglial nodules or inflammation; (2) discrete foci of parenchymal necrosis with cytomegalic cells and macrophages; and (3) microglial nodules, characterized by well-demarcated, dense cellular aggregates of macrophages, rod-shaped microglia, or both. Microglial nodules are more common in gray matter than in white matter, and they uncommonly contain CMV inclusions (visualized in only 7–12% of cases), although CMV DNA can be detected by in situ hybridization or PCR.

Diagnosis

CMV ventriculoencephalitis.

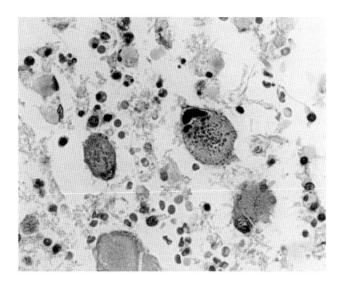

FIGURE 6-26. Examination of the enlarged cells seen in Figure 6-25 under higher-power magnification reveals prominent intranuclear inclusions and multiple, small intracytoplasmic inclusions, characteristic of cytopathic changes induced by cytomegalovirus infection (hematoxylin and eosin stain; original magnification, ×100).

HEMORRHAGIC INFARCTION

Clinical History

A 55-year-old man was admitted for evaluation of fever, cough, and diarrhea for 3 days. Fourteen months earlier, he was diagnosed with chronic lymphocytic leukemia, for which he had been treated with various chemotherapeutic agents. On physical examination, his temperature was 40°C, his pulse rate was 130 beats per minute, his respiratory rate was 20 breaths per minute, and his blood pressure was 135/85 mm Hg. His liver and spleen were enlarged, and numerous ecchymoses were present on all extremities. The remainder of the examination was noncontributory. Chest radiograph showed bilateral, diffuse alveolar infiltrates. Pertinent abnormal laboratory test results included a hemoglobin concentration of 8.3 g/dl, a white blood cell count of 2,400 cells per µl (36% neutrophils, 4% band forms, 58% lymphocytes, 2% monocytes), and a platelet count of 68,000 per µl. Blood was collected for bacterial cultures, and broad-spectrum antimicrobial therapy was initiated.

The following day, the microbiology laboratory reported that all blood cultures were positive for a gram-negative bacillus, which subsequently was identified as *E. coli*. Collection of a sputum specimen for bacterial, fungal, and mycobacterial stains and cultures was ordered the day of admission, but the patient was unable to produce an expectorated sample until hospital day 3. The

sputum KOH preparation was positive for budding yeast and nonseptate hyphae; therefore, antifungal agents were added to the antimicrobial regimen. Two days later, the patient was found unresponsive. His pupils were fixed and nonreactive to light, and corneal reflex was absent. A CT scan of the head showed findings consistent with acute hemorrhage in the right cerebellum. His condition continued to deteriorate, and he died later that day.

Pathologic Findings

At autopsy examination, the predominant findings were in the lungs and brain. In the right upper lobe of the lung, a hemorrhagic lesion 5 cm in diameter contained several thrombosed arteries. The brain was diffusely swollen, and tonsillar herniation had occurred. Areas of hemorrhagic infarction, the largest measuring 6 cm × 2.5 cm × 3.5 cm, were present in the right occipital lobe and the right cerebellum. H and E–stained sections of tissue from the areas of infarction in the lung and brain showed necrotic, thrombosed blood vessels and an extensive infiltrate of neutrophils (Figure 6-27). Examination of these sections under higher magnification revealed ribbonlike, nonseptate hyphae invading blood vessel walls (Figure 6-28) and within the thrombus material and necrotic brain parenchyma.

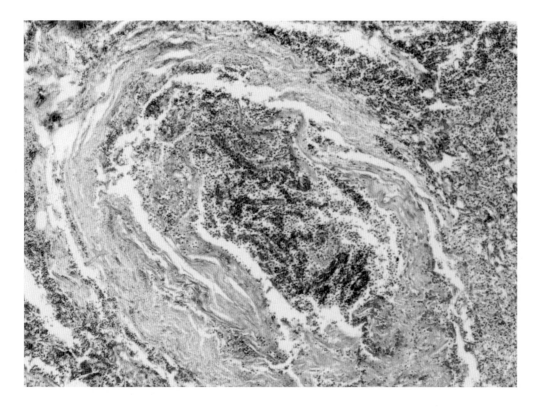

FIGURE 6-27. Section of brain tissue from an area of hemorrhagic infarction shows a blood vessel occluded by zygomycetes and an extensive inflammatory cell infiltrate composed almost completely of neutrophils (hematoxylin and eosin stain; original magnification, ×25). A premortem fungal culture of sputum grew *Mucor* species.

FIGURE 6-28. Higher-power magnification of the tissue section illustrated in Figure 6-27 shows ribbonlike, non-septate hyphae invading the blood vessel wall and within the vessel lumen (hematoxylin and eosin stain; original magnification, ×100).

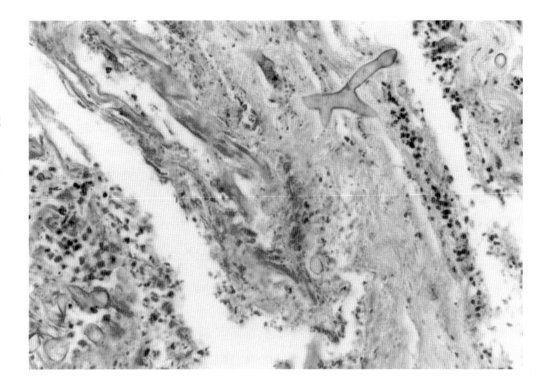

Differential Diagnoses

Organisms most commonly associated with vascular invasion and subsequent hemorrhagic infarction include the zygomycetes, *Aspergillus* species, and *Candida* species.

Microbiology

The fungal culture of the premortem sputum culture grew *Mucor* species.

Comment

Well-circumscribed areas of hemorrhagic infarction, which histologically show thrombosed blood vessels and an inflammatory cell infiltrate composed predominantly of neutrophils, are characteristic of the zygomycetes and aspergilli, although other hyaline moulds, such as *Fusarium* species or *Pseudallescheria boydii*, could induce these changes. It is important to remember, however, that in severely neutropenic patients, such as bone marrow transplant recipients, the prominent neutrophilic inflammatory infiltrate and tissue necrosis typically associated with zygomycosis frequently are absent (Figure 6-29).

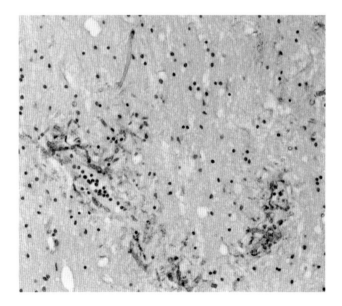

FIGURE 6-29. Section of cerebellum from a neutropenic patient with chronic lymphocytic leukemia shows zygomycetes hyphae invading blood vessel walls and the adjacent neuropil with no associated inflammation or necrosis (hematoxylin and eosin stain; original magnification, ×50). Fungal culture grew *Mucor* species.

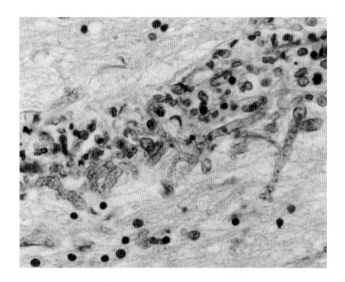

FIGURE 6-30. Section of brain tissue shows zygomycetes hyphae infiltrating a blood vessel wall (hematoxylin and eosin stain; original magnification, ×100). These hyphae are narrower than those illustrated in Figure 6-28, and a few septa appear to be present. In such cases, differentiation of zygomycetes and aspergilli is difficult, and fungal culture is necessary.

The presence of broad, nonseptate hyphae in this case confirms the diagnosis of zygomycosis, but fungal culture of involved tissue must be performed to determine which of the zygomycetes (i.e., *Mucor* species, *Rhizopus* species, *Absidia* species, or *Cunninghamella* species) is responsible. Typical ribbonlike hyphae, however, are not found in all cases of zygomycosis. Occasionally, the hyphae are more narrow and appear to have a few septa (Figure 6-30) resembling aspergilli; when this occurs, fungal culture is required for diagnosis. In rare cases of zygomycosis, sporangia may be found, thus allowing expert morphologic identification of the species and confirming the diagnosis.

Diagnosis

Zygomycosis.

INTRACRANIAL SPACE-OCCUPYING LESION IN A PREVIOUSLY HEALTHY MAN

Clinical History

A 25-year-old man with a history of intermittent ethanol abuse developed severe right-sided headaches followed 1 month later by a grand mal seizure that led to hospitalization. Physical examination revealed bilateral papilledema, retinal hemorrhages, left-central facial weakness, mild left hemiparesis, and bilateral Babinski's reflexes. Shortly after admission, he became unresponsive and had a dilated, fixed right pupil. Therefore, an emergency neuroradiologic procedure was performed, demonstrating a large right temporal mass with marked leftward displacement of the brain structures. He then underwent right temporal craniotomy with removal of a large multilocular abscess. Despite initial recovery of normal mental status, administration of antibacterial and antifungal agents, and placement of ventriculoperitoneal and intraventricular shunts, severe headaches returned, and he progressively deteriorated with unresponsiveness and seizures. He died on hospital day 34.

Pathologic Findings

The tissue removed at craniotomy consisted of multiple abscesses, encircled by a rim of fibroblasts and multinucleate giant cells and containing numerous brown septate-branching hyphae within a central zone of necrosis. At autopsy, the brain was markedly swollen with cerebellar tonsillar herniation, greenish-brown right temporal abscesses, ventriculitis, and periventriculitis (Figure 6-31). The abscesses contained many neutrophils, and septate-branching hyphae extended into surrounding viable tissue, including within multinucleate giant cells (Figure 6-32).

Differential Diagnoses

The differential diagnosis of a space-occupying lesion in this patient included bacterial and fungal abscess, actinomycosis, tuberculoma, primary neoplasm of the CNS, and metastatic malignant tumor.

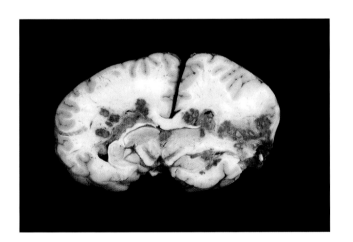

FIGURE 6-31. Cross section of the brain from a patient with phaeohyphomycotic cerebral abscesses shows numerous round, black, space-occupying lesions in both cerebral hemispheres.

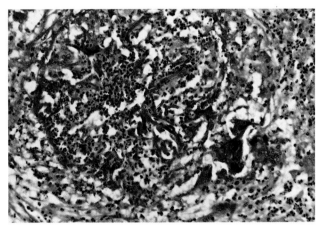

FIGURE 6-32. Photomicrograph of a brain with cerebral phaeo-hyphomycosis shows an intracranial abscess containing polymorphonuclear leukocytes admixed with epithelioid histiocytes and giant cells. Brown-pigmented septate hyphae are present within the central portion of the abscess and within multinucleate giant cell (hematoxylin and eosin stain; original magnification, ×50).

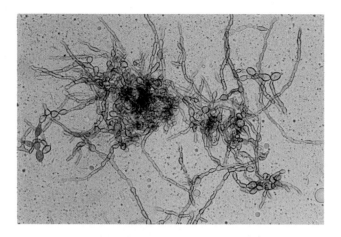

FIGURE 6-33. Digestion of the aspirated brain material with potassium hydroxide revealed brown-pigmented septate hyphae and chlamydospores consistent with the isolate *Cladophialophora bantiana* (unstained; high-power magnification).

Microbiology

Pus from the initial abscess material removed during surgery contained no bacteria detected by Gram stain or culture. Fungal culture subsequently grew *Cladophialophora* (formerly *Xylohypha* or *Cladosporium*) *bantiana*, and KOH preparation of abscess material revealed dematiaceous septate branching hyphae (Figure 6-33).

Comment

Brain abscess occurs after introduction of microorganisms into the brain from contiguous infected foci (e.g., otitis media, mastoiditis, paranasal sinusitis), hematogenous spread (e.g., from dental or thoracic foci), or trauma (e.g., after dural tear or neurosurgery). In 15–20% of cases, including cases of cerebral phaeohyphomycosis such as this, the route of entry and spread are not apparent but are presumed to represent subclinical pulmonary entry and hematogenous spread. Hematogenous abscesses typically occur in the distribution of the middle cerebral artery at the gray-white junction and are in some cases associated with right-to-left shunts (e.g., cyanotic congenital heart disease or pulmonary arteriovenous malformations). Before the advent of CT scans, the occurrence of multiple abscesses was considered to be rare. CT scanning and gadolinium-enhanced magnetic resonance imaging demonstrate the essential pathology, the central abscess with neutrophils and necrotic debris that are hypodense by CT, an enhancing rim representing the increased vascularity and vascular permeability of the developing capsule, and the surrounding edema that is hypodense by CT.

The most frequent etiologic agents of brain abscess are *Staphylococcus aureus*, gram-negative bacilli (e.g., *Proteus* species, *E. coli*, and *Pseudomonas aeruginosa* often as a mixed infection), anaerobic bacteria (e.g., *Bacteroides* and *Prevotella* species also often as a mixed infection), and *Streptococcus intermedius* group (commonly in the frontal lobe in association with sinusitis). A large variety of fungi comprise 10–15% of cases of brain abscess, with *C. bantiana* being the most frequent dematiaceous agent in previously normal persons.

Diagnosis

Phaeohyphomycotic cerebral abscesses.

SPACE-OCCUPYING LESION IN A PATIENT WITH ACQUIRED IMMUNODEFICIENCY SYNDROME

Clinical History

A 30-year-old man, diagnosed with AIDS 1 year earlier, was admitted for evaluation of weight loss of approximately 20 pounds during the past 6 weeks and "strange behavior" and seizures for 1 week. On physical examination, he was somnolent and afebrile. His pulse rate was 64 beats per minute, his respiratory rate was 14 breaths per minute, and his blood pressure was 138/78 mm Hg. He had right ptosis, disconjugate gaze, and his pupils were unequal in size (right, 5 mm; left, 2 mm). Extraocular movements could not be evaluated because of lack of patient cooperation. The remainder of the examination was noncontributory. Pertinent abnormal laboratory test results included a serum alkaline phosphatase level of 301 U per liter, lactate dehydrogenase of 342 IU per liter, and liver enzymes three times the upper limit of normal. A chest radiograph was normal. A CT scan of the head with and without contrast showed midline shift and a nonenhancing mass in the right frontal-parietal area. Based on the absence of ring-enhancement of the lesion, an infiltrative malignant process was considered to be a more likely diagnosis than brain abscess, cerebral toxoplasmosis, or a metastasis from a primary malignancy outside the CNS. Brain biopsy was scheduled for definitive diagnosis. On hospital day 3, he became comatose and required intubation and mechanical ventilation. He died the following day.

Pathologic Findings

At autopsy, the predominant findings were in the brain. The cerebral hemispheres were swollen, more on the right than the left, and herniation of the cingulate gyrus on the right side underneath the falx and grooving of the right uncus were evident. On sectioning, the white matter of the right hemisphere was expanded, and the junction of the gray and white matter was blurred. Well-demarcated areas of necrosis, the largest measuring 3 cm in diameter, were present in both hemispheres, four in the right and two in the left. The cerebellum and brain stem appeared grossly normal. Cytologic preparations of material aspirated from the largest cerebral lesion showed a few cysts of *Toxoplasma gondii* containing bradyzoites (Figure 6-34) and some aggregates of tachyzoites (Figure 6-35). H and E–stained sections of the cerebral lesions showed a perivascular accumulation of lymphocytes, marked necrosis and

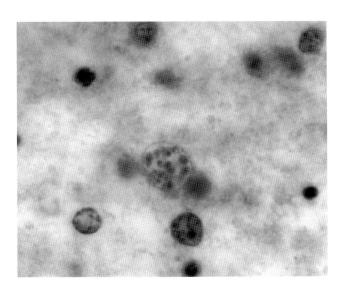

FIGURE 6-34. Cytologic preparation of material aspirated from a necrotic lesion in the frontal lobe of a patient with acquired immunodeficiency syndrome shows a cyst of *Toxoplasma gondii* containing many well-defined bradyzoites (Papanicolaou stain; original magnification, ×250).

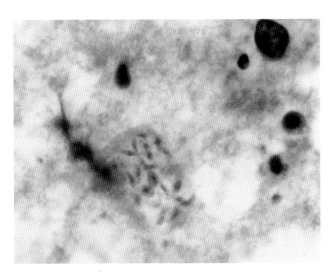

FIGURE 6-35. Another area of the cytologic preparation illustrated in Figure 6-34 shows an aggregate of *Toxoplasma gondii* tachyzoites (Papanicolaou stain; original magnification, ×250). In smears stained by the Papanicolaou method, the tachyzoite nucleus is purple-blue to red and the cytoplasm is gray, but when stained by the Giemsa method, the nucleus is blue and the cytoplasm is red.

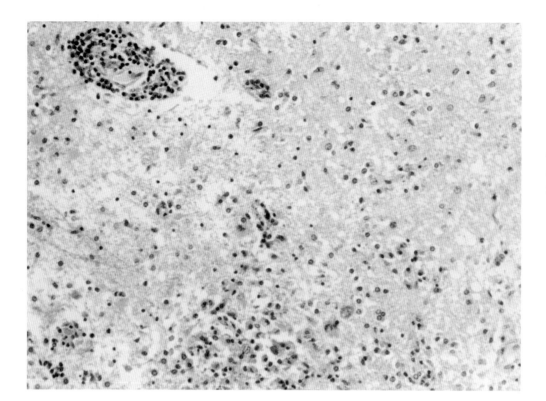

FIGURE 6-36. Section of the necrotic frontal lobe lesion shows a perivascular lymphocytic infiltrate, edema, and necrosis of the parenchyma with a diffuse lymphohistiocytic inflammatory cell infiltrate (hematoxylin and eosin stain; original magnification, ×50).

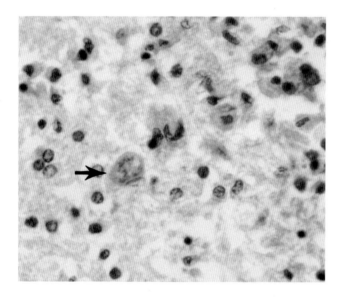

FIGURE 6-37. Higher-power magnification of the section illustrated in Figure 6-36 shows an area of necrosis that contains a *Toxoplasma gondii* cyst (*arrow*) and many lymphocytes and histiocytes (hematoxylin and eosin stain; original magnification, ×100).

Differential Diagnoses

T. gondii parasites may resemble those of *Trypanosoma cruzi* or *Leishmania*, especially in sites outside the CNS, but the lack of a kinetoplast distinguishes *T. gondii* organisms from the latter two. In skeletal muscle and myocardium, *T. gondii* cysts also must be differentiated from cysts of *Sarcocystis*, based on size, thickness of the cyst wall, and presence of compartments. Cysts of *Sarcocystis* are larger (21–51 μm in diameter) and have a thicker cell wall (1.5–3.0 μm) than those of *T. gondii*.

Comment

In cases of CNS toxoplasmosis, the brain generally is swollen, and signs of uncal, tonsillar, or cingulate herniation may be present. Coronal sections of the brain demonstrate multiple, well-circumscribed necrotic and sometimes hemorrhagic areas, measuring a few millimeters to several centimeters in diameter, in the basal ganglia and other central areas of the cerebrum, cerebellum, and spinal cord. The predominant microscopic features are the marked necrosis in different stages of evolution and a prominent vasculitis involving small, medium, and large vessels, often with thrombosis. Organisms frequently are difficult to identify because of the extensive necrosis; in such cases, immunohistochemical studies are useful (Figure 6-38). In patients with CNS toxoplasmosis who have been successfully treated but die months later of other causes, the lesions in the brain are indistinguishable from healed cavitated infarcts, and organisms are absent.

edema of the brain parenchyma, and a diffuse lymphohistiocytic inflammatory infiltrate (Figure 6-36). At high-power magnification, a few cysts of *T. gondii* were visualized (Figure 6-37), but organisms were difficult to identify because of the marked necrosis.

In tissue imprints stained by the Giemsa method, tachyzoites are crescentic in shape, with one end broader than the other, and measure 4–8 μm in length and 2–3 μm in width. The nucleus, located near the broader end, stains dark red, whereas the cytoplasm stains blue. Cysts vary in size up to 40 μm in diameter and contain many tachyzoites. In H and E–stained tissue sections, tachyzoites and cysts generally are smaller because of fixation and processing shrinkage, and the morphologic features of the tachyzoites are not as well defined.

Diagnosis

Cerebral toxoplasmosis.

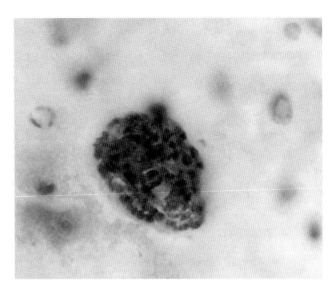

FIGURE 6-38. Immunohistochemical staining of a lesion in the basal ganglia of a patient with suspected toxoplasmosis accentuates the bradyzoites within a cyst, confirming the diagnosis (BioGenex peroxidase-antiperoxidase stain; original magnification, ×250).

NECROTIZING MASS LESIONS IN A HUMAN IMMUNODEFICIENCY VIRUS–INFECTED PATIENT

Clinical History

A 49-year-old man with a history of injection drug use for the previous 36 years was admitted for evaluation of recent onset of fever and change in mental status. He had been admitted elsewhere 1 month earlier for evaluation of a large left pleural effusion. A presumptive diagnosis of tuberculous pleuritis was made, and appropriate antituberculous therapy was initiated. He also was diagnosed with HIV infection during that admission.

On physical examination, he was uncooperative, lethargic, and disoriented to time and place, but no focal neurologic deficit was found. His temperature was 38°C, his pulse rate was 96 beats per minute, his respiratory rate was 20 breaths per minute, and his blood pressure was 115/80 mm Hg. Examination of the oral cavity showed thrush; the remainder of the examination was noncontributory. Lumbar puncture was performed, and the CSF showed a white blood cell count of 42 cells per µl with 88% lymphocytes and 12% neutrophils, protein concentration of 725 mg/dl, and a glucose concentration of 28 mg/dl (concomitant serum glucose concentration was 105 mg/dl). Magnetic resonance imaging of the brain revealed multiple infra- and supratentorial necrotizing mass lesions, reported as suggestive of toxoplasmosis or lymphoma. Antituberculous agents were continued, and antimicrobial therapy effective against *T. gondii* was begun. His mental status failed to improve, however, and he died 1 week after admission.

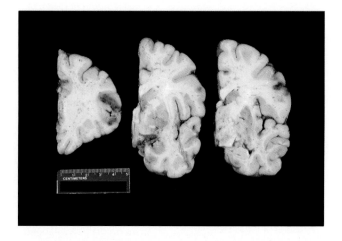

FIGURE 6-39. Coronal sections of a cerebral hemisphere of the patient with *Balamuthia mandrillaris* encephalitis shows multiple foci of hemorrhagic necrosis of the cerebral cortex.

Pathologic Findings

At autopsy, the predominant findings were in the brain. The cerebral hemispheres were swollen and edematous. Coronal sections demonstrated many necrotic and hemorrhagic areas measuring up to 3 cm in diameter involving the white and gray matter of the cerebellum and cerebral cortex (Figure 6-39). H and E–stained sections of these lesions showed marked hemorrhagic necrosis with a minimal inflammatory cell infiltrate (Figure 6-40). At higher magnification, amebae were seen throughout the necrotic tissue but were most numerous surrounding and within the walls of the medium- and large-sized blood vessels (Figure 6-41). The features of the amebic trophozoites and cysts (Figure 6-42) allow a differential diagnosis of *Acanthamoeba* and *Balamuthia*. The nucleus of the trophozoites has a large nucleolus that stains darkly with H and E, and the cysts are identified by their thick, irregular ectocyst containing the endocyst, which often appears shrunken. Immunofluorescence staining performed at the Centers for Disease Control and Prevention identified the etiologic agent as *Balamuthia mandrillaris* (Figure 6-43).

Differential Diagnoses

Parasites of *Acanthamoeba* and *Balamuthia* are differentiated from those of *Entamoeba histolytica* based on the nuclear characteristics of the organism (*E. histolytica* does not have a prominent nucleolus) and the presence of cysts, which are not found in tissue of cases of invasive infection with *E. histolytica*. *Acanthamoeba* and *Balamuthia* are distinguished from *Naegleria* based on the histologic pattern of the lesions: *Naegleria* causes primary meningoencephalitis, characterized by foci of hemorrhagic, microscopic necrosis, and an inflammatory cell infiltrate composed of mononuclear cells (predominantly lymphocytes) and neutrophils. *Acanthamoeba* and *Balamuthia*, in contrast, are associated with extensive necrosis and, in some cases, a granulomatous response.

Comment

Acanthamoeba species have been reported as the cause of more than 100 cases of granulomatous amebic encephalitis, and the more recently described *B. mandrillaris* as the cause of at least 63 cases. These protozoa infect immunocompromised persons and cause a disease that lasts for weeks or even months. In contrast, primary amebic meningoencephalitis caused by the free-living

FIGURE 6-40. Section of a lesion in the occipital lobe shows extensive hemorrhagic necrosis with only a few chronic inflammatory cells and a perivascular and intramural accumulation of protozoal parasites (hematoxylin and eosin stain; original magnification, ×100).

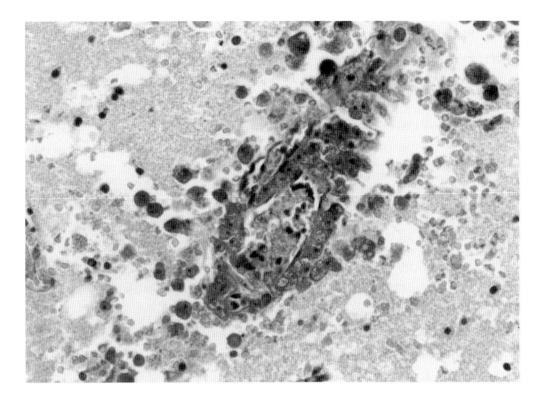

FIGURE 6-41. Higher-power magnification of the section illustrated in Figure 6-40 demonstrates the characteristic *Balamuthia mandrillaris* trophozoites, which have a prominent, dark nucleolus and vacuolated cytoplasm (hematoxylin and eosin stain; original magnification, ×250).

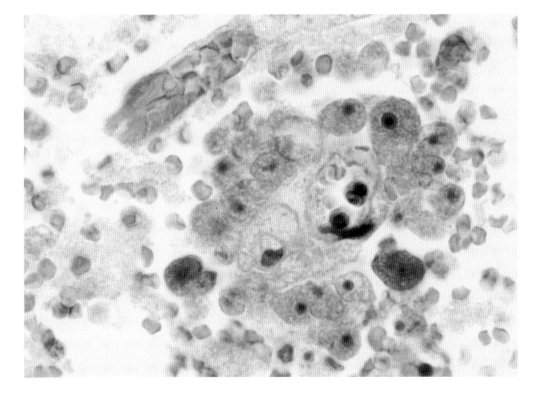

ameba of the genus *Naegleria* has affected at least 179 previously healthy persons; they were infected by exposure to contaminated freshwater, with entry of the parasites into the brain via the olfactory neuroepithelium. The course is fulminant, with involvement mainly of the olfactory bulbs and inferior frontal cortex, with death occurring after 3–7 days of illness. The gross features illustrated in this case are typical of granulomatous amebic encephalitis. The cerebral hemispheres are swollen and edematous, and evidence of increased intracranial pressure is often present. Coronal sections show necrotic, hemorrhagic lesions that resemble hemorrhagic infarcts.

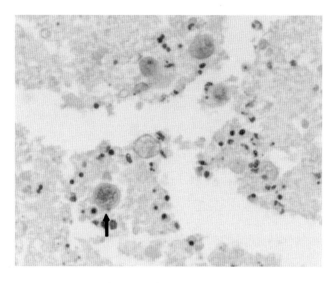

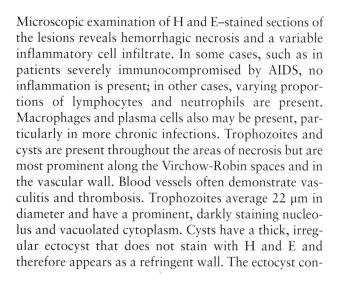

FIGURE 6-42. Another area of the section shown in Figure 6-40 reveals amebae, including a shrunken cyst (*arrow*; hematoxylin and eosin stain; original magnification, ×100).

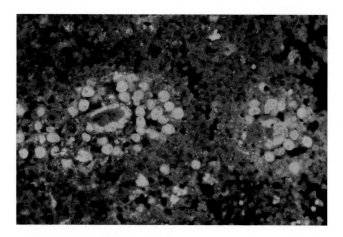

FIGURE 6-43. Photomicrograph of brain from this patient stained immunohistochemically with antibodies specific for *Balamuthia mandrillaris* demonstrates numerous protozoa in a perivascular distribution (specific anti–*B. mandrillaris* indirect immunofluorescence; magnification, ×250; courtesy of Dr. G. Visvesvara).

Microscopic examination of H and E–stained sections of the lesions reveals hemorrhagic necrosis and a variable inflammatory cell infiltrate. In some cases, such as in patients severely immunocompromised by AIDS, no inflammation is present; in other cases, varying proportions of lymphocytes and neutrophils are present. Macrophages and plasma cells also may be present, particularly in more chronic infections. Trophozoites and cysts are present throughout the areas of necrosis but are most prominent along the Virchow-Robin spaces and in the vascular wall. Blood vessels often demonstrate vasculitis and thrombosis. Trophozoites average 22 µm in diameter and have a prominent, darkly staining nucleolus and vacuolated cytoplasm. Cysts have a thick, irregular ectocyst that does not stain with H and E and therefore appears as a refringent wall. The ectocyst con-

tains an endocyst that typically is shrunken and appears as a dark mass.

Skin involvement has often been considered as a portal of entry, but might represent hematogenous spread as occurs to the brain and at times other organs. Cutaneous lesions may appear as nodules that break down and drain. *Acanthamoeba* may represent normal nasopharyngeal flora or may colonize the throat and sinuses, overgrow, and possibly cause symptoms.

Although generally an autopsy diagnosis, *Acanthamoeba* can be cultivated from CSF on non-nutrient agar with *E. coli*.

Diagnosis

Granulomatous amebic encephalitis.

CYSTIC MASS LESION OF THE FRONTAL LOBE

Clinical History

A 42-year-old woman was referred to a neurology clinic for evaluation of "abnormal behavior," which had begun approximately 3 months after returning from a 2-year period of travel in Southeast Asia. Her physical examination was noncontributory. A cranial CT scan revealed a mass lesion in the right frontal lobe. Open brain biopsy was performed, and a 2-cm fragment of brain tissue was removed.

Pathologic Findings

On cut section, the specimen consisted of a cyst filled with thick fluid and containing a white, amorphous fragment of tissue (Figure 6-44). Microscopic examination of an H and E–stained section of the amorphous tissue within the cyst revealed the inverted scolex of *Cysticercus cellulosae* (Figure 6-45) with two suction plates, a hooklet-armed rostellum, and a portion of the gastrodermis. Minimal inflammation was present in the surrounding tissue. Examination of the section under higher-power magnification revealed the characteristic round to oval calcareous corpuscles (Figure 6-46).

Differential Diagnoses

On gross examination, a viable cysticercus resembles a cyst or congenital cyst. Histologic examination, however, confirms the diagnosis of cysticercosis—in this case, infection with *C. cellulosae* (the cysticercus of the tapeworm *Taenia solium*), which is the most common cysticercus occurring in humans. The cysticercus of other species, however, such as *Taenia crassiceps* (a parasite of the red fox) and *Taenia saginata* (a parasite of cows), has rarely been reported in humans. The cysticercus of *T. crassiceps* (*Cysticercus longicollis*) is identified based on the rostel-

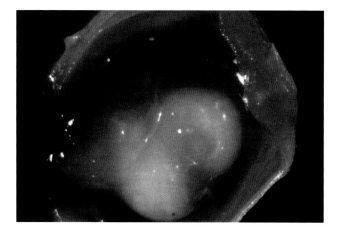

FIGURE 6-44. An opened cyst of *Cysticercus cellulosae* that was removed from the brain reveals the viable white scolex in clear cyst fluid. (Courtesy of Dr. William Luer.)

FIGURE 6-45. Section of the cystic lesion removed from the frontal lobe shows the scolex of *Cysticercus cellulosae* (hematoxylin and eosin stain; original magnification, ×25). The scolex is characterized by a tegument; the presence of suckers (*arrowhead*), which appear as a round to oval mass of smooth muscle cells; and the rostellum, which contains the hooklets (*arrow*). The rest of the helminth's mesenchyme is composed of lax fibers and connective tissue with many calcareous corpuscles, which are seen on the left side of the figure.

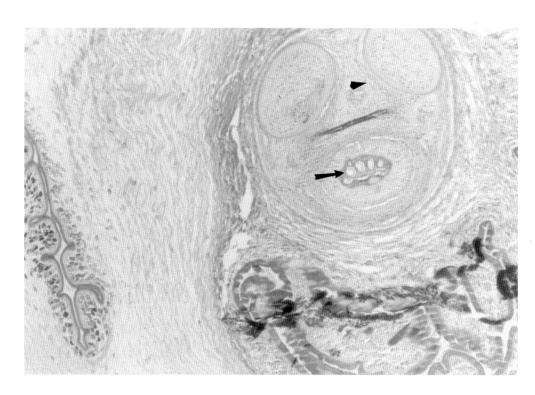

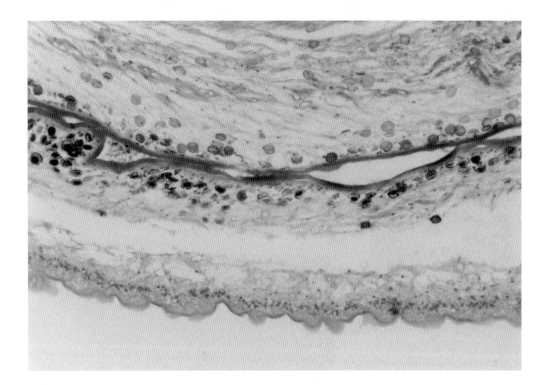

FIGURE 6-46. Higher-power magnification of the section illustrated in Figure 6-45 shows the external cuticular layer and multiple, oval calcareous corpuscles within the inner parenchymal layer (hematoxylin and eosin stain; original magnification, ×50).

lar hooklets and its asexual reproduction by exogenous and occasionally endogenous budding, typically at the opposite pole of the scolex. Differentiation of *Cysticercus bovis* (the cysticercus of *T. saginata*) from *C. cellulosae* is difficult. Hooklets are absent from the rostellum of *C. bovis*, but to demonstrate the absence of hooklets, the entire specimen must be sectioned serially. Additionally, *C. cellulosae* may not always contain hooklets.

Comment

Viable *C. cellulosae* have a characteristic histologic appearance. The bladder wall, which measures up to 80 µm thick, is composed of several layers. The outer layer consists of microvilli or hairlike processes that measure up to 6 µm long and are supported by a dense layer approximately 1 µm thick. Beneath the dense layer are the cells of the tegument, which have darkly staining nuclei and minimal cytoplasm. Between these nuclei are loosely arranged muscle fibers. The remainder of the bladder wall consists of loose connective tissue and fibers, with excretory ducts.

The scolex of *C. cellulosae* is a solid mass of mesenchymatous tissue characterized by the presence of suckers, which contain round-to-oval smooth muscle cells, and the rostellum, with its hooklets. The rest of the scolex is composed of connective tissue and the calcare-

ous corpuscles, which are an important histologic marker of larval or adult cestode tissue. The calcareous corpuscles are round to oval bodies generally less than 15 µm in diameter that usually are formed of concentric layers of calcium and phosphate; therefore, they stain positively with the von Kossa stain. The scolex and neck are covered by a tegument with a thick (up to 15 µm) external layer that stains deep red with H and E.

Cysticerci are often nonviable. In such cases, the structures described are in various stages of degeneration and disintegration; it is important to search for recognizable calcareous corpuscles, hooklets, or both. When extensive necrosis or complete resorption of the cysticercus occurs, however, diagnosis may be impossible. In contrast to viable cysticerci, dead cysticerci elicit a marked inflammatory reaction in the surrounding host tissue. In specimens containing a cysticercus that has recently died, neutrophils predominate; in cases where the cysticercus has been dead for a longer period, neutrophils are admixed with lymphocytes and macrophages. With extensive degeneration of the cysticercus, granulation tissue, fibrosis, and occasionally Charcot-Leyden crystals also are present.

Diagnosis

Cerebral cysticercosis.

PROGRESSIVE NEUROLOGIC IMPAIRMENT IN A PATIENT WITH ACQUIRED IMMUNODEFICIENCY SYNDROME

Clinical History

A 39-year-old man with AIDS had a cryptococcal infection for which he was receiving amphotericin B and fluconazole. His history included disseminated *M. avium* complex infection. When he developed altered mental status and became semicomatose, he was admitted to a hospital. He was unable to follow commands and was responsive only to painful stimuli. Laboratory evaluation revealed only mild leukocytosis (11,200 per μl) and a slightly decreased platelet count (146,000 per μl). He died after 1 week of intensive care and multiple antimicrobial agents.

Pathologic Findings

At necropsy, the main lesions were in the brain and lungs. Severe hemorrhagic *P. aeruginosa* bronchopneumonia and disseminated cryptococcal infection involving the pulmonary interstitium, peribronchial lymph nodes, meninges, and pituitary gland were present. The most important unexpected diagnosis was a multifocal primary large cell lymphoma involving the right thalamus, right visual cortex of the occipital lobe, and right lateral temporal lobe of the brain (Figure 6-47). Immunohistochemical staining for CD20 documented that the lymphoma was of B-lymphocyte phenotype. In situ hybridization demonstrated the presence of Epstein-Barr viral nucleic acid sequences (EBER 1) in the malignant lymphocytes.

Differential Diagnoses

Differential diagnoses included cryptococcal meningitis, tuberculous meningitis, progressive multifocal leukoencephalopathy, HIV-associated dementia, toxoplasmosis, and primary lymphoma of the brain.

Comment

Disease of the CNS, including HIV-associated encephalopathy, toxoplasmosis, cryptococcal meningitis, and progressive multifocal leukoencephalopathy (in decreasing order of frequency), affects a large fraction of AIDS patients. Approximately 1% of AIDS patients suffer from each of

the following: CNS lymphoma, tuberculous meningitis, and neurosyphilis. Lymphomas occur in 6% or more of AIDS patients, usually late in the course, a 120-fold greater incidence than in the general population. B-cell phenotypes,

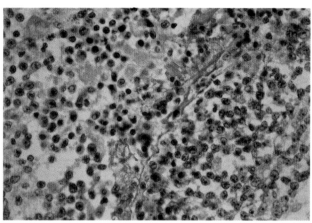

A

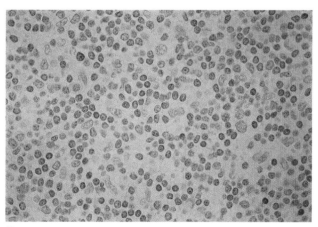

B

FIGURE 6-47. (**A**) Photomicrograph of a primary lymphoma of the central nervous system in the brain of a patient with acquired immunodeficiency syndrome. The lymphocytes show strong in situ hybridization with a probe that is specific for Epstein-Barr virus. (**B**) Lymphocytes appear negative in the control slide (high-power magnification).

either monoclonal or oligoclonal, are observed in approximately 90% of lymphomas occuring in AIDS patients. The types that occur in these patients are immunoblastic lymphoma (60%), Burkett's small noncleaved cell lymphoma (20%), and primary CNS lymphoma (20%). Although only one-half of these Burkett lymphomas contain Epstein-Barr viral DNA, most of the primary brain lymphomas do. Radiologically, CNS lymphoma and toxoplasmosis are difficult to distinguish, as both cause single or multiple ring-enhancing lesions. Periventricular spread, in which malignant lymphocytes diffusely involve the cerebral parenchyma and accumulate around the blood vessels, is a frequent occurrence in primary CNS lymphoma.

Diagnosis

Primary lymphoma of the CNS and cryptococcal meningitis.

RECOMMENDED READING

Bacterial Meningitis

Gray LD, Fedorko DP. Laboratory diagnosis of bacterial meningitis. Clin Microbiol Rev 1992;5:130.

Schuchat A, Robinson K, Wenger JD, et al. Bacterial meningitis in the United States in 1995. N Engl J Med 1997;337:970.

Tunkel AR, Scheld WM. Pathogenesis and pathophysiology of bacterial meningitis. Clin Microbiol Rev 1993;6:118.

Cryptococcus neoformans

Mitchell TG, Perfect JR. Cryptococcosis in the era of AIDS—100 years after the discovery of *Cryptococcus neoformans*. Clin Microbiol Rev 1995;8:515.

Powderly WG. Cryptococcal meningitis and AIDS. Clin Infect Dis 1993;17:837.

Mycobacteria

Kent SJ, Crowe SM, Yung A, et al. Tuberculous meningitis: a 30-year review. Clin Infect Dis 1993;17:987.

Viral Encephalitis

Deresiewicz RL, Thaler SJ, Hsu L, Zamani AA. Clinical and neuroradiographic manifestations of eastern equine encephalitis. N Engl J Med 1997;336:1867.

Whitley RJ. Viral encephalitis. N Engl J Med 1990;323:242.

Herpes Simplex Virus

Lakeman FD, Whitley RJ. Diagnosis of herpes simplex encephalitis: application of polymerase chain reaction to cerebrospinal fluid from brain-biopsied patients and correlation with disease. J Infect Dis 1995;171:857.

Whitley RJ, Lakeman F. Herpes simplex virus infections of the central nervous system: therapeutic and diagnostic considerations. Clin Infect Dis 1995;20:414.

Rabies

Noah DL, Drenzek CL, Smith JS, et al. Epidemiology of human rabies in the United States, 1980 to 1996. Ann Intern Med 1998;128:922.

Tepsumethanon V, Lumlertdacha B, Mitmoonpitak C, et al. Fluorescent antibody test for rabies: prospective study of 8,987 brains. Clin Infect Dis 1997;25:1459.

Malaria

Aikawa M, Iseki M, Barnwell JW, et al. The pathology of human cerebral malaria. Am J Trop Med Hyg 1990;43:30.

Riganti M, Pongponratn E, Tegoshi T, et al. Human cerebral malaria in Thailand: a clinico-pathologic correlation. Immunol Lett 1990;25:199.

Turner GD, Morrison H, Jones M, et al. An immunohistochemical study of the pathology of fatal malaria. Evidence for widespread endothelial activation and a potential role of intercellular adhesion molecule-1 in cerebral sequestration. Am J Pathol 1994;145:1057.

Progressive Multifocal Leukoencephalopathy

Berger JR, Kaszovitz B, Post MJD, Dickinson G. Progressive multifocal leukoencephalopathy associated with human immunodeficiency virus infection. Ann Intern Med 1987;107:78.

Fong IW, Toma E. The natural history of progressive multifocal leukoencephalopathy in patients with AIDS. Clin Infect Dis 1995;20:1305.

Major EO, Amemiya K, Tornatore CS, et al. Pathogenesis and molecular biology of progressive multifocal leukoencephalopathy, the JC virus-induced demyelinating disease of the human brain. Clin Microbiol Rev 1992;5:49.

Richardson EP Jr, Webster HF. Progressive multifocal leukoencephalopathy: its pathological features. Prog Clin Biol Res 1983;105:191.

Cytomegalovirus

Arribas JR, Storch GA, Clifford DB, Tselis AC. Cytomegalovirus encephalitis. Ann Intern Med 1996;125:577.

Kalayjian RC, Cohen ML, Bonomo RA, Flanigan TP. Cytomegalovirus ventriculoencephalitis in AIDS. A syndrome with distinct clinical and pathologic features. Medicine 1993;72:67.

McCutchan JA. Cytomegalovirus infections of the nervous system in patients with AIDS. Clin Infect Dis 1995;20:747.

Zygomycetes

Radner AB, Witt MD, Edwards JE Jr. Acute invasive rhinocerebral zygomycosis in an otherwise healthy patient: case report and review. Clin Infect Dis 1995;20:163.

Sugar AM. Mucormycosis. Clin Infect Dis 1992;14(suppl 1):S126.

Toxoplasma gondii

Bertoli F, Espino M, Arosemena JR, et al. A spectrum in the pathology of toxoplasmosis in patients with acquired immunodeficiency syndrome. Arch Pathol Lab Med 1995;119:214.

Luft BJ, Hafner R, Korzun AH, et al. Toxoplasmic encephalitis in patients with the acquired immunodeficiency syndrome. N Engl J Med 1993;329:995.

Luft BJ, Remington JS. Toxoplasmic encephalitis in AIDS. J Infect Dis 1988;157:1.

Porter SB, Sande MA. Toxoplasmosis of the central nervous system in the acquired immunodeficiency syndrome. N Engl J Med 1992;327:1643.

Acanthamoeba and *Balamuthia*

Denney CF, Iragui VJ, Uber-Zak LD, et al. Amebic meningoencephalitis caused by *Balamuthia mandrillaris*: case report and review. Clin Infect Dis 1997;25:1354.

Gardner HAR, Martinez AJ, Visvesvara GS, Sotrel A. Granulomatous amebic encephalitis in an AIDS patient. Neurology 1991;41:1993.

Ofori-Kwakye SK, Sidebottom DG, Herbert J, et al. Granulomatous brain tumor caused by *Acanthamoeba*. J Neurosurg 1986;64:505.

Cysticercosis

Bandres JC, White AC Jr, Samo T, et al. Extraparenchymal neurocysticercosis: report of five cases and review of management. Clin Infect Dis 1992;15:799.

White AC Jr. Neurocysticercosis: a major cause of neurological disease worldwide. Clin Infect Dis 1997; 24:101.

Brain Abscess

Chun CH, Johnson JD, Hofstetter M. Brain abscess. A study of 45 consecutive cases. Medicine 1986;65:415.

Mathisen GE, Johnson JP. Brain abscess. Clin Infect Dis 1997;25:763.

Epstein-Barr Virus Lymphoma

Chang KL, Flaris N, Hickey WF, et al. Brain lymphomas of immunocompetent and immunocompromised patients: study of the association with Epstein-Barr virus. Mod Pathol 1993;6:427.

Flinn IW, Ambinder RF. AIDS primary central nervous system lymphoma. Curr Opin Oncol 1996;6:373.

Guterman KSA, Hair LS, Morgello S. Epstein-Barr virus and AIDS-related primary central nervous system lymphoma. Clin Neuropathol 1996;15:79.

MacMahon EME, Glass JD, Hayward SD, et al. Epstein-Barr virus in AIDS-related primary central nervous system lymphoma. Lancet 1991;338:969.

O'Neill BP, Illig JJ. Primary central nervous system lymphoma. Mayo Clin Proc 1989;64:1005.

Infections of the Genitourinary System

Infections of the urinary tract and the female and male genitalia comprise a diverse group of diseases. Microorganisms enter via the urethral, vaginal, and hematogenous routes and cause infections localized at the portal of entry (e.g., genital ulcers of chancroid or trichomoniasis) or spread via the lymphatic vessels (e.g., lymphogranuloma venereum or granuloma inguinale), nerves (e.g., herpes simplex virus [HSV] type 2), urethra (e.g., cystitis, prostatitis, or epididymitis), or vagina (e.g., vaginitis, cervicitis, endometritis, chorioamnionitis, or salpingitis). The infectious agents are usually introduced into the genitourinary tract by sexual contact with an infected partner or by colonization of adjacent surfaces (e.g., urethral meatus) by fecal flora.

In most cases of genitourinary infection, the surgical pathologist is not the physician who establishes the etiologic diagnosis. The anatomic pathology of the urinary tract is usually assessed by computerized tomographic scanning, intravenous pyelography, or cystoscopy. The gross appearance of genital lesions is observed by the gynecologist, urologist, dermatologist, or primary care physician, and a careful description or photograph is seldom provided to the pathologist. Cytopathologists frequently diagnose herpesvirus infections, trichomoniasis, bacterial vaginosis, and candidiasis. Microscopic examination of urine assists in the diagnosis of cystitis and pyelonephritis, and examination of genital ulcer material by darkfield method assists in the diagnosis of primary syphilis. Microscopic examination of potassium hydroxide–digested material helps in the identification of Candida, dermatophytes, and pubic lice and the mites or larvae of scabies. Examination of material stained by Gram stain can detect gonococci, *Haemophilus ducreyi* (chancroid), and intracytoplasmic *Calymmatobacterium granulomatis* (donovanosis or granuloma inguinale), but immunocytochemical staining is usually necessary for specific identification. For detection and identification of *Chlamydia trachomatis* by microscopy, immunofluorescence staining is most effective.

Nevertheless, the vast majority of genitourinary infections are diagnosed by microbiological methods, including culture of urine and urethral and cervical exudates. The laboratory procedures are quite diverse, depending on whether the agent sought is a virus, chlamydia, aerobic or anaerobic bacterium, mycobacterium, mycoplasma, fungus, or protozoon. Infections with organisms that cannot be cultivated, such as *Treponema pallidium*, are diagnosed more often by serology than by morphologic detection.

Thus, the potential roles of the pathologist in the diagnosis of infectious diseases of the genitourinary tract are broad, and microscopic interpretation of organisms and cytopathologically altered cells in smears is as important as tissue changes in the cervix, endometrium, and other biopsies or resected organs. The suggestion of a particular infectious etiology (e.g., chlamydia in patients with plasma cells in the endometrium) may lead to clinical pursuit of the etiologic diagnosis by culture or serology.

FEVER AND SEVERE BACK PAIN
OF TWO WEEKS' DURATION

Clinical History

A 46-year-old woman was admitted to the hospital for evaluation of a 2-week history of fever, decreased appetite, and weight loss of approximately 12 pounds. Additional complaints included severe, off-and-on back pain for approximately 1 month, dysphagia, productive cough, weakness, and fatigue. On physical examination, she was thin and appeared depressed. Her blood pressure was 102/48 mm Hg, her pulse was 104 beats per minute, and her respirations were 18 breaths per minute. Examination of the oral cavity revealed gingivitis, thick yellow drainage in the posterior pharynx, and white deposits on her tongue consistent with thrush. On auscultation of the chest, there were diffuse rhonchi and decreased breath sounds bilaterally. Her abdomen was soft but tender, particularly in the right upper quadrant. The remainder of the examination was within normal limits.

Pertinent abnormal laboratory test results were as follows: hemoglobin, 8.1 g/dl; white blood cell count, 13,300 cells per μl; sodium, 121 mmol/liter; blood urea nitrogen, 168 mg/dl; creatinine, 6.43 mg/dl; and calcium, 8.2 mg/dl. Her urine was cloudy and contained red and white blood cells and bacteria but was negative for glucose and ketones. Results of her chest radiograph were normal. Blood and urine were collected for bacterial culture, and empiric antimicrobial therapy was initiated, but she did

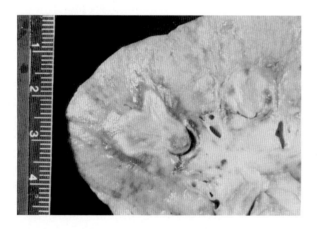

FIGURE 7-1. Photograph of the cut surface of a kidney from a patient with acute pyelonephritis and papillary necrosis shows small cortical abscesses and blunting, hemorrhage, and necrosis of the papillae.

not respond clinically. On the third hospital day, she developed disseminated intravascular coagulation and pulmonary edema. Despite intensive supportive care, she died the following day.

Pathologic Findings

At autopsy, the predominant findings were in the kidneys. The renal capsules stripped with difficulty, revealing a brown, soft, granular cortical surface with several microabscesses. When the kidneys were bisected, extensive renal papillary necrosis was evident and opaque, tan streaks extended from the medulla into the cortex (Figure 7-1). The ureters and urinary bladder were normal. Histopathologic examination of sections of the kidney showed marked acute and chronic tubulointerstitial inflammation with papillary necrosis (Figures 7-2 and 7-3), focal hemorrhage, microabscess formation, and botryomycosis (Figures 7-4 and 7-5). A Brown-Hopps stain of a section of the area of inflammation demonstrated numerous gram-negative bacilli (Figure 7-6) and aggregates of pointed crystals in the medullary regions. In addition to the renal abnormalities, abscesses were present throughout the pancreas and in the pericardium and anterior mediastinum.

Microbiology

Two days after admission, the microbiology laboratory reported that both blood and urine cultures had yielded growth of *Escherichia coli*.

Comment

Acute pyelonephritis, also called *acute infectious interstitial nephritis*, is an acute suppurative inflammation of the kidney caused by bacterial infection. Most cases are associated with predisposing conditions, including urinary tract obstruction, instrumentation of the urinary tract, pregnancy, preexisting renal lesions that have caused scarring and obstruction, diabetes mellitus, immunosuppression, and immunodeficiency. Gram-negative bacilli that are normal flora of the lower gastrointestinal tract are responsible for the majority of urinary tract infections. The most common pathogen is *E. coli*, followed by *Proteus* species, *Klebsiella* species, and *Enterobacter* species. Morphologically, the hallmarks of acute

FIGURE 7-2. Section of the kidney illustrated in Figure 7-1 shows tubules containing polymorphonuclear leukocytes and foci of liquefactive necrosis (hematoxylin and eosin stain; original magnification, ×100).

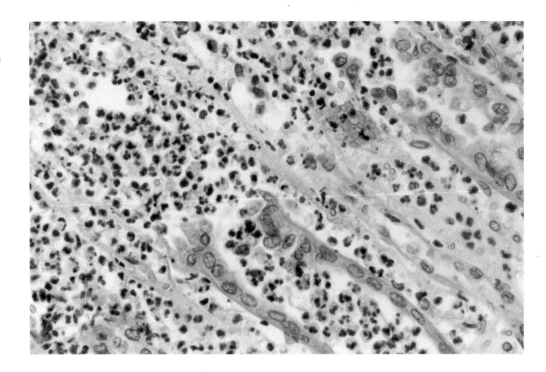

FIGURE 7-3. Section of a renal papilla of the kidney illustrated in Figure 7-1 reveals marked necrosis and focal aggregates of inflammatory cells (hematoxylin and eosin stain; original magnification, ×25).

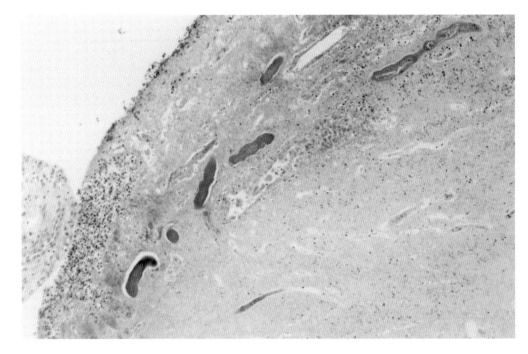

pyelonephritis are patchy interstitial and intratubular suppurative inflammation, which may occur as focal abscesses in one or both kidneys or as large, wedge-shaped areas of coalescent suppuration. Medullary abscesses are associated with ascending infection, whereas abscesses confined to the cortices are a result of

hematogenous seeding. Infection may spread to the kidney via the ascending route with intrarenal reflux from the calyces or via the hematogenous route, as illustrated in Figures 7-7, 7-8, and 7-9. Early in the infection, the infiltrate of neutrophils involves only the interstitial tissue, but it soon spreads to the tubules, producing an

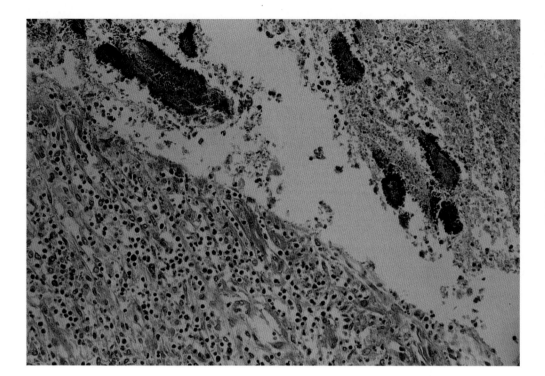

FIGURE 7-4. Section of the kidney illustrated in Figure 7-1 shows necrosis of a renal papilla and features of a botryomycotic abscess (i.e., granules, representing colonies of bacteria, surrounded by radiating clublike structures; hematoxylin and eosin stain; original magnification, ×50).

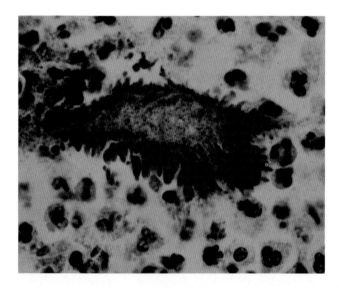

FIGURE 7-5. Higher-power magnification of a granule shown in Figure 7-4 demonstrates the classic Splendore-Hoeppli reaction (i.e., a necrotic cluster of bacteria is surrounded by eosinophilic to amphophilic, clublike structures, presumably composed of immunoglobulins; hematoxylin and eosin stain; original magnification, ×250).

abscess. Aggregates of neutrophils often extend along the involved nephron into the collecting tubules. The glomeruli usually are resistant to the infection, except in cases of severe necrosis and with fungal infections.

Possible complications of acute pyelonephritis include pyonephrosis, which occurs with complete or nearly complete obstruction of the urinary tract, especially obstructions that are high, perinephric abscess (in which the suppurative inflammatory process extends through the renal capsule into the perinephric tissue) and papillary necrosis, as were present in this case. Papillary necrosis occurs predominantly in persons with diabetes mellitus or obstruction of the urinary tract. It usually is bilateral but may be unilateral, and in the involved kidney, one or all of the pyramids may be affected. Morphologically, the tips or distal two-thirds of the pyramids manifest ischemic coagulative necrosis with preservation of the outlines of the tubules and a neutrophilic infiltrate at the junctions between viable and necrotic tissue.

Botryomycosis is an inflammatory process caused by bacteria in which one or more abscesses contain microcolonies of bacteria that appear as basophilic granules (see Figure 7-5) in an acellular matrix that is

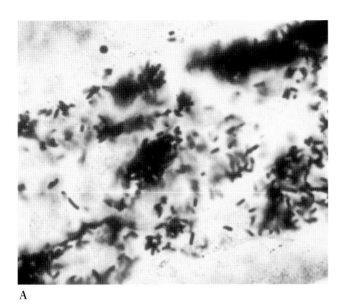

A

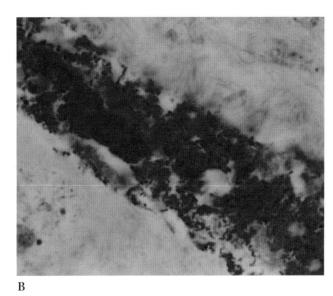

B

FIGURE 7-6. (A) Section of the kidney illustrated in Figure 7-1 and stained with a silver impregnation method shows numerous rod-shaped bacteria within a tubule (Steiner stain; original magnification, ×250). (B) A tissue Gram stain of this same section shows that the bacteria are gram-negative bacilli (Brown-Hopps stain; original magnification, ×250).

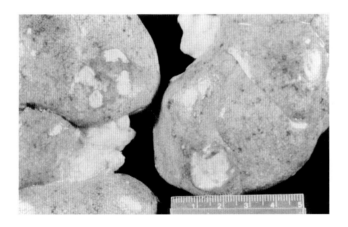

FIGURE 7-7. Photograph of kidneys from a patient with *Staphylococcus aureus* sepsis illustrates several cortical abscesses.

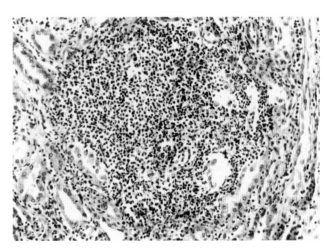

FIGURE 7-8. Section of the kidney illustrated in Figure 7-7 shows a microabscess, characterized by an aggregate of neutrophils and histiocytes, with intact renal tubules at the abscess periphery (hematoxylin and eosin stain; original magnification, ×50).

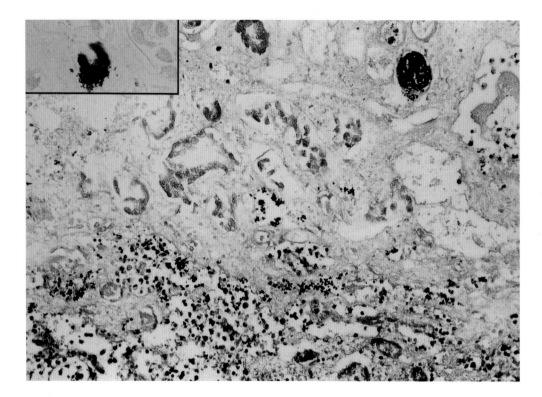

FIGURE 7-9. Section of the kidney illustrated in Figure 7-7 shows remnants of necrotic tubules, degenerating acute inflammatory cells, and an aggregate of bacteria (hematoxylin and eosin stain; original magnification, ×50). *Inset*: Staining the section with a tissue Gram stain demonstrates that the bacteria are gram-positive cocci, as expected in a patient with *Staphylococcus aureus* sepsis (Brown-Brenn stain; original magnification, ×100).

rich in immunoglobulins. These structures resemble actinomycotic granules from which they must be distinguished. Botryomycotic abscesses occur most frequently in deep, subcutaneous tissue; other sites include the liver, kidneys, lung, prostate, and lymph nodes. *Staphylococcus aureus* is the bacterium most commonly isolated from botryomycotic abscesses, but other bacteria, such as *E. coli* and *Pseudomonas aeruginosa*, have also been implicated.

Diagnosis

Acute pyelonephritis with papillary necrosis and botryomycosis caused by infection with *E. coli*.

GENITAL ULCERS

Clinical History

An 18-year-old woman presented to her family physician with complaints of vulvar pain and burning and vaginal discharge. Examination of the vulva revealed three variably sized areas of ulceration, the largest measuring 3 cm in maximal diameter (Figure 7-10). Scrapings collected from the edge of one ulcer were submitted for cytologic examination and for viral culture, and a biopsy was submitted for histologic studies.

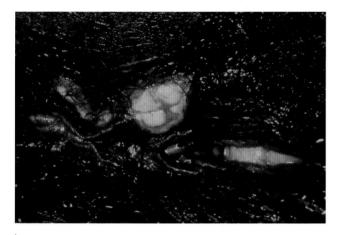

FIGURE 7-10. Photograph illustrates vulvar ulcerations caused by infection with herpes simplex virus. (Courtesy of Dr. Tung Dinh.)

Pathologic Findings

The cytologic preparation showed cells demonstrating characteristic cytopathic effects of infection with HSV (i.e., multinucleate giant epithelial cells, closely packed nuclei that tended to indent or mold the adjacent nucleus, nuclear chromatin that had marginated to the nuclear periphery, and a ground-glass appearance of the nuclei; Figure 7-11). Sections of the lesion showed ulceration of the surface and cells with cytopathic effects consistent with HSV infection (Figure 7-12).

Differential Diagnoses

Infectious causes of genital ulcers include HSV type 2, *T. pallidum*, *H. ducreyi*, *C. trachomatis*, and *C. granulomatis*. They uncommonly include *Mycobacterium tuberculosis*, *Histoplasma capsulatum*, *Entamoeba histolytica*, *Neisseria gonorrhoeae*, and *Francisella tularensis*.

Microbiology

Viral culture of the ulcer scrapings yielded HSV type 2.

Comment

The most common cause of genital ulcers in the United States is HSV, followed by *T. pallidum*. Chancroid (caused by infection with *H. ducreyi*), which is diagnosed

Figure 7-11. Cytologic preparation of cells scraped from the edge of a vulvar ulcer caused by herpes simplex virus illustrates the cytopathic effects elicited by infection with this virus: a multinucleate giant cell with nuclei that are closely apposed, causing indentation or molding of the adjacent nucleus, and nuclear chromatin that has marginated to the periphery of the nucleus, resulting in a ground glass appearance (Papanicolaou stain; original magnification, ×250). Viral culture of the scrapings grew herpes simplex virus type 2.

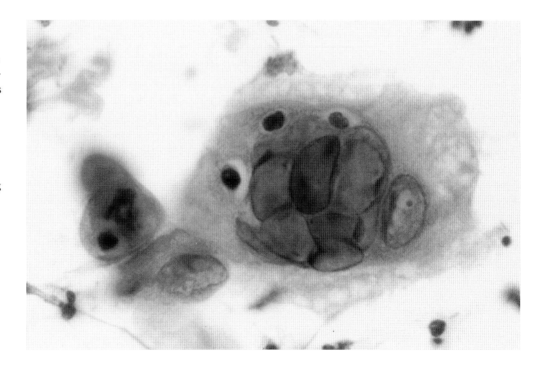

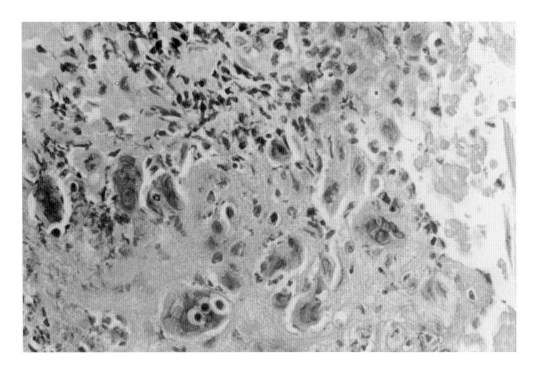

FIGURE 7-12. Section of a vulvar ulcer shows ulceration of the epithelium and several multinucleate giant cells with nuclear molding and margination of the peripheral chromatin—changes consistent with the cytopathic effects of herpes simplex virus infection (hematoxylin and eosin stain; original magnification, ×100).

in 40–90% of patients with genital ulcers in Africa and India, is becoming more common in major metropolitan areas of the United States. Lymphogranuloma venereum, caused by C. trachomatis serotypes L₁–L₃, is much more common in Africa and the Far East than in the United States. Donovanosis (i.e., granuloma inguinale), caused by infection with C. granulomatis, is endemic in India, Papua-New Guinea, the West Indies, and some parts of Africa and South America.

Clues to the etiology of genital ulcers may be provided by the physical examination. HSV typically produces multiple, painful ulcerations, generally of uniform size, in groups surrounded by an erythematous border. The classic chancre of syphilis is a solitary, nontender, indurated lesion with a clean base, but more than one ulcer, usually similar in size, is not uncommon; tenderness is present in up to 30% of patients. The ulcers of chancroid (also called soft chancre, because the edge is not indurated) are painful, usually ragged with a necrotic base, and often vary in size. Lesions of donovanosis are nontender. The edge of the ulcer is thickened, giving it a rolled appearance, and the granulation tissue at the base produces beefy red lesions that often become large, friable, ulcerated masses projecting above the skin.

Histologic examination of a biopsy of the ulcer, preferably taken from the edge of the lesion, may be useful for diagnosis. The syphilitic chancre is characterized by a subepithelial infiltrate of lymphocytes and plasma cells, concentric proliferation of the vascular endothelium, and obliterative endarteritis. Lesions of chancroid

show erosion of the epithelium, collections of neutrophils in epidermal pustules, and a perivascular mononuclear cell infiltrate and proliferating endothelial cells in the dermis. Lymphogranuloma venereum is characterized by necrotizing granulomas, similar in appearance to those caused by infection with Yersinia enterocolitica (see Chapter 3). Lesions of donovanosis show pseudoepitheliomatous hyperplasia and a marked inflammatory cell infiltrate in the dermis composed of vacuolated macrophages containing Donovan bodies (pink-staining, rod-shaped bacteria), plasma cells, some neutrophils, and few (if any) lymphocytes (Figures 7-13 and 7-14).

The diagnosis of genital HSV may be determined by direct examination of a smear of material scraped or aspirated from the edge of the lesion. The smear should be stained with the Wright, Giemsa, or Papanicolaou stain for detection of cells demonstrating the cytopathic effects of HSV infection, as illustrated in this case. These morphologic changes, however, are not pathognomonic of HSV; infection with varicella-zoster virus (VZV) produces identical cytopathic effects, but VZV genital infection is much less common than HSV. Additionally, this technique provides a diagnosis in less than half of culture-proven cases. Immunohistochemical and immunocytochemical studies, such as staining a smear with monoclonal antibodies to HSV types 1 and 2, are more sensitive than the nonspecific stains, providing a diagnosis in about 75% of cases, and will identify the specific pathogen. Histopathologic examination of a biopsy of the lesion also may provide a diagnosis of HSV or VZV, but as with smears, the cytopathic changes of HSV cannot be distinguished from those of VZV. Viral culture is the most sensitive and specific diagnostic test. Cultures are most likely to be positive in primary, vesicular lesions and least likely to be positive after the lesion becomes crusted.

Diagnosis

Vulvar ulcers caused by HSV type 2.

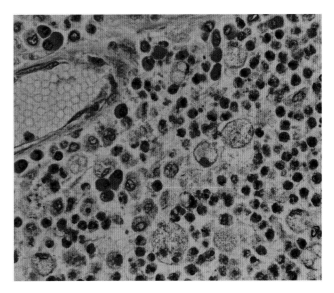

FIGURE 7-13. Section of a genital ulcer from a patient with granuloma inguinale shows an inflammatory infiltrate composed of vacuolated histiocytes, plasma cells, and neutrophils (hematoxylin and eosin stain; original magnification, ×100).

FIGURE 7-14. Higher-power magnification of the lesion illustrated in Figure 7-13 shows multiple rod-shaped bacteria in the vacuolated cytoplasm of the histiocytes (hematoxylin and eosin stain; original magnification, ×250).

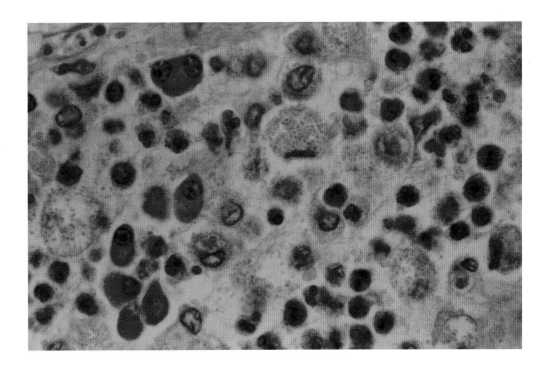

ABNORMAL GENITAL CYTOPATHOLOGY

Clinical History

A 22-year-old, single, sexually active woman visited her family physician for her annual gynecologic examination. She was healthy, with no problems relating to the genitourinary tract. Her physical examination was normal. Five days after the visit, her physician received the results of her Papanicolaou smear: epithelial cell abnormality consistent with low-grade squamous intraepithelial lesion. Based on this report, she was referred to a gynecologist for colposcopy and endocervical biopsy.

Pathologic Findings

Examination of the cervical Papanicolaou smear showed mature squamous cells illustrating the cytopathic effects typical of infection with human papillomavirus (HPV): enlarged, hyperchromatic nuclei, binucleation, and sharply circumscribed perinuclear halos (Figure 7-15). Similar changes were observed in the endocervical biopsy (Figure 7-16).

Differential Diagnoses

The main differential diagnosis of a low-grade squamous intraepithelial lesion is a nonspecific inflammatory reaction.

Comment

Papillomaviruses are small, nonenveloped DNA viruses that belong in the Papovaviridae family. These viruses are classified on the basis of the host species, the site they infect, and their degree of nucleic acid homology. HPVs that share less than 50% nucleic acid sequence homology with previously characterized types are given a new number, whereas types that share more than 50% homology are divided into subsets under the same number. More than 60 types of HPV have been identified as of 1998, of which 20 types have been isolated from the female genital tract.

Genital HPVs have been divided into three oncogenic risk groups: (1) Low risk (including mainly HPV 6 and 11), intermediate risk (including 31, 33, 35, 51, and 52), and high risk (including mainly HPV 16, 18, 45, and 56). HPV infections are often latent, and, as such, neither replicate as complete virions nor cause cytopathic changes. When latency is lost, cervical cellular changes are seen. Low-risk HPVs are typically associated with low-grade squamous intraepithelial lesions (LSIL), including condyloma accuminatum (Figures 7-17, 7-18, and 7-19), flat condyloma, and mild dysplasia/cervical intraepithelial neoplasia I. In LSIL, HPV DNA is typically episomal, and viral infection is productive, with presence of complete virions and viral cytopathic effect within the superficial cervical squamous epithelial cells; progression to invasive carcinoma is uncommon. High and intermediate-risk HPVs may be associated with

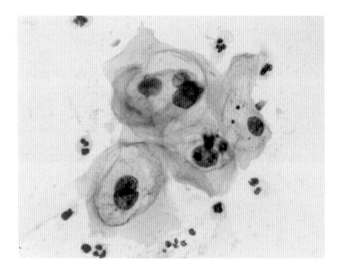

FIGURE 7-15. Cytologic preparation of cells collected from the cervix shows a cluster of mature squamous cells that illustrate the classic cytopathic effects of infection with human papillomavirus: enlarged, hyperchromatic nuclei, binucleation, and sharply circumscribed perinuclear halos (Papanicolaou stain; original magnification, ×100).

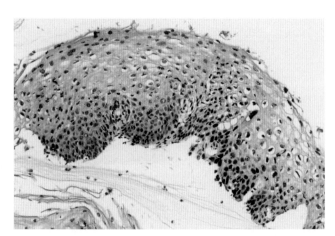

FIGURE 7-16. Section of an ectocervical biopsy shows findings characteristic of a flat condyloma/cervical intraepithelial neoplasia grade I. Nuclei of cells above the basal layer of the epithelium are moderately enlarged and hyperchromatic, and the chromatin has a smudged appearance. Several cells have prominent, well-defined perinuclear halos, and some cells are binucleate (hematoxylin and eosin stain; original magnification, ×50).

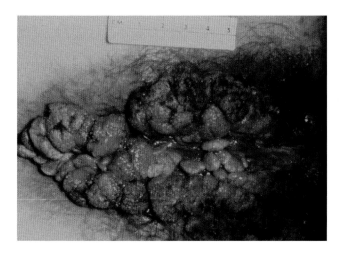

FIGURE 7-17. Photograph of a large, exophytic condyloma acuminatum involving the vulvoperineal area. (Courtesy of Dr. Ramon Sanchez.)

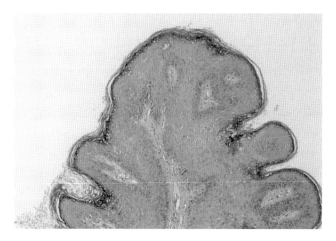

FIGURE 7-18. Section of a biopsy of the exophytic lesion illustrated in Figure 7-17 shows a squamous papillary frond with a keratinizing squamous epithelium (hematoxylin and eosin stain; original magnification, ×25).

LSIL, high-grade squamous intraepithelial lesions (HSIL), and invasive carcinoma. The high risk viral infections are those most often, but not inevitably, progressing to invasive carcinoma. Non-HPV cofactors are thought to be required for transformation to squamous cell carcinoma. Although the HPV DNA may be episomal or integrated in HSIL, in invasive carcinoma, viral DNA is typically integrated into the host cell genome. Methods available for identifying HPV type include Southern blot and slot blot hybridization, in situ hybridization, and the polymerase chain reaction.

The morphologic features of LSIL include those of a condyloma, either a flat or exophytic lesion, and mild dysplasia. Histologic characteristics of a condyloma are varying degrees of papillomatosis, acanthosis, koilocytotic atypia (i.e., squamous cells with nuclear pleomorphism, hyperchromasia, perinuclear halos, binucleate/multinucleate forms, and thickening and irregularity of the nuclear membrane), and in some cases mild nuclear atypia. Binucleate cells are an important feature of HPV infection, but they also can be found in reactive lesions that are negative for HPV.

Koilocytosis represents the classic HPV cytopathic effect, is associated with productive viral infections, and is typically seen in cells composing the superficial one-third of the cervical squamous epithelium. Nonspecific reactive change involves the more basal and intermediate cell layers and is associated with mild nuclear enlargement, presence of nucleoli, and absence of hyperchromasia. In mild dysplasia, nuclear enlargement and hyperchromasia, usually associated with koilocytosis, are found in the superficial layers, and an abnormal basal cell layer occupies no more than one-third of the height of the squamous epithelium.

HSIL includes moderate and severe dysplasia and, in the older terminology, carcinoma in situ. Koilocytosis is usually not found in HSIL, and the degree of nuclear hyperchromasia, irregularity, and mitotic activity

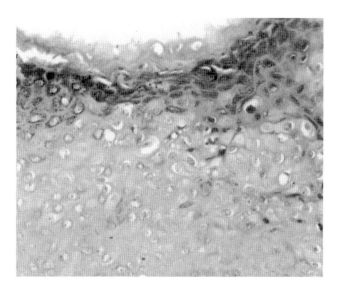

FIGURE 7-19. Higher magnification of the epithelium of the lesion illustrated in Figure 7-18 shows a granular layer, superficial keratinization, and focal koilocytosis (i.e., perinuclear vacuolation) consistent with the cytopathic effect induced by infection with human papilloma virus (hematoxylin and eosin stain; original magnification, ×100).

is higher than that seen in LSIL. In HSIL, abnormal basal-type cells and mitotic activity are present above the lower one-third of the squamous epithelium. In general, the more severe the lesion, the more superficially located is the undifferentiated layer of abnormal basal-type cells.

Diagnosis

Low-grade squamous intraepithelial lesion of the endocervix due to HPV infection.

PREMATURE RUPTURE OF MEMBRANES WITH INFECTION OF THE AMNIOTIC FLUID

Clinical History

A 35-year-old woman (gravida III, para II) at 32 weeks' gestation by dates presented to an emergency department complaining of contractions every 10–15 minutes and vomiting. She denied fever, chills, and dysuria. On physical examination, she was afebrile and had a blood pressure of 127/60 mm Hg, a pulse rate of 94 beats per minute, and a respiratory rate of 20 breaths per minute. Her cervix was dilated to 2 cm, and the fetal heart rate was 140 beats per minute. Results of the remainder of the physical examination were within normal limits. A urinalysis showed a moderate amount of blood and a few white blood cells. A diagnosis of premature rupture of membranes was made, and antibiotic prophylaxis was begun. Amniocentesis was performed, and fluid was submitted for fetal lung maturity studies, Gram stain,

and bacterial culture. The gram-stained smear showed neutrophils and many gram-positive bacilli. Labor progressed, and a male infant was delivered vaginally on day 3 of hospitalization.

Pathologic Findings

The placenta was submitted for pathologic studies. It was ovoid, measured 17 cm × 13 cm × 2.3 cm, and weighed 410 g. The umbilical cord was 15 cm in length and 1 cm in diameter. The fetal surface was dull and yellow-green, and the fetal membranes were dull and yellow-brown. Sections stained with hematoxylin and eosin (H and E) demonstrated chorioamnionitis (Figure 7-20), and the Brown-Brenn stain revealed many gram-positive bacilli (Figure 7-21).

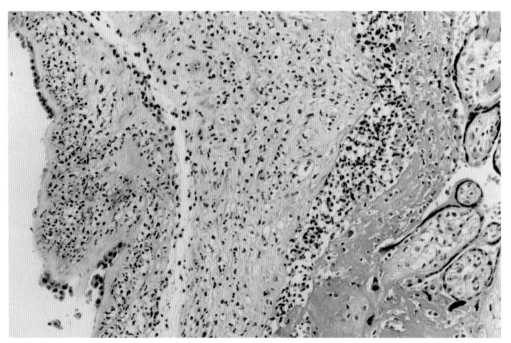

FIGURE 7-20. (A) Section of placenta from a woman with chorioamnionitis shows an acute inflammatory infiltrate, predominantly located within the amnion and chorion, with minimal superficial involvement of the villi (hematoxylin and eosin stain; original magnification, ×50).

A

Differential Diagnoses

The agents most commonly associated with chorioamnionitis are anaerobes, genital mycoplasmas, *Streptococcus agalactiae*, and *E. coli. Listeria monocytogenes*, a gram-positive bacillus, is a less frequent cause.

Microbiology

Bacterial cultures of the amniotic fluid grew *L. monocytogenes*.

Comment

Chorioamnionitis, also called *intra-amniotic infection syndrome*, is an infection of the uterus and its contents during pregnancy. It occurs in 1–2% of term patients and in as many as 25% of women with preterm labor. Most cases are ascending in origin. Infrequently, chorioamnionitis results from hematogenous transplacental spread in mothers who are bacteremic, particularly with *L. monocytogenes*, as occurred in this case.

Listeria bacteremia may occur any time during pregnancy but is most common during the third trimester. Typically, patients present with fever and chills and occasionally may complain of back pain. Physical examination generally is noncontributory. Fever and chills may resolve with or without therapy; the only clue to diagnosis may be positive results of blood culture. In some cases, the fetus is unaffected by the bacteremia, whereas in others, the infection appears to precipitate labor, which may result in premature birth of a dead or infected baby.

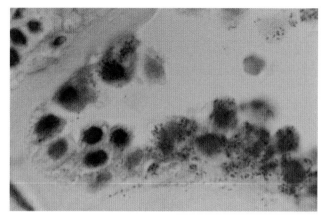

B

FIGURE 7-20. *Continued.* (**B**) Under higher-power magnification, short bacilli are visible (hematoxylin and eosin stain; original magnification, ×250).

Risk factors for ascending-route chorioamnionitis are prolonged duration of labor or rupture of membranes, multiple vaginal examinations, young age, low socioeconomic status, nulliparity, and preexisting bacterial vaginosis. The diagnosis usually is based on clinical manifestations, but amniotic fluid Gram stain and culture, increased leukocyte esterase activity, and low glucose concentration are useful in supporting the clinical impression. Clinical management includes antimicrobial treatment and delivery of the fetus.

Diagnosis

Chorioamnionitis due to *L. monocytogenes*.

FIGURE 7-21. Staining with a tissue gram stain shows that the organisms seen in the hematoxylin and eosin–stained section are short, gram-positive bacilli (culture of the amniotic fluid grew *Listeria monocytogenes*; Brown-Brenn stain; original magnification, ×250).

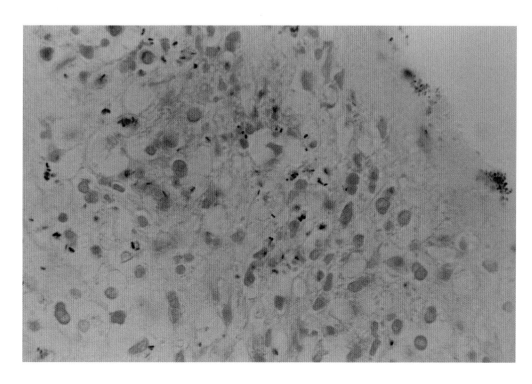

STILLBORN INFANT SECONDARY TO INTRAUTERINE INFECTION

Clinical History

A 21-year-old pregnant woman at 28 weeks' gestation by dates was admitted to the hospital for care regarding intrauterine fetal demise, which had been diagnosed during a routine prenatal clinic visit. She reported last feeling fetal movements 2 weeks earlier. Examination of a cervical smear showed organisms consistent with *Trichomonas vaginalis* and many white blood cells. A nucleic acid probe test, performed on an endocervical swab specimen, detected *C. trachomatis*, and the RPR (serologic test for syphilis) revealed antibodies at a titer of 1:640. Additional serologic tests showed that she had IgG antibodies to HSV, cytomegalovirus, rubella virus, and *Toxoplasma gondii*; tests for IgM antibodies to these same agents were negative.

The day after admission, a stillborn male infant was delivered after oxytocin (Pitocin) induction. The pla-

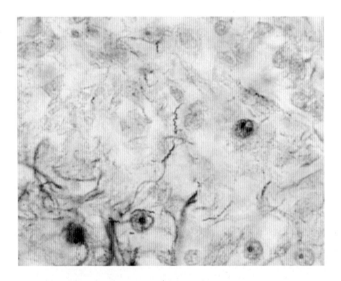

FIGURE 7-22. Section of lung from a stillborn fetus with congenital syphilis shows spirochetes with loose coils, consistent with *Treponema pallidum* (Steiner stain; original magnification, ×250).

centa could not be easily extracted manually; therefore, the mother was taken to the operating room where the placenta was removed by sharp curettage.

Pathologic Findings

The male infant was macerated, weighed 820 g (expected for gestational age, 640–1,030 g), and had a crown-rump length of 24 cm (expected, 24.2 ± 2.5 cm). With the exception of maceration, the external examination was normal. All organs were autolyzed, but their weights were within the expected ranges. The placenta weighed 150 g (expected, 170–330 g), and the umbilical cord was 37 cm in length, which was within the expected limits. The only pertinent histologic findings were in the umbilical cord and the lung. All sections of the umbilical cord showed marked autolysis and inflammatory cells (predominantly mononuclear cells with occasional neutrophils) within the vessel walls and in Wharton's jelly, most prominently near the placental disc. Focal necrosis, mineralization, and neovascularization were also present in Wharton's jelly. Tissue Gram stain of sections of the cord that showed inflammation and necrosis revealed no organisms, but the Steiner stain demonstrated numerous spirochetes. Spirochetes also were present in sections of lung (Figure 7-22).

Comment

The spectrum of congenital syphilis includes late abortion or stillbirth, as occurred in this case, and early and late congenital syphilis. The criteria for diagnosis of congenital syphilis are as follows. A confirmed case is an infant in whom *T. pallidum* spirochetes are identified by dark-field microscopy, fluorescent antibody, or other specific stains performed on specimens from lesions, placenta, umbilical cord, amniotic fluid, or autopsy material. A presumptive case is either of the following: (1) an infant whose mother had untreated or inadequately treated syphilis at delivery, regardless of the findings in the infant, or (2) an infant or child who has a reactive treponemal test for syphilis and any evidence of congenital syphilis on physical examination or long bone radiograph, a reactive cerebrospinal fluid (CSF) VDRL, an elevated CSF cell count or protein concentration without other cause, or quantitative nontreponemal serologic titers at birth that are fourfold higher than the mother's at the same time. A syphilitic stillbirth is death of a fetus that weighs more than 500 g or has a gestational age higher than 20 weeks and whose mother had untreated or inadequately treated syphilis at birth.

In cases of late abortion or stillbirth, the infected placenta usually is paler, thicker, and larger than normal. A finding regarded as characteristic of congenital syphilis is necrotizing funisitis, which was present in this case and may provide a clue to the diagnosis if syphilis had not been considered previously. Sections of the placenta typically show focal villositis, enlarged villi, and an increased amount of connective tissue around the capillaries in the stroma. Spirochetes may be found in sections of umbilical cord and placenta by staining with a silver impregnation method, such as the Steiner or Warthin-Starry method. A stillborn syphilitic fetus often is macerated, as in this case. The liver and spleen may be enlarged due to increased extramedullary hematopoiesis, and radiographs of the long bones frequently show evidence of osteochondritis and periostitis.

Diagnosis

Syphilitic stillbirth.

NONFUNCTIONING KIDNEY AFTER NEPHROLITHIASIS AND RECURRENT URINARY TRACT INFECTIONS

Clinical History

A 56-year-old woman, with a history of recurrent urinary tract infections, bilateral nephrolithiasis (including a right staghorn calculus), and a draining sinus on her right flank, was seen at a urology clinic. Other medical problems included diabetes mellitus and hypertension, both of which were controlled with medication. Several years before, she had undergone right percutaneous nephrolithotomy and placement of a nephrostomy tube in an attempt to relieve the stone burden. After removal of the tube, a sinus tract developed and drained purulent material intermittently since that time. During the current visit, a nuclear medicine renal scan was performed and showed that the right kidney was nonfunctioning. Based on this information, a right nephrectomy was performed. No specimens were submitted for microbiologic studies.

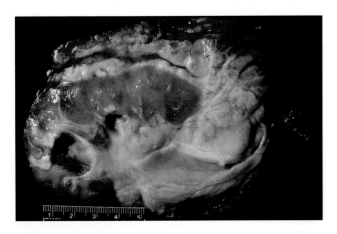

FIGURE 7-23. Photograph of a kidney removed from a patient with xanthogranulomatous pyelonephritis. (Courtesy of Dr. Eduardo Eyzaguirre.)

Pathologic Findings

The kidney weighed 220 g, measured 12.5 cm × 9 cm × 5 cm, and was surrounded by firmly adherent adipose tissue. Removal of the adipose tissue revealed a granular cortical surface that varied from red to tan. The cut surface of the renal parenchyma was pale with an poorly defined corticomedullary junction (Figure 7-23). An ill-defined, slightly nodular, yellow-tan, firm mass measuring 4.5 cm × 3 cm × 4 cm, and extending into the adjacent perirenal adipose tissue was present in the lower pole. In addition, multiple similar-appearing smaller nodules, ranging from 0.3 to 1.0 cm in diameter, were scattered throughout the parenchyma. Histologic examination of sections of the nodules showed aggregates of vacuolated macrophages admixed with mononuclear cells, fibroblasts, foci of neutrophils, and a few multinucleate giant cells (Figures 7-24, 7-25, and 7-26).

Differential Diagnoses

Based on the gross appearance of the kidney, xanthogranulomatous pyelonephritis and carcinoma should be considered in the differential diagnosis. The histologic findings, however, exclude carcinoma. The differential diagnosis of aggregates of foamy histiocytes with or without granulomas includes xanthogranulomatous pyelonephritis and mycobacterial infections, particularly *Mycobacterium avium* complex in a patient infected with human immunodeficiency virus. Fungal infection, such as with *H. capsulatum*, is also possible but is less likely.

Comment

Xanthogranulomatous pyelonephritis is an uncommon, aggressive type of chronic pyelonephritis that typically

FIGURE 7-24. Section of renal medulla from the kidney illustrated in Figure 7-23 shows an aggregate of vacuolated histiocytes admixed with mononuclear cells and fibroblasts and one residual renal tubule (hematoxylin and eosin stain; original magnification, ×25).

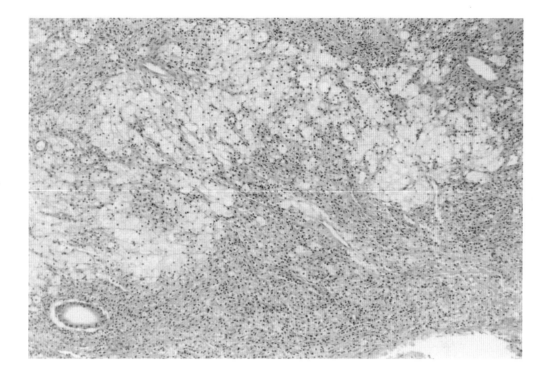

FIGURE 7-25. Higher-power magnification of the section illustrated in Figure 7-24 shows the vacuolated histiocytes, lymphocytes, fibroblasts, and collagen (Movat stain; original magnification, ×100).

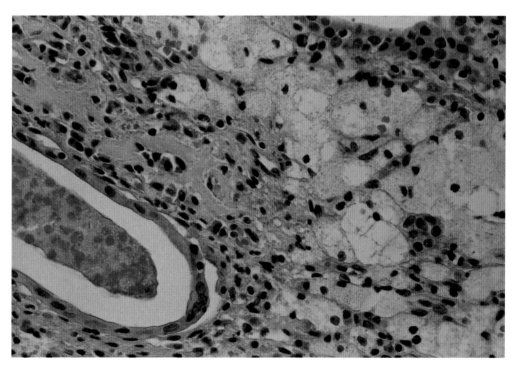

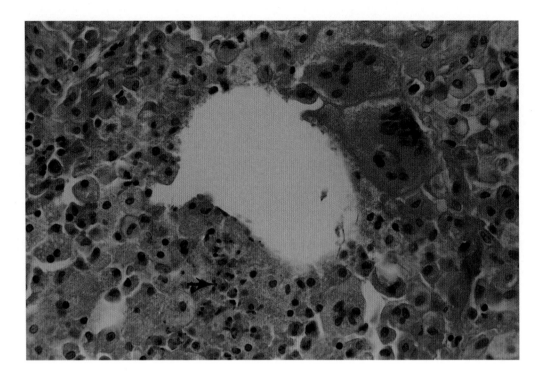

FIGURE 7-26. Another area of the section illustrated in Figure 7-24 shows a focus of neutrophils (*arrow*) and a few multinucleate giant cells (hematoxylin and eosin stain; original magnification, ×100).

affects middle-aged women but has been reported in men and women and in all age groups, including infants. The process usually involves only one kidney and can penetrate deeply into perirenal tissue and even extend to adjacent organs. Potential pathogenetic factors include ureteral obstruction (as was present in this case), infection (most commonly with *E. coli* or *Proteus mirabilis*), or both.

Xanthogranulomatous pyelonephritis evolves from a focus of pericalyceal necrosis with a predominant neutrophilic inflammatory cell reaction and a few foamy his-tiocytes through a stage characterized by sheets of foamy histiocytes, often with cholesterol crystals and granulomas, and varying numbers of lymphocytes and plasma cells. Special stains for mycobacteria and fungi are negative. Multiple stages may be present in the involved kidney, but a correlation between the histologic stage and the extent or clinical course of the disease does not seem to exist.

Diagnosis

Xanthogranulomatous pyelonephritis.

DIFFICULTY IN URINATION AND AN ENLARGED, NODULAR PROSTATE GLAND

Clinical History

A 63-year-old man presented to a family medicine clinic with a 2-week history of increasing difficulty of urination, frequency, and nocturia. Physical examination was non-contributory except for an enlarged, nodular prostate gland. Urinalysis revealed 3–6 white blood cells per low-power field and no red blood cells. Urine was collected for bacterial culture, and biopsy of the prostate gland was performed.

Pathologic Findings

Three fragments of tan tissue, each measuring 5.4 cm × 0.1 cm, were submitted for histopathologic examination. Sections of the fragments showed an inflammatory infiltrate composed of aggregates of macrophages admixed with a few lymphocytes, which in some areas completely replaced the normal prostatic architecture (Figures 7-27 and 7-28), and occasional Michaelis-Gutmann bodies (Figures 7-29 and 7-30). These histopathologic features are characteristic of malakoplakia.

Differential Diagnoses

The differential diagnoses include neoplastic and inflammatory disorders characterized by histiocytic infiltrates, such as fibrous histiocytoma and mycobacterial infections.

Microbiology

The urine culture grew more than 10^5 colonies of *E. coli*.

Comment

Malakoplakia is a rare inflammatory process, predominantly affecting the genitourinary tract, that is characterized by aggregates of histiocytes, some of which contain round, basophilic, calcific, frequently concentrically laminated structures, termed *Michaelis-Gutmann bodies*. The most common location of malakoplakia is the urinary bladder, although the process has been reported in the urethra, ureter, kidney, prostate (as in this case), epididymis, testis, vagina, broad ligament, and other pelvic organs. Malakoplakia also has been described in various

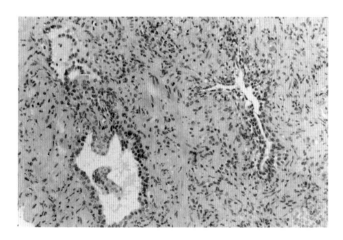

FIGURE 7-27. Section of prostate gland from a patient with malakoplakia shows a few glands and focal aggregates of histiocytes (hematoxylin and eosin stain; original magnification, ×50).

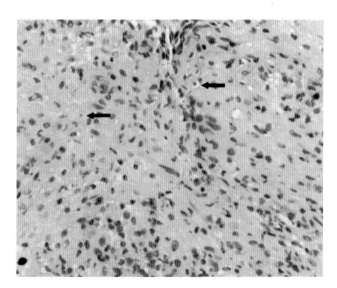

FIGURE 7-28. In other areas of the tissue obtained from the patient with malakoplakia, the normal architecture of the prostate gland has been effaced by aggregates of histiocytes, a few of which contain Michaelis-Gutmann bodies (*arrows*; hematoxylin and eosin stain; original magnification, ×50).

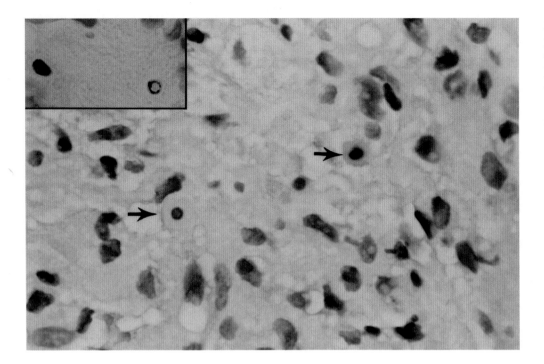

FIGURE 7-29. Higher-power magnification of the section illustrated in Figure 7-28 demonstrates the Michaelis-Gutmann bodies (*arrows*), which consist of basophilic cores surrounded by pale pink halos (hematoxylin and eosin stain; original magnification, ×250). *Inset*: Michaelis-Gutmann bodies typically contain calcium and sometimes iron salts; they therefore appear dark brown in sections stained with the von Kossa stain (von Kossa stain; original magnification, ×250).

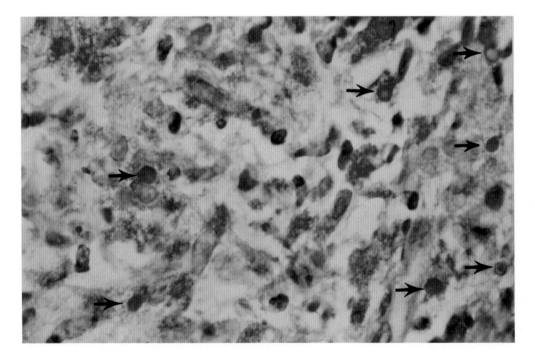

FIGURE 7-30. Staining sections with the periodic acid-Schiff stain shows positively staining granular material within histiocytes and several intracellular Michaelis-Gutmann bodies (*arrows*) in varying stages of development (periodic acid-Schiff stain; original magnification, ×250).

extrapelvic and extraurinary locations, including the gastrointestinal tract (most commonly the colon and rectum), lymph nodes, lungs, bone, adrenal glands, brain, skin, subcutaneous tissues, and conjunctiva.

Fewer than 20 cases of malakoplakia of the prostate have been reported. The age of the patients at diagnosis ranged from 49 to 85 years (mean, 64.5 years). More than half of the patients presented with obstructive lower urinary tract symptoms, as this patient did. In most cases, malakoplakia involved the prostate gland only; in a few cases, the urinary bladder also was affected; in one patient, the testis, kidney, retroperitoneum, and prostate were involved. In all cases in which bacterial cultures of urine were performed, including this patient, *E. coli* was recovered in significant numbers.

Diagnosis

Malakoplakia of the prostate gland.

RECOMMENDED READING
General

Centers for Disease Control and Prevention. 1998 Guidelines for treatment of sexually transmitted diseases. MMWR Morb Mortal Wkly Rep 1998;47:1.

Genital Ulcers

DiCarlo RP, Martin DH. The clinical diagnosis of genital ulcer disease in men. Clin Infect Dis 1997;25:292.

Hart G. Donovanosis. Clin Infect Dis 1997;25:24.

Leiman G, Markowitz S, Margolius KA. Cytologic detection of cervical granuloma inguinale. Diagn Cytopathol 1986;2:138.

Richens J. The diagnosis and treatment of donovanosis (granuloma inguinale). Genitourin Med 1991;67:441.

Sehgal VN, Shyamprasad AL, Beohar PC. The histopathological diagnosis of donovanosis. Br J Vener Dis 1984;60:45.

Trees DL, Morse SA. Chancroid and *Haemophilus ducreyi*: an update. Clin Microbiol Rev 1995;8:357.

Whitley RJ, Kimberlin DW, Roizman B. Herpes simplex viruses. Clin Infect Dis 1998;26:541.

Human Papillomavirus

Crum CP, Barber S, Roche JK. Pathobiology of papillomavirus-related cervical diseases: prospects for immunodiagnosis. Clin Microbiol Rev 1991;4:270.

Meisels A, Fortin R. Condylomatous lesions of the cervix and vagina. I. Cytologic patterns. Acta Cytol 1976;20:505.

Meisels A, Fortin R, Roy M. Condylomatous lesions of the cervix. II. Cytologic, colposcopic and histopathologic study. Acta Cytol 1977;21:379.

Prasad CJ. Pathobiology of human papillomavirus. Clin Lab Med 1995;15:685.

Botryomycosis

Winslow DJ. Botryomycosis. Am J Pathol 1959;35:153.

Winslow DJ, Chamblin SA. Disseminated visceral botryomycosis. Am J Clin Pathol 1960;33:42.

Syphilis

Larsen SA, Steiner BM, Rudolph AH. Laboratory diagnosis and interpretation of tests for syphilis. Clin Microbiol Rev 1995;8:1.

Rawstron SA, Vetrano J, Tannis G, Bromberg K. Congenital syphilis: detection of *Treponema pallidum* in stillborns. Clin Infect Dis 1997;24:24.

Tramont EC. Syphilis in adults: from Christopher Columbus to Sir Alexander Fleming to AIDS. Clin Infect Dis 1995;21:1361.

Young SA, Crocker DW. Occult congenital syphilis in macerated stillborn fetuses. Arch Pathol Lab Med 1994;118:44–47.

Xanthogranulomatous Pyelonephritis

Clapton WK, Boucaut HAP, Dewan PA, et al. Clinicopathological features of xanthogranulomatous pyelonephritis in infancy. Pathology 1993;25:110.

D'Costa GF, Nagle SB, Wagholikar UL, Nathani RR. Xanthogranulomatous pyelonephritis in children and adults—an 8 year study. Indian J Pathol Microbiol 1990;33:224.

Goodman M, Curry T, Russell T. Xanthogranulomatous pyelonephritis (XGP): a local disease with systemic manifestations: report of 23 patients and review of the literature. Medicine (Baltimore) 1979;58:171.

Levy M, Baumal R, Eddy AA. Xanthogranulomatous pyelonephritis in children. Etiology, pathogenesis, clinical and radiologic features, and management. Clin Pediatr (Phila) 1994;33:360.

Moller JC, Kristensen IB. Xanthogranulomatous pyelonephritis: a clinicopathological study with special reference to pathogenesis. Acta Pathol Microbiol Scand 1980;88:89.

Parsons MA, Harris SC, Longstaff AJ, Grainger RG. Xanthogranulomatous pyelonephritis: a pathological, clinical and etiological analysis of 87 cases. Diagn Histopathol 1983;6:203.

Malakoplakia

Damjanov I, Katz SM. Malakoplakia. Path Annu 1981;16:103.

Kawamura N, Murakami Y, Okada K. Three cases of malakoplakia of prostate. Urology 1980;15:77.

McClure J. Malakoplakia of the prostate: a report of two cases and a review of the literature. J Clin Path 1979;32:629.

Sarma HN, Ramesh K, Al Fituri O, et al. Malakoplakia of the prostate gland—report of two cases and review of the literature. Scand J Urol Nephrol 1996;30:155.

CHAPTER 8

Infections of the Hematopoietic System

Infections of the hematopoietic system are often life-threatening. All are characterized by hematogenous or lymphatic dissemination with targets of infection that include the bone marrow, the mononuclear phagocytic system (spleen, liver, lymph nodes, and adrenal glands), the vascular system (blood vessels and cardiac valves), and the bloodstream. The clinical presentation of these illnesses varies from the classically defined fever of unknown origin (an illness of 1 month or more that has failed to yield a diagnosis after the initial workup) to acute flulike illness with early, nonspecific symptoms of fever, headache, myalgia, and malaise. Accurate, timely diagnosis is often further impeded, because many of the etiologic organisms grow slowly (most mycobacteria and many fungi); are fastidious, requiring special media; or are obligately intracellular or even noncultivable agents. In many instances, the etiologic agents cannot be diagnosed by cultivation meth-

ods available in the typical clinical microbiology laboratory. Immunocompetent and immunocompromised patients are susceptible to many of these microorganisms, although the course, host responses, and outcome of the infection usually differ surprisingly.

Many of these cryptogenic diseases yield a diagnosis by microscopic evaluation of a bone marrow biopsy or a peripheral blood smear. Frequently, serology (usually in the convalescent stage) is the commonly used method for establishing a specific diagnosis (e.g., rickettsial vascular infection, Q fever endocarditis, ehrlichiosis, cat-scratch disease, tularemia, and brucellosis). Many of these illnesses are zoonoses or are transmitted by hematophagous insects and ticks. Very few of the infectious agents require humans for their survival in nature (e.g., malaria, *Mycobacterium tuberculosis*, and parvovirus B19). In most instances, human infection is incidental.

FEVER AND SPLENOMEGALY IN A CENTRAL AMERICAN IMMIGRANT

Clinical History

A 22-year-old Latin American woman (gravida III, para II) arrived in the United States from El Salvador 4 days before the onset of chills, fever, headache, myalgias, and passing dark urine. When she presented for medical care, her physical examination revealed pregnancy of 15 weeks' gestation, hypotension (blood pressure of 77/47 mm Hg), pulse of 113 beats per minute, respiratory rate of 27 breaths per minute, a temperature of 37.2°C, splenomegaly, and mild icterus. Laboratory evaluation demonstrated leukopenia (2,500 per µl), anemia (hemoglobin, 6.4 g/dl), thrombocytopenia (37,000 per µl), hyperbilirubinemia (2.6 mg/dl), elevated serum lactate dehydrogenase (836 U/liter), and hypoalbuminemia (2.5 g/dl). On the second hospital day, her temperature spiked to 39.8°C. Examination of a peripheral blood smear was requested.

Pathologic Findings and Microbiology

The diagnosis of *Plasmodium vivax* malaria was established by the detection of plasmodia in thick and thin smears stained by the Giemsa method in the clinical parasitology laboratory. Typical of vivax malaria, the blood smears showed not only ring forms but also trophozoite and schizont parasites within larger than average red blood cells (reticulocytes; Figure 8-1). Many of the infected erythrocytes also contained cytoplasmic Schüffner's dots.

Differential Diagnoses

Because this patient had a fever and had been in an endemic area, malaria was a prominent consideration in the differential diagnosis, which also included influenza; viral hepatitis; typhoid fever; leptospirosis; relapsing fever; dengue fever; yellow fever; arenaviral, hantaviral, and filoviral hemorrhagic fevers; rickettsioses; and traveler's diarrhea.

Comment

Malaria comprises infection with any of four protozoan parasites: *Plasmodium falciparum*, *P. vivax*, *Plasmodium ovale*, and *Plasmodium malariae*. The most severe infection, falciparum malaria, may result in death owing to (1) obstruction of the cerebral microcirculation by heavily parasitized erythrocytes (Figure 8-2) that develop knobs on their surface that adhere to thrombospondin, CD36, and ICAM-1 on the endothelial cell surfaces, (2) anemia associated with hemolysis and defective production of erythrocytes, or a combination of both. In falciparum malaria, development of mature trophozoites and schizogony take place in these sequestered red blood cells, and only early ring-form trophozoites appear in the circulation. Often, multiple ring-shaped formations are present in individual red blood cells, a phenomenon that occurs in babesiosis but in no other type of malaria. A diagnostic

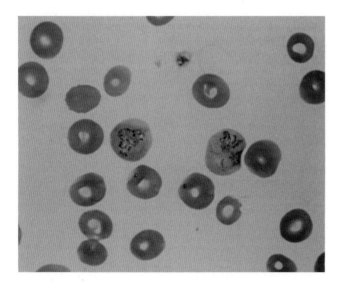 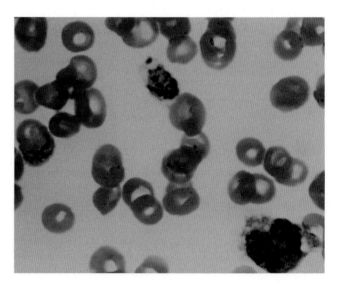

FIGURE 8-1. Two fields from a peripheral blood smear from a patient with *Plasmodium vivax* malaria show amoeboid trophozoites and a schizont (Giemsa stain; original magnification, ×250).

FIGURE 8-2. A thin blood smear shows heavy parasitization with numerous intraerythrocytic ring-forms (trophozoites) of *Plasmodium falciparum*. A red blood cell at the upper left contains two identical ring-shaped organisms (*arrow*) with blue cytoplasm and a dense purple nucleus (Giemsa stain; original magnification, ×250).

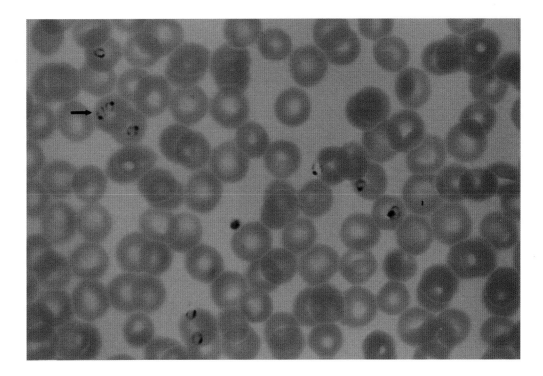

test for falciparum malaria is a rapid dipstick that detects histidine-rich protein 2 of *P. falciparum* trophozoites.

In contrast to *P. falciparum*, *P. vivax* and *P. ovale* develop into mature trophozoites and schizonts in circulating erythrocytes that can be identified in peripheral blood smears. These two plasmodial species also have hypnozoite forms that persist in hepatocytes and result in recurring relapses for months or even years after leaving the endemic zone.

Although methods for antigen detection, serology, DNA hybridization, and detection of the protozoal DNA by the polymerase chain reaction (PCR) have been developed, the simplest and least expensive method for diagnosis of malaria is routine microscopy. Excellent sensitivity is achieved by examination of a drop of blood in which the red blood cells have been lysed, leaving highly concentrated parasites that maintain their characteristic morphology when stained with the Giemsa method (thick smear). Thin smears allow the evaluation of the erythrocytes for their size and for Maurer's clefts (falciparum malaria), Schüffner's dots (vivax and ovale malaria), or Zieman's stippling (*P. malariae* infection). Attention should be paid to the occasional occurrence of simultaneous infection with two types of malaria.

Diagnosis

P. vivax malaria.

ELDERLY ASPLENIC STEROID-TREATED PATIENT WITH FEVER AND THROMBOCYTOPENIA

Clinical History

A 73-year-old, moderately obese woman, who had undergone splenectomy 21 years previously for chronic idiopathic thrombocytopenic purpura, presented with complaints of fever, chills, night sweats, myalgia, mild headache, nausea, fatigue, and weakness for 2 weeks. These symptoms appeared during tapering of steroids that had been given for a recurrence of thrombocytopenia. She recalled a tick bite a few days before the illness began. Physical examination was unremarkable. Pertinent laboratory test results included normal red and white blood cell counts, an erythrocyte sedimentation rate of 53 mm per hour, a platelet count of 12,000 per μl, serum bilirubin of 1.7 mg/dl, albumin of 2.9 g/dl, and haptoglobin below the limits of detection. Blood and urine were submitted for bacterial culture. Examination of a peripheral blood smear was requested.

Differential Diagnoses

The diagnostic considerations included gram-negative sepsis, ehrlichiosis, Rocky Mountain spotted fever, babesiosis, and idiopathic thrombocytopenic purpura complicated by an intercurrent infection.

Pathologic Findings

Peripheral blood smears stained by the Giemsa method showed intraerythrocytic ring forms of protozoa suggestive of *Babesia microti* or *Plasmodium falciparum* and a few Howell-Jolly bodies (Figure 8-3). Extensive examination failed to detect the tetrad form that is diagnostic of babesiosis.

Microbiology

Because of the pathologic findings, blood was sent to a reference laboratory for detection of *B. microti* DNA by PCR and antibodies to *B. microti* by indirect immunofluorescence assay. Babesia DNA was present, and the antibody titer was equal to or greater than 1:2,048. All routine cultures of blood and urine yielded no growth of organisms.

Comment

B. microti is maintained in the same *Ixodes scapularis* tick–*Peromyscus leucopus* mammalian cycle as Lyme borreliosis and human granulocytotropic ehrlichiosis and is transmitted to humans by the bite of these ticks in the

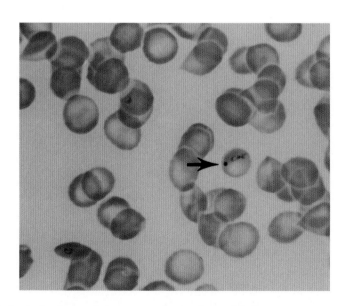

Figure 8-3. Two fields from a blood smear from a patient with babesiosis. One to four protozoal organisms of *Babesia microti* are present within some erythrocytes, including one containing a Howell-Jolly body (*arrow*), a reflection that the patient is asplenic (Giemsa stain; original magnification, ×250). (Courtesy of Dr. Johann Bakken.)

northeastern and upper Midwestern states. Transfusion-transmitted and transplacental infections have also been documented. Based on serosurveillance data, a high proportion of infections are subclinical or undiagnosed. Risk factors for symptomatic illness and for severe illness (i.e., old age, asplenia, and immunosuppression) were all present in this case. The patient's hemolysis was manifested by mild hyperbilirubinemia, undetectable haptoglobin, and polychromasia, but not by anemia. The patient was treated with the combination of clindamycin and quinine, which caused fever to rise to 38.4°C during the second and third hospital days; she remained afebrile thereafter. A substantial decrease in parasitemia and a rise in platelet count occurred during the first 10 days of treatment. Thrombocytopenia, attributed initially to chronic idiopathic thrombocytopenic purpura in this patient, occurs frequently in babesiosis.

At least two other species of *Babesia* cause human disease: strain WA-1 (closely related to the canine pathogen *Babesia gibsoni*) and *Babesia divergens* (a bovine pathogen that has caused severe febrile hemolytic disease in asplenic patients in Europe). Strain WA-1 was isolated from a patient from the Pacific northwest with an intact spleen and a normal immune system, and closely related babesiae have caused severe, life-threatening illness in asplenic patients in California. A fatal case in an elderly, asplenic man from Missouri was shown to be caused by an organism genetically closely related to *B. divergens*, an organism that had not been thought to occur naturally in the United States.

Diagnosis of babesiosis is most often established by examination of thick and thin blood smears stained by Romanovsky's method, but PCR, hamster inoculation, and serology are also used, particularly in cases where parasitemia is very low or a possibility of falciparum malaria exists. In this case, a travel history revealed that the patient had never been outside of the upper Midwest region of the United States.

Diagnosis

Babesiosis.

RECURRENT EPISODES OF FEBRILE FLULIKE ILLNESS

Clinical History

A 25-year-old college student experienced abrupt onset of fever, headache, and myalgia; the episode was associated with nausea, vomiting, and blurred vision and lasted for 3 days. Four days after recovery, an illness nearly identical, but not quite as severe, recurred with resolution after 2–3 days. When a third episode began 4 days later, the student sought medical attention. Evaluation revealed an erythrocyte sedimentation rate of 43 mm per hour and normal blood counts (with the exception of monocytosis), serum chemical assays, and chest radiograph. Examination of a peripheral blood smear was requested.

In all, he suffered five febrile periods of 2–3 days each before an infectious disease specialist was consulted. A petechial rash occurred on his legs during the last febrile episode. Further history obtained by the infectious disease physician revealed that the patient had twice been studying rattlesnakes in a cave in central Texas for approximately 1.5 hours per visit, 7 and 21 days, respectively, before the onset of illness. A course of doxycycline was given, and the illness resolved with no further relapses. Two other persons who accompanied him into the cave also had suffered similar febrile illnesses and had recovered.

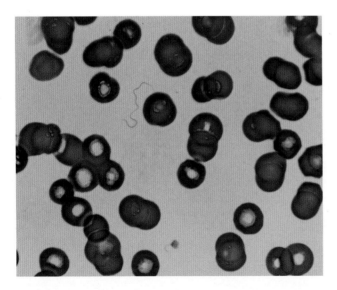

FIGURE 8-4. A blood smear shows a thin, loosely coiled, darkly stained borreliae (center of the field) in the plasma between red blood cells (Giemsa stain; original magnification, ×250).

Pathologic Findings

Review of a peripheral blood smear prepared at the time of his third febrile period revealed the presence of borreliae (Figure 8-4).

Microbiology

All cultures and serologic assays from the patient were nondiagnostic. Investigation of the cave by personnel of the Texas Department of Health revealed *Ornithodoros turicata* ticks from which *Borrelia turicatae* were isolated.

Comment

Three species of tick-borne *Borrelia* are found in the United States, each in its own soft-bodied ticks: *O. turicata* ticks transmit *B. turicatae* in the southwestern states, and *Ornithodoros hermsii* and *Ornithodoros parkeri* transmit *Borrelia hermsii* and *Borrelia parkeri*, respectively, in the western states. Other *Ornithodoros* species transmit other *Borrelia* species in other parts of the world. Typically, *B. turicatae* is transmitted by a tick bite occurring in a cave, and *B. hermsii* is transmitted while the person is sleeping in a mountain cabin that has rodent nests containing ticks. These ticks can survive without a blood meal for more than a decade, and the borreliae can survive within the tick for a similar period. The borreliae are maintained in nature by transovarian transmission in the tick and are transmitted to humans during rapid, painless, generally nocturnal feeding. After an average incubation period of 7 days, the first febrile attack begins abruptly and lasts for a mean of 3 days. After an afebrile interval averaging 8 days, a relapse of the illness occurs. A mean of three relapses, with as many as 13 episodes, are of 2–3 days' duration and are usually progressively less severe. The mechanism for the relapses is that the borreliae switch to the expression of genes that encode different surface proteins, enabling these organisms to evade the established immune response. The fatality rate for tick-borne relapsing fever is approximately 2%, although louse-borne epidemics caused by *Borrelia recurrentis* have case-fatality rates as high as 40%. The last reported epidemic occurred during World War II in North Africa with 50,000 deaths, but evidence of *B. recurrentis* infection has been associated with the war in Burundi.

The laboratory diagnosis is established by identification of borreliae, usually 10–20 µm long and 0.3–0.5 µm wide, with four to six spiral coils, in thick and thin smears of peripheral blood stained by Giemsa, Wright, or acridine orange stain. Organisms are detected only during febrile episodes, at which time the sensitivity of examining smears is approximately 70%. Blood counts are usually normal except for monocytosis, which in this case was 20% and 21% during the second and third relapses, respectively; automated hematology analysis can account for not visualizing the borreliae microscopically. Often, an astute laboratory technologist makes the diagnosis by manual blood smear examination even before the primary physician has considered the possibility.

Diagnosis

Tick-borne relapsing fever caused by *B. turicatae*.

HYDROPS FETALIS WITH INCLUSIONS IN BONE MARROW HEMATOPOIETIC CELLS

Clinical History

A 14-year-old girl (gravida I) at an estimated gestational age of 25 weeks was taken to a hospital by her mother when the girl admitted that she had noticed decreased fetal movements for the previous 3 weeks. An ultrasound study confirmed fetal demise. Labor was induced medically, and a stillborn male infant with severe hydrops was delivered vaginally 20 hours later.

Pathologic Findings

The infant weighed 597 g and was 31 cm long, with a crown-rump length of 22 cm. The head circumference was 20 cm, the thoracic circumference was 17 cm, and the abdominal circumference was 19 cm. Straw-colored, blood-tinged fluid was present in all body cavities: 50 ml in the peritoneum, 27 ml in both thoracic cavities, and 2 ml in the pericardial sac. Sections of the bone marrow showed enlarged erythroid precursors with intranuclear inclusions. Erythroid precursors with intranuclear inclusions were also found in foci of extramedullary hematopoiesis in sections of the liver (Figure 8-5), spleen, and adrenal gland and in vessels in sections of placenta (Figures 8-6 and 8-7), kidney, and lungs.

Differential Diagnoses

Differential diagnoses of hydrops fetalis include chronic anemia (e.g., isoimmunization disorder, homozygous alpha-thalassemia, fetomaternal or fetofetal transfusions), cardiac or pulmonary failure due to causes other than anemia (e.g., large arteriovenous malformation, premature closure of the foramen ovale, cystic adenomatoid malformation, pulmonary lymphangiectasia), perinatal tumors (e.g., neuroblastoma, chorioangioma), achondroplasia, renal disorders (e.g., congenital nephrosis, renal vein thrombosis), and infectious diseases (e.g., parvovirus B19, syphilis, cytomegalovirus, toxoplasmosis, congenital hepatitis, and rubella).

Comment

Congenital anomalies and tumors were excluded based on the gross findings at autopsy. The presence of erythroid precursors with intranuclear inclusions is characteristic of infection with parvovirus B19. These cells are not found in any of the other possible causes of hydrops fetalis.

The most common presentation of infection with parvovirus B19 is erythema infectiosum, a mild, self-

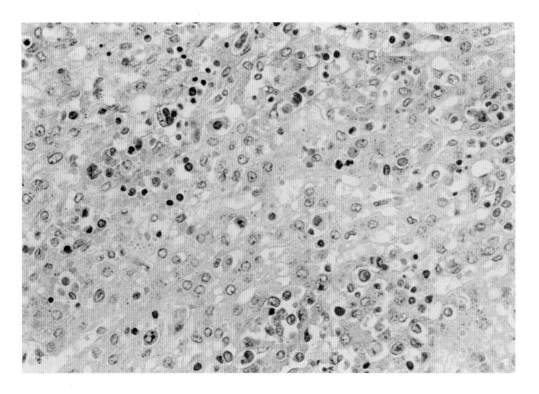

FIGURE 8-5. Section of liver from a stillborn fetus that died of hydrops fetalis caused by congenital parvovirus B19 infection shows erythrophagocytosis and many nucleated red blood cell precursors within the hepatic sinusoids. Within some of these erythrocyte precursors are well-defined intranuclear inclusions, consistent with parvovirus B19 infection (hematoxylin and eosin stain; original magnification, ×100).

FIGURE 8-6. Section of placenta from a stillborn fetus that died of hydrops fetalis caused by congenital parvovirus B19 infection shows many nucleated red blood cells within the fetal capillaries (hematoxylin and eosin stain; original magnification, ×100).

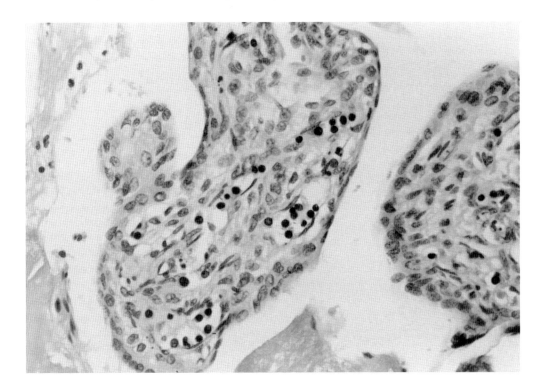

FIGURE 8-7. Higher-power magnification of the section illustrated in Figure 8-6 shows smudgy intranuclear inclusions consistent with B19 infection within the nucleated red blood cell precursors (hematoxylin and eosin stain; original magnification, ×250).

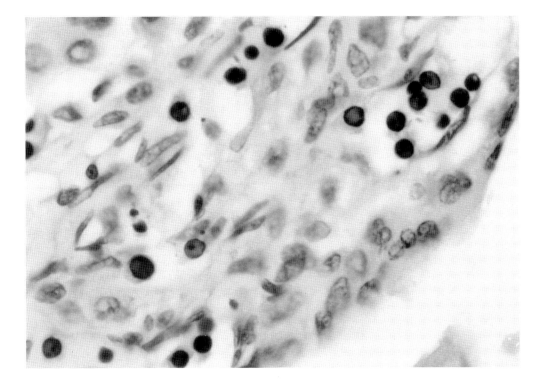

limited illness of children 4–15 years of age manifested by a facial rash with a "slapped-cheek" appearance (Figure 8-8) accompanied by or followed in a few days by a morbilliform, annular, or confluent rash on the extremities. In adults, especially women, a prominent feature of infection with parvovirus B19 is arthropathy without rash. Parvovirus B19 may cause aplastic crisis in persons who have chronic hemolytic anemia, and in immunocompromised persons, such as those infected with the human immunodeficiency virus (HIV), parvovirus B19 infection may become chronic, causing continuous lysis of red blood cell precursors and, eventually, severe persistent anemia. If parvovirus B19 infection is acquired during pregnancy, the virus may be transmitted to the

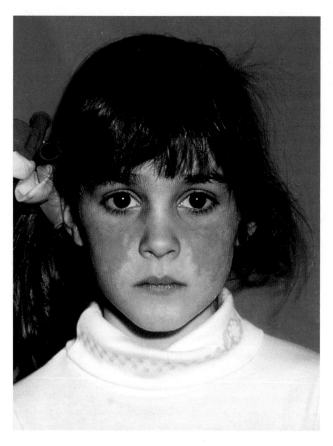

FIGURE 8-8. Photograph shows a 6-year-old girl who has the typical facial rash (described as having a "slapped cheek" appearance) of erythema infectiosum due to infection with parvovirus B19. (Courtesy of Dr. Joan Barenfanger.)

fetus, producing a persistent fetal infection with anemia and subsequent congestive heart failure, generalized edema (hydrops fetalis), and death, as occurred in this case. The occurrence of hydrops fetalis, however, is rare; maternal infection with parvovirus B19 usually does not result in fetal demise.

Infection with parvovirus B19 is usually diagnosed by detecting specific antibodies in the serum. The most useful diagnostic test is the detection of specific immunoglobulin (Ig) M, which is present early in the illness, declines 1–2 months after the onset, and generally disappears 2–3 months later. IgG antibodies generally persist for life. Diagnosis can also be made histopathologically. Infection with parvovirus B19 causes specific changes in the bone marrow of persons with aplastic crisis and in the tissues of congenitally infected fetuses. In bone marrow, the number of erythroid precursors is significantly decreased, and those that are present show megaloblastic changes with intranuclear changes (lantern cells). Nuclei are eosinophilic, enlarged, ballooned, and have marginal inclusions. Identical-appearing erythroblasts are found in many tissues of congenitally infected fetuses, especially in the capillaries but also in the sinusoids of the liver, spleen, and bone marrow. Localization of the virus can be demonstrated by immunohistochemistry and in situ hybridization. Additionally, the virus can be detected in serum by nucleic acid amplification tests, such as PCR.

Diagnosis

Hydrops fetalis due to congenital parvovirus B19 infection.

OVERWHELMING INFECTION WITH MONOCYTIC CELLS CONTAINING CYTOPLASMIC INCLUSIONS IN BONE MARROW

Clinical History

A 36-year-old field biologist and naturalist sought medical attention for a nonproductive cough, fever, chills, myalgia, and lethargy of 3 weeks' duration. Previously, he had been healthy and had been running 4 miles each day. Laboratory evaluation revealed antibodies to HIV, a CD4 lymphocyte count of 18 per µl, neutropenia (468 per µl), thrombocytopenia (15,000 per µl), markedly elevated hepatic enzymes, and serum bilirubin of 3.2 mg/dl. He developed acute renal failure and died on the third hospital day. A bone marrow aspirate and biopsy had been performed earlier that day.

Pathologic Findings

The bone marrow aspirate contained monocytic cells with 1–3 µm cytoplasmic inclusions that appeared to be composed of smaller units (less than 0.5 µm in diameter) and were stained blue with Wright stain (Figure 8-9). The bone marrow biopsy and spleen, Peyer's patches, kidneys, and lymph nodes collected at necropsy contained mononuclear phagocytes with cytoplasmic aggregates stained by specific immunohistochemistry for antigens of *Ehrlichia chaffeensis*.

Microbiology

None of the cultures or serologic tests performed antemortem on this patient revealed the unsuspected diagnosis.

Comment

Humans are infected by *E. chaffeensis* via the bite of *Amblyomma americanum* and possibly other ticks, which acquire the ehrlichiae while feeding on white-tailed deer and possibly dogs, both of which are found to be naturally infected. Seasonal tick exposure, particularly in May through July, and laboratory evidence of leukopenia, thrombocytopenia, and elevated hepatic enzymes usually are the only diagnostic clues. Visualization of cytoplasmic vacuoles containing clusters of ehrlichiae, predominantly in monocytes, is achieved in fewer than 10% of cases in which careful examination of peripheral blood smears is performed. The tissues of severely immunocompromised patients (such as this HIV-infected, CD4 lymphocyte-depleted man) contain much higher quantities of ehrlichiae than in the usual immunocompetent patient with human monocytotropic ehrlichiosis (HME).

Most cases of HME are diagnosed by demonstration of a fourfold or greater rise in serum IgG antibodies to *E. chaffeensis* with a titer of 1:128 or greater by indirect immunofluorescence assay. Nucleic acid amplification by PCR specific for *E. chaffeensis* detects ehrlichial DNA in blood samples, providing a sensitive, specific, and timely diagnosis.

The pathologic lesions include myeloid hyperplasia and megakaryocytosis of the bone marrow, granulomas in the bone marrow and liver, perivascular lymphohistiocytic infiltrates in the brain and meninges where infected macrophages have been detected, interstitial pneumonia associated with adult respiratory distress syndrome, hepatocellular apoptosis, and splenic and lymph nodal necrosis. Immunohistologic or PCR identification of *E. chaffeensis* offers the possibility of a specific postmortem diagnosis in such cases.

Diagnosis

HME.

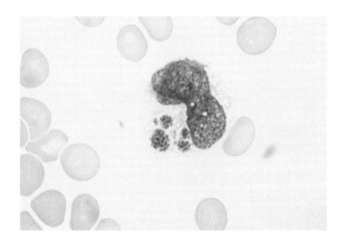

FIGURE 8-9. Aspirate of bone marrow from an acquired immunodeficiency disease patient with opportunistic overwhelming human monocytotropic ehrlichiosis shows a monocyte precursor containing four morulae within which individual purple-stained ehrlichiae are observed (Wright stain; original magnification, ×250). (Reprinted with permission from J Barenfanger, PG Patel, JS Dumler, DH Walker. Identifying human ehrlichiosis. Lab Med 1996;27:372.)

FEVER AND PANCYTOPENIA IN A PREVIOUSLY HEALTHY MAN

Clinical History

A 78-year-old man from northwestern Wisconsin was admitted to the hospital with an illness of five days' duration characterized by fever, chills, myalgias, headache, malaise, nausea, and diarrhea. On admission, he had a temperature of 40.5°C and bilateral roentgenographic interstitial pneumonia. His white blood cell count was 2,900 per μl (47% neutrophils, 33% bands, 15% lymphocytes, 5% monocytes), and he had a hemoglobin of 10.5 g/dl, a platelet count of 34,000 U/μl, serum albumin of 1.9 g/dl, creatinine of 1.9 mg/dl, and aspartate aminotransferase of 165 U/liter. After microscopic examination of a blood smear 48 hours after admission, doxycycline was given with defervescence within 24 hours.

Pathologic Findings

Examination of the peripheral blood smear revealed that 10% of the neutrophils contained cytoplasmic aggregates of basophilic structures 0.5 μm in diameter (Figure 8-10).

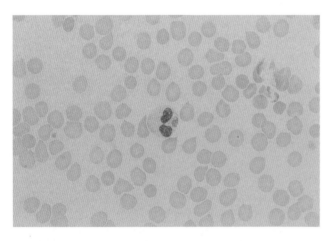

FIGURE 8-10. Smear of peripheral blood from a patient with human granulocytotropic ehrlichiosis shows a band neutrophil with a cytoplasmic morula containing numerous ehrlichiae (Wright-Giemsa stain; original magnification, ×250).

These morulae are clusters of gram-negative coccobacilli inside cytoplasmic vacuoles. The vacuolar microcolony is called a *morula*, the Latin word for mulberry, which the aggregate of *Ehrlichia* species organisms resembles.

Microbiology

Routine blood cultures were negative. PCR with generic primers for the 16S rRNA gene amplified a DNA product that was the source of the original sequence of the human granulocytotropic ehrlichiosis. The convalescent serum contained (IgG) antibodies to *Ehrlichia equi* at a titer of 1:80.

Comment

Human granulocytotropic ehrlichiosis is transmitted by the bite of the black-legged tick *I. scapularis* and is maintained in a zoonotic cycle involving the white-footed mouse *Peromyscus leucopus*. It is an emerging infectious disease that shares the same epidemiology and ecology as Lyme borreliosis. The ehrlichia is an obligately intracellular bacterium and thus is not cultivated by usual approaches. Because the majority of patients do not have a diagnostic antibody titer at the time of presentation for medical care, diagnosis must be based on clinical suspicion (fever, tick exposure, leukopenia with or without thrombocytopenia, and elevated serum levels of hepatic enzymes) or detection of ehrlichial morulae in circulating neutrophils in a peripheral blood smear examined carefully by visual microscopy rather than by relying solely on the automated differential leukocyte count. Molecular diagnostics offer substantially greater sensitivity, as PCR identifies 75–90% of patients. In contrast, peripheral smears are diagnostic in only 25–80%.

Diagnosis

Human granulocytotropic ehrlichiosis.

PANCYTOPENIA AND MULTISYSTEM FEBRILE ILLNESS IN A HUMAN IMMUNODEFICIENCY VIRUS–INFECTED PATIENT

Clinical History

A 27-year-old man from east Texas, who had been diagnosed with HIV infection 4 years earlier, was admitted for evaluation of fever of 2 weeks' duration, decreased appetite, nausea and vomiting, and night sweats for 1 week. On physical examination, his temperature was 38°C, his pulse was 104 beats per minute, his respiratory rate was 20 breaths per minute, and his blood pressure was 90/60 mm Hg. Auscultation of the chest revealed decreased breath sounds and expiratory wheezes in all lung fields. The remainder of the examination was noncontributory. Pertinent abnormal laboratory test results included a white blood cell count of 800 cells per µl, a hemoglobin concentration of 4.4 mg/dl, and a platelet count of 108,000 per µl. Chest radiograph showed diffuse reticulonodular infiltrates.

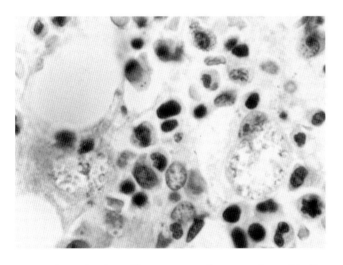

FIGURE 8-11. Section of bone marrow from a patient with disseminated histoplasmosis shows small yeast cells in the cytoplasm of enlarged histiocytes (hematoxylin and eosin stain; original magnification, ×250).

Organisms considered to be the most likely cause of this patient's illness were *Mycobacterium tuberculosis*, *Mycobacterium avium* complex (MAC), and *Histoplasma capsulatum*. Blood was collected for bacterial, fungal, and mycobacterial cultures, and an induced sputum specimen was obtained for fungal and mycobacterial stains and cultures. No organisms were visualized in the sputum smear stained with auramine O (for acid-fast bacilli [AFB]) or in the KOH preparation. Bone marrow biopsy and aspiration were performed to evaluate the pancytopenia; samples were submitted to the hematopathology laboratory for histologic examination and to the microbiology laboratory for fungal and mycobacterial cultures.

Pathologic Findings

The bone marrow biopsy specimen contained several well-formed granulomas composed of epithelioid histiocytes, some of which contained yeast cells within their cytoplasm (Figure 8-11). Stains for AFB were negative, but small, intracellular, budding yeast cells (consistent with *H. capsulatum*) were visualized in sections stained by the methenamine silver method. Yeast cells also were seen within cytoplasm of histiocytes and neutrophils in the smear prepared from the bone marrow aspirate (Figure 8-12).

Differential Diagnoses

The differential diagnoses of infectious causes of epithelioid granulomas in the bone marrow include disseminated infection with mycobacteria, especially *M. tuberculosis* (Figure 8-13) or MAC, but also other nontuberculous mycobacteria, or fungi, such as *H. capsulatum*, *Cryptococcus neoformans*, *Coccidioides immitis*, (Figures 8-14 and 8-15) or *Blastomyces dermatitidis*. Based on this dif-

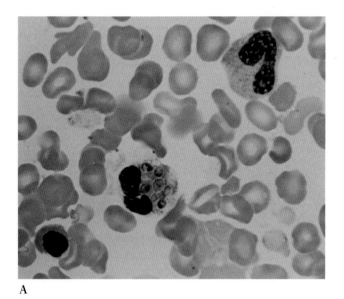
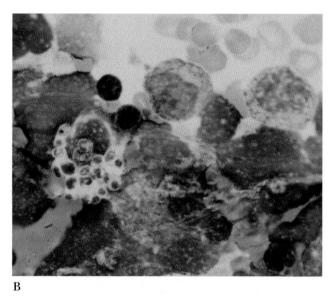

A   B

FIGURE 8-12. Smear of bone marrow aspirated from a patient with disseminated histoplasmosis. (**A**) Segmented neutrophil with several yeast cells, one of which is budding, in its cytoplasm. (**B**) Histiocyte with intracellular yeast cells surrounded by a narrow halo that represents protoplasmic retraction from the cell wall rather than a true capsule (Wright-Giemsa stain; original magnification, ×250).

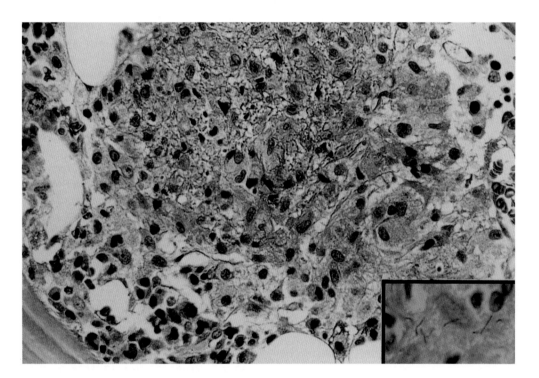

FIGURE 8-13. Section of bone marrow from a patient with disseminated tuberculosis demonstrates a nodular aggregate of histiocytes admixed with fibrin (hematoxylin and eosin stain; original magnification, ×100). *Inset*: Many acid-fast bacilli (Ziehl-Neelsen stain; original magnification, ×250). Cultures eventually grew *Mycobacterium tuberculosis*.

ferential diagnosis, special stains for AFB and fungi should be performed, and material should be submitted for culture, because the responsible agent may be isolated even when special stains for organisms are negative. In this case, stains for AFB were negative, and the methenamine silver stain showed small, budding yeast cells consistent with the diagnosis of histoplasmosis. In some cases, bacterial causes of bone marrow granulomas (e.g., brucellosis) are diagnosed most effectively by culture or serology, which is the usual method for diagnosing granulomatous diseases, such as Q fever and human monocytotropic ehrlichiosis.

FIGURE 8-14. Section of bone marrow from a patient with disseminated coccidioidomycosis shows a granuloma containing a giant cell with a mature spherule in its cytoplasm (hematoxylin and eosin stain; original magnification, ×50). Fungal cultures of the bone marrow aspirate grew *Coccidioides immitis*.

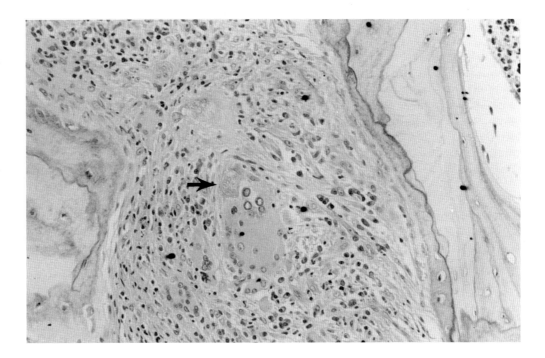

FIGURE 8-15. Higher-power magnification of another area of the section illustrated in Figure 8-14 shows many immature spherules and one mature spherule containing endospores (*arrow*; hematoxylin and eosin stain; original magnification, ×100).

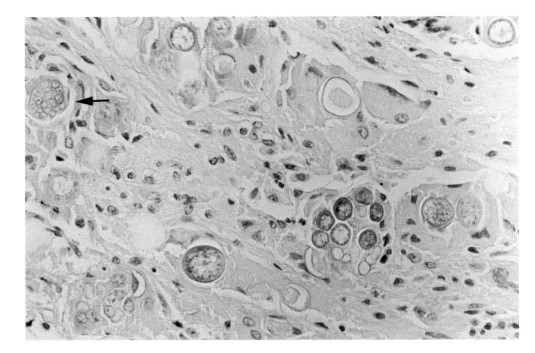

Microbiology

The bone marrow culture ultimately grew *H. capsulatum*.

Comment

Disseminated histoplasmosis is a common opportunistic infection in patients infected with HIV, generally developing in those whose illness is far advanced and who have CD4 lymphocyte counts less than 200 per μl. It was recognized as a complication of acquired immunodeficiency syndrome (AIDS) as early as 1981 but was not considered an AIDS-defining infection until 1987. Disseminated histoplasmosis occurs most frequently in patients living in areas endemic for *H. capsulatum* (i.e., Mississippi, Ohio, and Missouri River valleys) but has also been reported in those who live in areas nonendemic for the fungus.

The typical presentation of disseminated histoplasmosis in an HIV-infected patient is that of a febrile and wasting illness with marked weight loss. Only approximately half of the patients have respiratory symptoms, and some have diarrhea. Involvement of the central nervous system is uncommon. Frequent findings on physical examination are hepatosplenomegaly, followed by skin or mucous membrane lesions and enlarged lymph nodes. Laboratory abnormalities are nonspecific and include pancytopenia and markedly elevated serum lactate dehydrogenase levels. Many patients who present with manifestations of septic shock have evidence of disseminated intravascular coagulopathy. Results of the initial chest roentgenogram are normal in approximately one-third of patients; the most common abnormality, occurring in nearly half of the cases, is diffuse interstitial or reticulonodular infiltrates, reflecting miliary (hematogenous) involvement of the lungs.

Diagnosis of disseminated histoplasmosis is based on recovery of the fungus in culture or visualization of the yeast cells in tissue or aspirated material. Histologic examination of a bone marrow biopsy and aspirate appears to be the most sensitive and specific method that can provide a rapid diagnosis. Biopsies, aspirates, or both of enlarged lymph nodes, skin, or mucosal lesions, if present, also are potential sources of material for visual detection of the etiologic agent. However, fungal culture also should be performed on the tissue or aspirated material, because organisms are not always visualized. Occasionally, intracellular yeast cells are seen in the peripheral blood smear. Fungal culture of blood using the lysis-centrifugation technique, respiratory secretions, or both is an easy and effective way to recover *H. capsulatum*, but the cultures often require 2–4 weeks before growth is detected.

Diagnosis

Disseminated histoplasmosis.

RECURRENT FEVER AND GRANULOMATOUS INFECTION OF HEMATOPOIETIC TISSUE

Clinical History

A 51-year-old-man was admitted for evaluation of periodic fever and shaking chills that began 2 months earlier. Fever occurred in approximately weekly cycles, started at night, rose to levels of 40°C, and recurred for several days. He had lost 20 pounds in weight over this time, but had no localizing symptoms except for arthralgias. On admission, he had a fever of 40°C rectally, but other vital signs were normal. No palpable lymphadenopathy was present. The edge of the liver, which was firm, smooth, and nontender, was felt 2 cm below the right costal margin. Results of liver function tests were abnormal, with elevated values for serum alkaline phosphatase, gamma glutamyl transpeptidase, and conjugated bilirubin, suggesting an element of biliary obstruction. An ultrasound examination demonstrated multiple echolucent areas in the liver and spleen that were suspicious for lymphoma or metastatic disease. Computed tomography demonstrated an enlarged spleen with a large calcified lesion and adjacent hypodense areas (Figure 8-16). Blood was collected for routine bacterial culture.

The patient was quizzed about his occupational history. He had worked in a local abattoir 28 years earlier and had developed acute brucellosis with recurrent fever and chills, which was appropriately treated. Shortly thereafter, he quit his job at the abattoir, and he had not had recurrent fevers since then. Based on additional information, the patient was treated with antimicrobial therapy appropriate for brucellosis.

Pathologic Findings

The bone marrow aspirate and biopsy contained a normocellular bone marrow with a small number of non-caseating granulomas (Figure 8-17). No mycobacteria or fungi were demonstrated in special stains.

Microbiology

The blood culture was reported positive for small gram-negative coccobacilli. Subsequently, three out of seven cultures were found to contain *Brucella suis*. Serologic studies demonstrated a titer of 1:80 or higher for IgG antibodies to *Brucella* species.

Comment

This case demonstrates the remarkable ability of some bacteria to lie dormant in the body before reactivation of

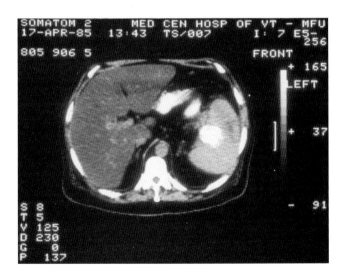

FIGURE 8-16. A well-defined mass in the spleen was documented by computed tomography. These lesions, which eventually calcify, have been particularly associated with *Brucella suis* infections.

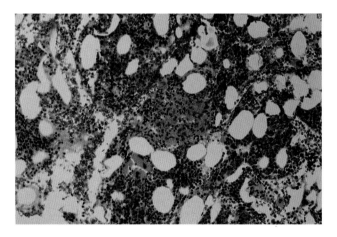

FIGURE 8-17. Several small, well-formed, non-caseating granulomas are present in this bone marrow biopsy. The granulomas have no distinguishing features and cannot be defined etiologically without microbiological studies (hematoxylin and eosin stain; medium-power magnification).

Table 8-1. Animals Associated with *Brucella* Species

Brucella Species	Primary Animal Host	Other Hosts and Comments
Brucella abortus	Cattle	Buffalo, camels, yaks
Brucella melitensis	Goats, sheep	Camels
Brucella suis, biovars 1–3	Domestic and wild swine	—
B. suis, biovar 4	Reindeer, caribou	—
Brucella canis	Dogs (especially kennel-raised)	Rare cause of human disease

active infection and clinical disease. The present illness almost certainly represents a reactivation of the infection that was contracted almost 30 years earlier. Calcified lesions (probably granulomas) in the spleen have been described in healed infections with *B. suis*, and the hypodense lesions in the computed tomographic scan probably represent current infection with active granulomas, as were seen in the bone marrow.

Brucellosis is contracted by humans after exposure to animal secretions, milk, or products made from contaminated milk. Workers in slaughterhouses have traditionally been at substantial risk. Aggressive immunization campaigns in livestock have virtually eliminated this infection from the United States. A current political-scientific-environmental issue is the concern for ranchers in Idaho and Montana that *Brucella*-infected bison (a population that is difficult to immunize) from Yellowstone National Park will infect domestic cattle when they wander onto private ranch lands. Epidemics may be associated with uncooked (or unpasteurized) food products (e.g., cheese) derived from infected animals. Meat products are usually not vehicles because of the small numbers of organisms and extensive cooking.

Brucellae are facultative intracellular pathogens that grow on agar media in the laboratory but proliferate in association with macrophages in the body. The ability to persist for long periods in a dormant state is shared by other facultative intracellular pathogens, such as *M. tuberculosis*. Four species of *Brucella* associated with different animal species are shown in Table 8-1.

Brucellosis is primarily a disease of the mononuclear phagocytic system. The clinical manifestation is, accordingly, a nonspecific febrile disease, evoking a wide differential diagnosis unless the exposure history is elicited. In some cases, the pathology may be concentrated in one organ, including the liver, brain, lung, and eye. Endocarditis is a rare but usually fatal complication.

The diagnosis of brucellosis usually is made serologically. No single diagnostic titer exists, although most patients have antibody at a titer of 1:160 or greater. Isolation of the bacterium can be difficult, especially in cases of chronic infection. Additionally, some identification systems do not include *Brucella* in the database; the organism may be misidentified as *Moraxella* species, another small, gram-negative coccobacillus that is (biochemically) inert. The bacteria, if isolated, should be treated with great care, because laboratory-acquired infections occur.

Diagnosis

Brucellosis (undulant fever).

SPINDLE-CELL MASS IN THE SPLEEN

Clinical History

A 61-year-old man presented with a history of unexplained weight loss and fatigue for 1 year and recent onset of dysphagia. The only notable physical finding was splenomegaly (spleen palpable 4 cm below the costal margin). He was anemic (hemoglobin, 9.4 g/dl) and leukopenic (3,500 cells per μl). Radiographic studies of the esophagus revealed a hiatal hernia with ulceration at the esophageal-gastric junction. He underwent surgical repair of the hiatal hernia, during which time splenectomy also was performed. Bone marrow biopsy was submitted for histopathologic examination and mycobacterial and fungal cultures. A serologic test performed after receipt of the surgical pathology report for the splenectomy specimen revealed the presence of antibodies to HIV.

Pathologic Findings

The spleen weighed 350 g and measured 14 cm × 10.8 cm × 3.6 cm. The capsular surface was smooth. Sectioning revealed nine light-brown, soft nodules measuring 0.3–1.0 cm in diameter. Histologically, the nodules were composed of clusters of spindle cells with pale eosinophilic cytoplasm and oval vesicular nuclei separated by compressed splenic red pulp sinusoids (Figure 8-18). Occasional mitoses were present, but no pleomorphism or areas of necrosis were found. In addition to the spindle cells, focal aggregates of lymphocytes and occasional histiocytes were discovered. Immunohistochemical studies showed that the spindle cells stained strongly with KP1 and Mac 387, indicating a monocytic/histiocytic origin; the lymphocytes were predominantly T cells. Ziehl-Neelsen staining revealed AFB (Figure 8-19), both within the spindle cells and extracellularly.

Differential Diagnoses

The differential diagnoses based on the hematoxylin and eosin (H and E)–stained sections include mycobacterial spindle-cell pseudotumor; Kaposi's sarcoma (KS); inflammatory pseudotumor; primary malignant fibrous histiocytoma; rare primary vascular neoplasms, such as epithelioid and spindle-cell hemangioendothelioma and hemangiopericytoma; and metastatic spindle-cell amelanotic melanoma. Based on the results of the Ziehl-Neelsen stain, the diagnosis of mycobacterial spindle-cell pseudotumor was made. Mycobacterial culture, however, is required to identify the mycobacterium causing the infection.

Microbiology

Results of mycobacterial and fungal cultures of the bone marrow aspirate were negative. Unfortunately, tissue from the splenic lesions was not submitted for culture.

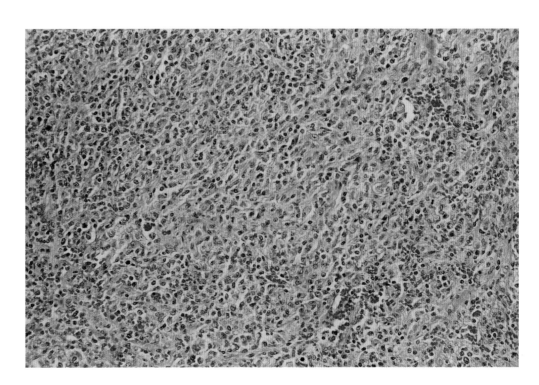

FIGURE 8-18. Section of a nodule in the spleen of a patient infected with human immunodeficiency virus shows clusters of spindle cells with pale eosinophilic cytoplasm and oval vesicular nuclei (hematoxylin and eosin stain; original magnification, ×50).

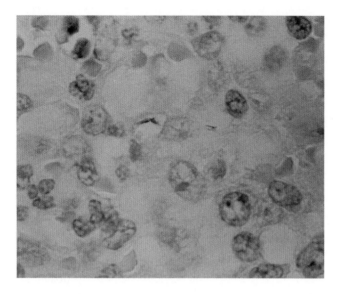

FIGURE 8-19. Acid-fast stain showed occasional intracellular and extracellular acid-fast bacilli, thus allowing a diagnosis of spindle-cell pseudotumor of the spleen (Ziehl-Neelsen stain; original magnification, ×250).

Comment

Mycobacterial spindle-cell tumors are rare. Almost all patients have been HIV seropositive. The majority of cases have involved lymph nodes, and most have been caused by infection with MAC. There have been only a few reports of mycobacterial spindle-cell pseudotumors of the spleen (including the case described here), and at least one case, caused by *M. tuberculosis*, involving the lung. Additionally, a subcutaneous spindle cell reaction due to infection with *Mycobacterium leprae*, termed *histoid*, has been described.

A critical aspect of the mycobacterial spindle-cell tumor is its resemblance to various neoplastic conditions.

Because virtually all patients are infected with HIV, the most important differential diagnosis is KS. In KS lesions, fascicles of spindle cells are admixed with erythrocytes and other inflammatory cells, which is similar to the appearance of mycobacterial spindle-cell tumors. In contrast to KS, however, mycobacterial spindle-cell tumors lack vascular slits, mitotic activity, and hyaline globules, and those involving the spleen typically do not show areas of fibrosis surrounding the small arteries of malpighian corpuscles, as are frequently described in KS lesions of the spleen. Less commonly encountered malignant conditions to consider in the differential diagnosis are primary malignant fibrous histiocytoma, a few primary vascular neoplasms, and metastatic spindle-cell melanoma. These lesions differ from mycobacterial spindle-cell pseudotumor as follows: Primary malignant fibrous histiocytomas and metastatic melanomas have more marked cellular pleomorphism, nuclear atypia, and a high mitotic rate. Additionally, the cells of malignant melanoma are negative for monocytic-histiocytic cell markers but show a strongly positive reaction with antibodies against S-100 protein. Cells of the epithelioid and spindle-cell hemangioendothelioma are positive for vascular endothelial markers and negative for monocytic-histiocytic markers. Hemangiopericytomas have a distinctive vascular pattern with prominent branching, staghorn vascular spaces among the spindle cells.

A benign entity to consider in the differential diagnosis is the inflammatory pseudotumor of the spleen. This condition has a prominent spindle cell component, similar to the mycobacterial spindle-cell pseudotumor, but it also shows foci of necrosis, nonspecific granulomatous changes, numerous plasma cells, and foamy macrophages, which generally are absent in the mycobacterial spindle-cell pseudotumor. Moreover, the inflammatory pseudotumor of the spleen presents as a single lesion, in contrast to the multinodular mycobacterial spindle-cell pseudotumors.

Diagnosis

Mycobacterial spindle-cell pseudotumor of the spleen.

LYMPHADENITIS WITH NECROTIZING GRANULOMAS AFTER CAT-INDUCED TRAUMA

Clinical History

The patient was a 7-year-old girl who developed a painful, enlarged, fluctuant lymph node in the left axilla at the lateral aspect of the pectoralis muscle. Otherwise, the patient was afebrile and felt well. After the lymphadenopathy persisted for 2 weeks, surgical excision of the lesion was performed. The family owned an adult cat, which had scratched her 2 weeks earlier. The scratch had been slow to heal, and the patient was treated with cephalexin. Two aspirations of the node were performed, and antibiotics were changed, but the lymph node continued to enlarge. A purified protein derivative skin test was negative at 48 hours. Finally, incisional biopsy was undertaken. Serum

TABLE 8-2. Results of Serologic Studies in a Case of Cat-Scratch Disease

Pathogen	Antibody Class	Titer
Bartonella henselae	IgG	1:1024
	IgM	1:80
Afipia felis	IgG	Less than 1:64
	IgM	Less than 1:20

IgG = immunoglobulin G; IgM = immunoglobulin M.

was sent to a reference laboratory for detection of antibodies to *Bartonella* species and *Afipia felis*.

Microbiology

One of the two aspirates yielded growth of a *Corynebacterium* species. Gram stain detected no organisms. The biopsy yielded no pathogens after culture for bacteria, mycobacteria, and fungi. Results of the serologic studies are shown in Table 8-2.

Pathologic Findings

The involved lymph nodes were hyperplastic and contained multiple granulomas that involved follicular and interfollicular areas. The granulomas were of varying size and shape. As these necrotizing granulomas enlarge, coalesce, or do both, they develop an irregular, "geographic" appearance that is referred to as *stellate necrosis* (Figure 8-20). Most lesions contained central necrosis that was composed of disintegrating, mononuclear phagocytes and polymorphonuclear neutrophils. Other granulomas contained central eosinophilic necrotic material, more closely resembling caseous necrosis (Figure 8-21). The inflammatory response extended focally through the capsule into the surrounding fat. A few clusters of short,

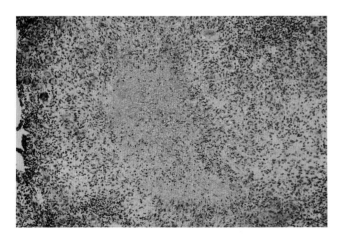

FIGURE 8-20. The normal architecture of the lymph node has been obliterated by a large, irregular (stellate) necrotizing granuloma, surrounded by extensive chronic inflammation. The differential diagnosis of such a lesion must include tuberculosis, histoplasmosis, and infections that produce typical stellate granulomas (hematoxylin and eosin stain; low-power magnification).

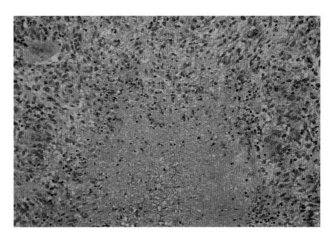

FIGURE 8-21. A higher-power view of one of the granulomas demonstrates the central necrosis and the extensive surrounding chronic infiltrate, which includes multinucleated giant cells. Portions of the periphery of this granuloma and that depicted in Figure 8-20 contain macrophages that have aligned themselves in a linear fashion around the edge of the necrosis (epithelioid cells; hematoxylin and eosin stain; medium-power magnification).

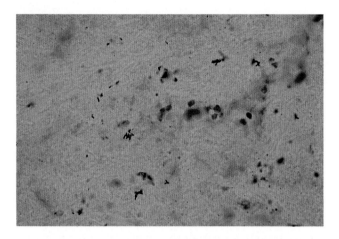

FIGURE 8-22. A cluster of bacilli is demonstrated with a Warthin-Starry stain. The morphology of the bacteria, which are thin, gram-negative bacilli when stained with Gram stain, is obscured by the deposition of silver salts (Warthin-Starry stain; high-power magnification).

plump bacilli were demonstrated with a Warthin-Starry stain (Figure 8-22); other special stains for bacteria, mycobacteria, and fungi were negative.

Comment

Cat-scratch disease has been transformed by the all-important process of establishing the etiologic agent. For decades, it was a clinical and pathologic entity that was considered likely to have an infectious cause. Cat-scratch lymphadenitis is now recognized as part of a spectrum of local and disseminated infections caused by a previously unrecognized bacterium. The discovery of the etiology began with the demonstration of bacilli in the involved lymph nodes using sensitive silver impregnation stains, such as the Warthin-Starry method. The bacteria were found most commonly adjacent to small blood vessels rather than in the center of the granulomas. Bacteria with similar morphologies were identified at the site of cat scratches and in granulomatous lesions of visceral organs.

Shortly thereafter, evidence leading to the identification of the bacterial etiology began to accumulate. An organism, subsequently identified as *A. felis*, was isolated from a patient with cat-scratch disease, but it does not appear to be an important cause of cat-scratch disease. The next clues came from very different clinical diseases. Investigators identified bacterial gene sequences in tissue of HIV-infected patients with a vasoproliferative disease known as *bacillary angiomatosis* and subsequently from a similar visceral process called *peliosis*. The DNA sequences matched most closely *Rochalimaea quintana*, the etiologic agent of trench fever. Concurrently, other investigators isolated a new bacterium from the blood of HIV-infected patients, later designated as *Rochalimaea henselae*. This spectrum of clinical disease is reminiscent of infections in South America caused by *Bartonella bacilliformis*. The two *Rochalimaea* species have now been reclassified as *Bartonella* species. A fourth pathogenic species, *Bartonella elizabethae*, has been described in a case of bacterial endocarditis, which may also be caused by *Bartonella quintana* and *B. henselae*.

B. henselae appears to be the primary cause of cat-scratch disease. A high proportion of cats are infected by this bacterium; these cats are characteristically bacteremic in the absence of clinical symptoms. The organism has been repetitively identified by PCR in involved lymph nodes and viscera, as well as in batches of the cat-scratch skin test antigen, which contains no DNA of *A. felis*. More than 90% of affected patients develop antibodies to *B. henselae*, as did this patient. The visceral granulomatous lesions have been associated with both *B. henselae* and *B. quintana*. Bacillary angiomatosis and peliosis hepatis have been most often reported in association with *B. quintana*. Bacteremia and bacteremic disease have been caused by both species.

The association of disease with cats has been known for decades. Kittens appear to be more likely to spread the infection than adult cats. Approximately two-thirds of patients recognize a previous scratch, and a residual scratch or skin papule may still be evident at the time lymphadenopathy develops. The differential diagnosis of necrotizing granulomas with stellate necrosis includes the lymphogranuloma venereum serotypes of *Chlamydia trachomatis*; *Yersinia pestis*, *Yersinia pseudotuberculosis*, and *Yersinia enterocolitica*; and *Francisella tularensis*. Although the granulomas of brucellosis are usually noncaseating, suppurative lesions have been described in the liver and spleen. Early lesions, in which only poorly delineated inflammation occurs, are followed by suppurative granulomas and ultimately caseating granulomas that resemble those of mycobacterial and fungal infection. Performing AFB stains for mycobacteria and methenamine silver stains for fungi is always prudent in the evaluation of granulomatous lesions that do not have a clearly established etiology. Bartonellae are detected much more often in the early lesions than in well-established granulomas.

Efficacy of therapy of cat-scratch disease is not well defined. Although oral erythromycin or doxycycline have been recommended for AIDS patients infected with *B. henselae*, immunocompetent patients usually recover just as soon without antimicrobial therapy. In most cases, symptomatic therapy is adequate.

Diagnosis

Cat-scratch disease.

LYMPHADENOPATHY WITH LARGE AGGREGATES OF HISTIOCYTES

Clinical History

A 36-year-old man diagnosed with AIDS 4 years previously presented with complaints of fever, malaise, nausea, and vomiting for 3 days and weight loss of 15 pounds over the preceding 2 months. Notable findings on physical examination were a temperature of 38°C, generalized lymphadenopathy, hepatosplenomegaly, and scleral icterus. Pertinent laboratory test results revealed pancytopenia, prolonged prothrombin and partial thromboplastin times, and elevated serum bilirubin and alkaline phosphatase levels. Blood was collected for bacterial, mycobacterial, and fungal cultures. Endoscopic studies of the upper gastrointestinal tract revealed multiple small mucosal erosions in the esophagus, stomach, and duodenum. Histologic examination of biopsies of these lesions showed aggregates of histiocytes filled with AFB in the lamina propria. Therapy for presumed disseminated MAC disease was begun, and he was discharged from the hospital.

He was admitted 2 months later for altered mental status and seizures. Cerebrospinal fluid and blood were submitted for bacterial, mycobacterial, and fungal cultures, and empiric broad-spectrum antimicrobial therapy was begun. He continued to deteriorate, however, and died 10 days after admission.

Pathologic Findings

At autopsy, marked enlargement of the abdominal and thoracic lymph nodes, spleen (weight, 1,230 g), and liver (weight, 3,120 g) was evident. The lymph nodes were rubbery; on cut section, some demonstrated foci of necrosis. Histologically, the normal parenchyma was replaced almost completely by sheets of histiocytes with granular cytoplasm (Figure 8-23A). Sections stained by the Ziehl-Neelsen method showed numerous AFB within the histiocyte cytoplasm (Figure 8-23B). In addition, foci of caseous necrosis surrounded by histiocytes and Langhans' giant cells were evident. In both the liver and spleen, several miliary nodules, shown histologically to be composed of aggregates of histiocytes filled with AFB, were present throughout the parenchyma. Histiocytes laden with AFB also were present in the lamina propria and submucosal region of the small intestine and appendix, lungs, and bone marrow. Additionally, the patient had disseminated cytomegalovirus infection involving the gastrointestinal tract, lungs, kidneys, adrenal glands, and testes.

Differential Diagnoses

The histologic findings in H and E–stained sections suggest a disseminated mycobacterial infection or dissemi-

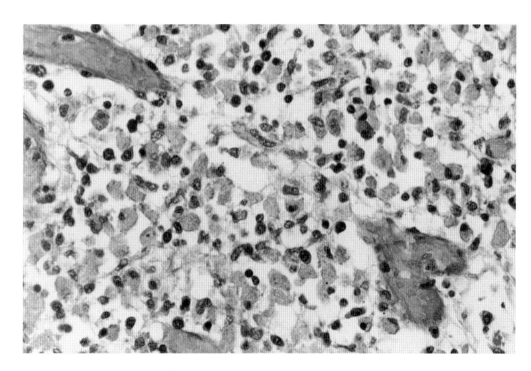

FIGURE 8-23A. Section of an enlarged retroperitoneal lymph node from an acquired immunodeficiency syndrome patient with disseminated *Mycobacterium genavense* infection shows effacement of the normal architecture by a diffuse infiltrate of histiocytes (hematoxylin and eosin stain; original magnification, ×100).

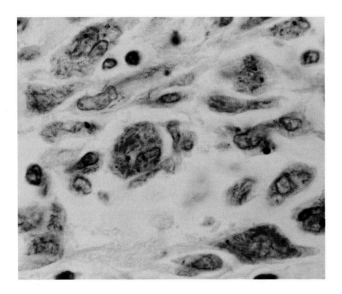

FIGURE 8-23B. Acid-fast stain of the section illustrated in **A** shows numerous acid-fast bacilli within the histiocyte cytoplasm (Ziehl-Neelsen stain; original magnification, ×250).

nated histoplasmosis, although if *H. capsulatum* were the responsible pathogen, yeast cells would likely have been visible in H and E–stained sections. In Whipple's disease (see Chapter 3), lymph nodes may show clusters (not a diffuse infiltrate) of histiocytes with pale cytoplasm, but noncaseating granulomas also are present. Moreover, the clinical history of this patient is not consistent with the diagnosis of Whipple's disease. Based on the most likely

differential diagnoses, stains for AFB and fungi should be performed. In this case, Ziehl-Neelsen staining confirmed infection with a mycobacterium. Mycobacteria that are associated with aggregates of histiocyte include MAC, *Mycobacterium genavense*, and *Mycobacterium leprae* in cases of lepromatous leprosy (see Chapter 5).

Microbiology

After approximately 8 weeks of incubation, both premortem mycobacterial blood cultures grew a mycobacterium, based on the presence of AFB in smears prepared from the culture broth and stained by a Kinyoun carbol fuchsin stain. Attempts to recover the mycobacterium by subculturing the broth to a solid medium, however, were unsuccessful.

Comment

In a patient with AIDS, MAC is the most common cause of disseminated mycobacterial infection. The inflammatory response most commonly seen in such cases is a diffuse infiltrate of histiocytes, although MAC infection also may be associated with mature granulomas or a diffuse infiltrate composed predominantly of giant cells with admixed mononucleate histiocytes (Figure 8-24). In addition to MAC, *M. genavense* causes clinical manifestations identical to those of disseminated MAC infection, and the associated inflammatory response almost always is diffuse infiltrates of histiocytes. Identification of the responsible mycobacterium requires mycobacterial culture.

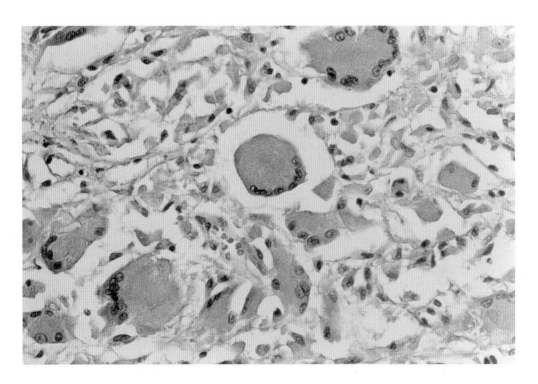

FIGURE 8-24. Section of lymph node from an acquired immunodeficiency syndrome patient with disseminated infection with *Mycobacterium avium* complex shows effacement of the normal architecture by a diffuse infiltrate of multinucleate giant cells admixed with mononuclear histiocytes (hematoxylin and eosin stain; original magnification, ×100).

M. genavense is a recently characterized, nontuberculous mycobacterium that uncommonly causes disease in severely immunocompromised patients with AIDS. Patients typically present with a syndrome of fever, anorexia, weight loss, abdominal pain, diarrhea, splenomegaly, and anemia. No uniformly accepted chemotherapeutic regimen exists, although most have included a macrolide. Survival after therapy has ranged from 2 months to over 1 year. It is difficult, however, to assess how infection with *M. genavense* contributes to a shortened life span, because most persons infected with this organism have other opportunistic infections as well.

In patients who have died with disseminated *M. genavense*, autopsy has shown massive involvement of the small intestine, spleen, liver, and abdominal lymph nodes, as occurred in this patient. The small intestine typically has a coarsened mucosal surface due to a marked infiltrate of granular histiocytes filled with AFB in the mucosa. The spleen and liver are enlarged and contain variably-sized nodules composed of large aggregates of granular histiocytes; focal spindle-cell proliferations may be present in the spleen. In involved lymph nodes, the normal tissue is replaced by granular histiocytes with numerous AFB in their cytoplasm.

Small aggregates of histiocytes often are present in the bone marrow.

Based on the described findings, a diagnosis of disseminated mycobacterial infection is possible. Microbiologic studies, however, are needed to determine the specific pathogen. Premortem, mycobacterial broth cultures of blood and bone marrow are useful for diagnosis; postmortem, involved tissue should be cultured. *M. genavense* tends to grow more slowly than the more commonly encountered mycobacteria, and it does not grow on the solid media generally used for mycobacterial culture. Therefore, if this is a suspected pathogen, specimens must be inoculated into a broth medium (e.g., BACTEC 13A or 12B), and cultures should be incubated for up to 10 weeks. *M. genavense* should be suspected when growth of AFB is detected in the broth medium but no organism is recovered in subcultures to a solid medium. Definitive identification requires 16S rRNA gene sequencing, which is available only in certain research laboratories.

Diagnosis

Disseminated mycobacterial infection in a patient with AIDS, most likely due to *M. genavense*.

POSTOPERATIVE ILLNESS WITH RECURRENT CARDIORESPIRATORY MANIFESTATIONS

Clinical History

A 54-year-old man, who had been discharged 4 days earlier, after a prolonged hospitalization during which time he underwent small bowel resection and repair of small bowel fistulae that occurred secondary to a gunshot wound, was readmitted for evaluation of acute onset of fever and chills. His white blood cell count was elevated, and a chest radiograph showed a left pleural effusion. The initial diagnosis was pneumonia, for which he was treated with broad-spectrum antimicrobial agents. He also underwent thoracentesis, which removed 2,500 cells per µl of serosanguinous fluid. Over the following few weeks, his condition improved, with the exception of the development of a large sacral decubitus ulcer that required surgical débridement.

On hospital day 34, the patient again became febrile. His white blood cell count rose to 28,200 cells per µl. Blood and sputum were submitted for bacterial culture, and empiric broad-spectrum antimicrobial agents were initiated. He developed respiratory distress requiring intubation and mechanical ventilation. Despite aggressive supportive therapy, his condition deteriorated, and he died on day 46 of hospitalization.

Pathologic Findings

At autopsy, the heart weighed 400 g. Small abscesses were present on the epicardial surface and in the subendocardium of the left ventricle (Figure 8-25), and microabscesses were observed in the interventricular septum (Figure 8-26). On the mitral valve, there was a 3 cm × 1 cm friable, brown vegetation at the site of perforation and destruction of the underlying mitral valve leaflet (Figure 8-27). Histologically, the valvular architecture was destroyed and replaced by fibrin, cellular debris, and clusters of gram-positive cocci (Figure 8-28). In addition to the findings in the heart, metastatic abscesses and septic infarcts in the liver, spleen, kidneys, brain, adrenal glands, pancreas, and thyroid gland were present.

Differential Diagnoses

The differential diagnoses include organisms that typically cause acute infective endocarditis: *Staphylococcus aureus, Streptococcus pneumoniae,* group B streptococci, *Streptococcus anginosus,* facultative gram-negative bacilli, *Pseudomonas aeruginosa,* and fungi. Of these, *S. aureus* is responsible for most cases of acute infective endo-

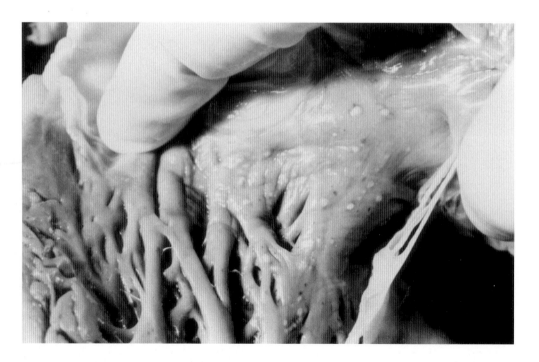

FIGURE 8-25. Photograph of the left ventricle of a patient who died of *Staphylococcus aureus* infective endocarditis shows multiple myocardial abscesses.

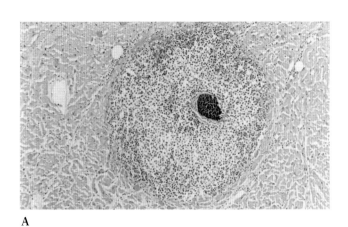

A

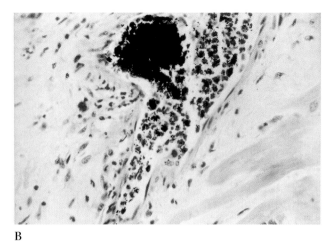

B

FIGURE 8-26. (A) Section of the left ventricle of the heart illustrated in Figure 8-25 shows a well-circumscribed aggregate of neutrophils surrounding a microcolony of bacteria (hematoxylin and eosin stain; original magnification, ×25). (B) Tissue Gram stain of a section of the left ventricle illustrated in A shows an infiltrate of neutrophils and a microcolony of gram-positive cocci within a small blood vessel (Brown-Hopps stain; original magnification, ×250).

FIGURE 8-27. Photograph of the mitral valve of the heart illustrated in Figure 8-25 shows a large vegetation and perforation of the valve leaflet.

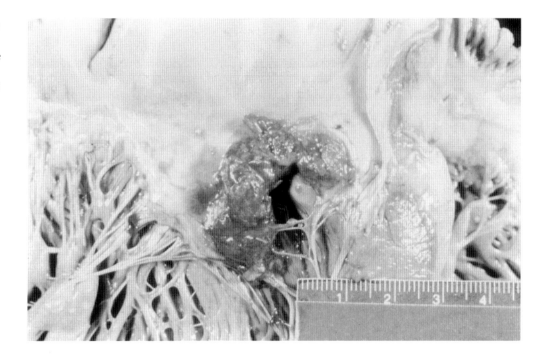

carditis. The first four organisms listed are gram-positive cocci, which were visualized in the valve tissue and microabscesses.

Microbiology

Premortem cultures of blood grew *S. aureus*.

Comment

Infective endocarditis is estimated to account for approximately 1 case per 1,000 hospital admissions. More than half of patients with infective endocarditis are older than age 50; the disease is uncommon in children. The mean age for men is 6–7 years older than that for women, and men are more commonly affected. The heart valve involved by the infection varies in each published series, ranging from 28% to 45% for the mitral valve, 5% to 36% for the aortic valve alone, and 0% to 35% for both aortic and mitral valves. The tricuspid valve is involved in only 0–6% of cases, and the pulmonic valve even less often (<1%). Virtually any type of structural disease predisposes to infective endocarditis, including rheumatic heart disease and various congenital heart diseases.

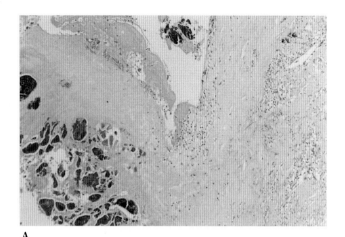

A

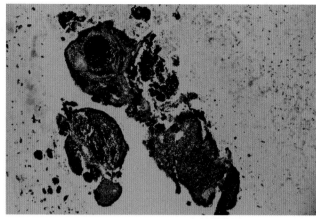

B

FIGURE 8-28. (A) Section of the mitral valve of the heart illustrated in Figure 8-25 shows many microcolonies of bacteria admixed with fibrin and necrotic debris on the external surface and minimal inflammation, predominantly in the area adjacent to the myocardium (hematoxylin and eosin stain; original magnification, ×25). (B) Tissue Gram stain of a section of the mitral valve illustrated in A shows microcolonies of gram-positive cocci on the valve surface (Brown-Hopps stain; original magnification, ×250).

Degenerative lesions, such as calcified mitral annulus, calcific nodular lesions secondary to arteriosclerotic cardiovascular disease, and postmyocardial infarction thrombus, which are most common in patients older than age 60 years, are important in the 30–40% of patients who have no demonstrable underlying valvular disease. Other conditions, such as syphilitic heart disease, arteriovenous fistulas, hemodialysis shunts or fistulas, intracardiac pacemaker wires, and intracardiac prostheses, also may predispose to endocarditis.

Staphylococci account for 20–30% of cases of infective endocarditis, of which 80–90% are due to *S. aureus*, the pathogen in this case. *S. aureus* attacks apparently normal valves in approximately one-third of endocarditis patients. The illness often is fulminant with widespread metastatic infection, resulting in death of the patient in approximately 40% of cases. Myocardial abscesses, purulent pericarditis, and valve ring abscesses are more common in *S. aureus* endocarditis than in infections caused by other organisms. Metastatic abscesses and septic infarcts involving the brain, kidney, spleen, lung, and other organs occur in more than 40% of patients with *S. aureus* endocarditis, including this patient. The mortality rate often exceeds 50% in patients older than age 50 years, particularly when the infection is nosocomially acquired.

Diagnosis

S. aureus infective endocarditis with metastatic abscesses and septic infarcts involving many peripheral organs.

RECOMMENDED READING

General

Abarca M, Garcia-Diaz JD. Significance of granulomas in bone marrow: a study of 40 cases. Eur J Haematol 1988;41:12.

Nichols L, Florentine B, Lewis W, et al. Bone marrow examination for the diagnosis of mycobacterial and fungal infections in the acquired immunodeficiency syndrome. Arch Pathol Lab Med 1991; 115:1125.

Malaria

Braunstein H, Tull ME. Detection of malarial parasites in routine Wright-stained blood smears. Am J Clin Pathol 1980;74:227.

Caraballo A, Ache A. The evaluation of a dipstick test for *Plasmodium falciparum* in mining areas of Venezuela. Am J Trop Med Hyg 1996;5:482.

Connor DH, Neafie RC, Hockmeyer WT. Malaria. In CH Binford, DH Connor (eds), Pathology of Tropical and Extraordinary Diseases. Vol. 1. Washington, DC: Armed Forces Institute of Pathology, 1976;273.

Craig MH, Sharp BL. Comparative evaluation of four techniques for the diagnosis of *Plasmodium falciparum* infections. Trans R Soc Trop Med Hyg 1997; 91:279.

Singh N, Singh MP, Sharma VP. The use of a dipstick antigen-capture assay for the diagnosis of *Plasmodium falciparum* infection in a remote forested area of central India. Am J Trop Med Hyg 1997; 56:188.

Weiss JB. DNA probes and PCR for diagnosis of parasitic infections. Clin Microbiol Rev 1995;8:113.

Babesiosis

Falagas ME, Klempner MS. Babesiosis in patients with AIDS: a chronic infection presenting as fever of unknown origin. Clin Infect Dis 1996;22:809.

Herwaldt BL, Springs FE, Roberts PP, et al. Babesiosis in Wisconsin: a potentially fatal disease. Am J Trop Med Hyg 1995;53:146.

Meldrum SC, Birkhead GS, White DJ, et al. Human babesiosis in New York state: an epidemiological description of 136 cases. Clin Infect Dis 1992; 15:1019.

Persing DH, Herwaldt BL, Glaser C, et al. Infection with a babesia-like organism in northern California. N Engl J Med 1995;332:298.

Quick RE, Herwaldt BL, Thomford JW, et al. Babesiosis in Washington state: a new species of *Babesia*? Ann Intern Med 1993;119:284.

Tick-Borne Relapsing Fever

Boyer KM, Munford RS, Maupin GO, et al. Tick-borne relapsing fever: an interstate outbreak originating at Grand Canyon National Park. Am J Epidemiol 1977;105:469.

Dupont HT, La Scola B, Williams R, Raoult D. A focus of tick-borne relapsing fever in Southern Zaire. Clin Infect Dis 1997;25:139.

Horton JM, Blaser MJ. The spectrum of relapsing fever in the Rocky Mountains. Arch Intern Med 1985;145:871.

Le CT. Tick-borne relapsing fever in children. Pediatrics 1980;66:963.

Rawlings JA. An overview of tick-borne relapsing fever with emphasis on outbreaks in Texas. Texas Med 1995;91:56.

Southern PM Jr, Sanford JP. Relapsing fever. A clinical and microbiological review. Medicine 1969;48:129.

Parvovirus B19

Schwarz TF, Nerlich A, Hottentrager B, et al. Parvovirus B19 infection of the fetus histology and in situ hybridization. Am J Clin Pathol 1991;96:121.

Human Monocytotropic Ehrlichiosis

Barenfanger J, Patel PG, Dumler JS, Walker DH. Identifying human ehrlichiosis. Lab Med 1996;27:372.

Dumler JS, Dawson JE, Walker DH. Human ehrlichiosis: hematopathology and immunohistologic detection of *Ehrlichia chaffeensis*. Human Pathol 1993;24:391.

Everett ED, Evans KA, Henry RB, McDonald G. Human ehrlichiosis in adults after tick exposure. Diagnosis using polymerase chain reaction. Ann Intern Med 1994;120:730.

Fishbein DB, Dawson JE, Robinson LE. Human ehrlichiosis in the United States, 1985 to 1990. Ann Intern Med 1994;120:736.

Ratnasamy N, Everett ED, Roland WE, et al. Central nervous system manifestations of human ehrlichiosis. Clin Infect Dis 1996;23:314.

Walker DH, Dumler JS. Human monocytic and granulocytic ehrlichiosis. Discovery and diagnosis of emerging tick-borne infections and the critical role of the pathologist. Arch Pathol Lab Med 1997;121:785.

Histoplasma capsulatum

Sarosi GA, Johnson PC. Disseminated histoplasmosis in patients infected with human immunodeficiency virus. Clin Infect Dis 1992;14(suppl 1):S60–S67.

Wheat LJ, Connolly-Stringfield PA, Baker RL, et al. Disseminated histoplasmosis in the acquired immune deficiency syndrome: clinical findings, diagnosis and treatment, and review of the literature. Medicine 1990;69:361.

Human Granulocytotropic Ehrlichiosis

Aguero-Rosenfeld ME, Horowitz HW, Wormser GP, et al. Human granulocytic ehrlichiosis: a case series from a medical center in New York State. Ann Intern Med 1996;125:904.

Bakken JS, Krueth J, Wilson-Nordskog C, et al. Clinical and laboratory characteristics of human granulocytic ehrlichiosis. JAMA 1996;275:199.

Chen S-M, Dumler JS, Bakken JS, Walker DH. Identification of a granulocytotropic Ehrlichia species as the etiologic agent of human disease. J Clin Microbiol 1994;32:589.

Roland WE, McDonald G, Caldwell CW, Everett ED. Ehrlichiosis—a cause of prolonged fever. Clin Infect Dis 1995;20:821.

Walker DH, Dumler JS. Emergence of the ehrlichioses as human health problems. Emerg Infect Dis 1996;2:18.

Brucellosis

Al-Eissa YA, Kambal AM, Al-Nasser MN, et al. Childhood brucellosis—A study of 102 cases. Pediatr Infect Dis 1990;9:74.

Blankenship RM, Sanford JP. Brucella canis: a cause of undulant fever. Am J Med 1975;59:424.

Buchanan TM, Faber LC, Feldman RA. Brucellosis in the United States 1960–1972. An abattoir-associated disease. Part 1. Clinical features and therapy. Medicine (Baltimore) 1974;53:403.

Hunt AC, Bothwell PW. Histological findings in human brucellosis. J Clin Pathol 1967;20:267.

Schirger A, Nichols DR, Martin WJ, et al. Brucellosis—Experience with 224 patients. Ann Intern Med 1960;52:827.

Spink WW, Hoffbauer FW, Walker WW, Green RA. Histopathology of the liver in human brucellosis. J Lab Clin Med 1949;34:40.

Wise RI. Brucellosis in the United States. Past, present and future. JAMA 1980;244:2318.

Young EJ. Human brucellosis. Rev Infect Dis 1983;5:821.

Mycobacteria

Bessesen MT, Shlay J, Stone-Venohr B, et al. Disseminated Mycobacterium genavense infection: clinical and microbiological features and response to therapy. AIDS 1993;7:1357.

Gaynor CD, Clark RA, Koontz FP, et al. Disseminated Mycobacterium genavense infection in two patients with AIDS. Clin Infect Dis 1994;18:455.

Hill AR, Premkumar S, Brustein S, et al. Disseminated tuberculosis in the acquired immunodeficiency syndrome era. Am Rev Respir Dis 1991;144:1164.

Kumar S, Kumar D, Cowan DF. Mycobacterial spindle cell pseudotumor of the spleen. Am J Clin Pathol 1994;102:863.

Maschek H, Georgil A, Schmidt RE, et al. Mycobacterium genavense autopsy findings in three patients. Am J Clin Pathol 1994;101:95.

Nadal D, Caduff R, Kraft R, et al. Invasive infection with Mycobacterium genavense in three children with the acquired immunodeficiency syndrome. Eur J Clin Microbiol Infect Dis 1993;12:37.

Suster S, Moran CA, Blanco M. Mycobacterial spindle-cell pseudotumor of the spleen. Am J Clin Pathol 1994;101:539.

Tortoli E, Simonetti MT, Dionisio D, Meli M. Cultural studies on two isolates of Mycobacterium genavense from patients with acquired immunodeficiency syndrome. Diagn Microbiol Infect Dis 1994;18:7.

Wolf DA, Wu CD, Medeiros LJ. Mycobacterial pseudotumors of lymph node. A report of two cases diagnosed at the time of intraoperative consultation using touch imprint preparations. Arch Pathol Lab Med 1995;119:811.

Cat-Scratch Disease

Delahoussaye PM, Osborne BM. Cat-scratch disease presenting as abdominal visceral granulomas. J Infect Dis 1990;161:71.

English CK, Wear DJ, Margileth AM, et al. Cat-scratch disease: isolation and culture of the bacterial agent. JAMA 1988;259:1347.

Margileth AM, Hayden GF. Cat scratch disease. N Engl J Med 1993;329:53–54.

Margileth AM, Wear DJ, English CK. Systemic cat scratch disease: report of 23 patients with prolonged or recurrent severe bacterial infection. J Infect Dis 1987;155:390–402.

Maurin M, Raoult D. Bartonella (Rochalimaea) quintana infections. Clin Microbiol Rev 1996;9:273.

Miller-Catchpole R, Variakojis D, Vardiman JW, et al. Cat scratch disease. Identification of bacteria in seven cases of lymphadenitis. Am J Surg Pathol 1986;10:276.

Schwartzman WA. Infections due to Rochalimaea: the expanding clinical spectrum. Clin Infect Dis 1992;15:893.

Stastny JF, Wakely PE Jr, Frable WJ. Cytologic features of necrotizing granulomatous inflammation consistent with cat-scratch disease. Diagn Cytopathol 1996;15:108.

van den Oord JJ, de Wolf Peeters C, Desmet VJ. Cellular composition of suppurative granulomas: an immunohistochemical study of suppurative granulomatous lymphadenitis. Human Pathol 1985;16:1009.

Zangwill KM, Hamilton DH, Perkins BA, et al. Cat scratch disease in Connecticut—epidemiology, risk factors, and evaluation of a new diagnostic test. N Engl J Med 1993;329:8.

Endocarditis

Bayer AS. Infective endocarditis. Clin Infect Dis 1993; 17:313.

Bayer AS, Theofilopoulos AN. Immunopathogenetic aspects of infective endocarditis. Chest 1990;97:204.

Viral Cytopathic Effects

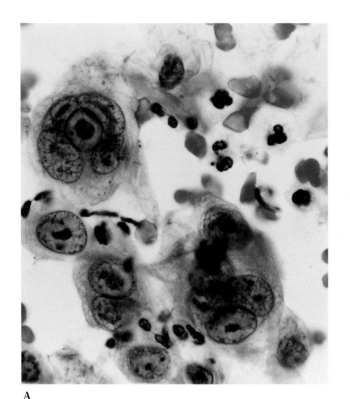

FIGURE A-1. (**A**) Cervical Papanicolaou smear shows characteristic cytopathic effects induced by infection with herpes simplex virus (HSV; changes induced by varicella-zoster virus [VZV] are identical, but VZV is a rare pathogen in the endocervix): multinucleated squamous epithelial cells, molding of the nuclei against each other, and a prominent, dense intranuclear inclusion surrounded by a clear zone and clumped nuclear chromatin at the margin (Papanicolaou stain; original magnification, ×250). (**B**) Section of esophagus illustrates HSV cytopathic effects in tissue (diagnosis in this case was confirmed by recovery of HSV type 1 in viral culture). Multinucleate giant cells and nuclear molding are present. Instead of the dense intranuclear inclusions present in the infected endocervical cells, the infected cells in this esophagus have an intranuclear inclusion that has a ground-glass appearance and fills the nucleus, pushing the chromatin to the margin (hematoxylin and eosin stain; original magnification, ×100).

A

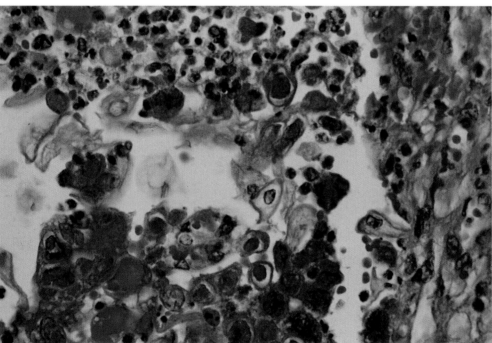

B

FIGURE A-2. (**A**) Smear of bronchial epithelial cells collected by brushing shows viral cytopathic effects that are typical of infection with a herpes virus. The nuclei are enlarged, peripheral margination of the chromatin is evident, and prominent Cowdry type A intranuclear inclusions are present. The viral culture grew varicella-zoster virus (Papanicolaou stain; original magnification, ×250). (**B**) Section of skin from a patient with zoster shows intraepithelial bullae, at the periphery of which are many epithelial cells with intranuclear inclusions (as described for herpes simplex virus; hematoxylin and eosin stain; original magnification, ×100).

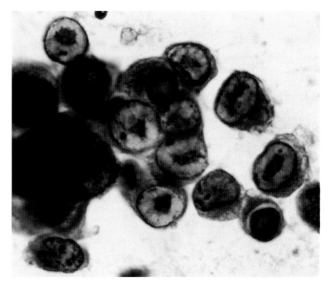

A

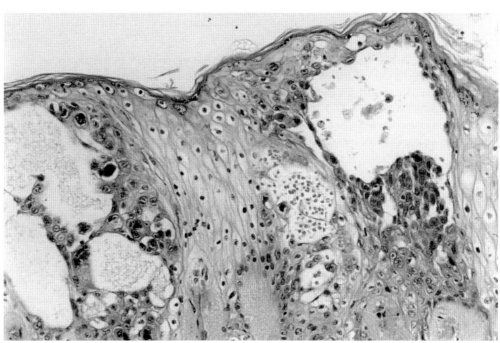

B

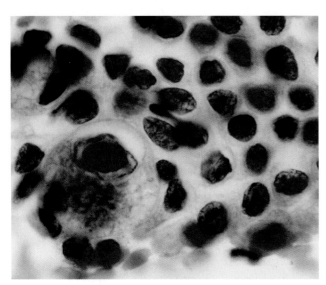

A

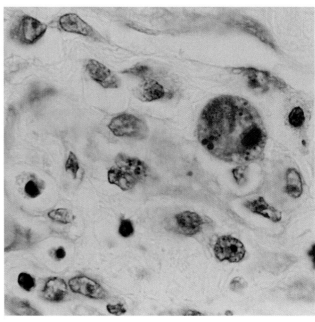

B

FIGURE A-3. (**A**) Cervical Papanicolaou smear shows characteristic cytopathic effects associated with infection with cytomegalovirus (CMV): enlargement of the virus-infected cell; a prominent large, oval intranuclear inclusion with peripheral margination of the nuclear chromatin, producing a clear space or halo around the inclusion; and less–well-defined granular intracytoplasmic inclusions (Papanicolaou stain; original magnification, ×250). (**B**) Section of an ulcer of the small intestine shows an enlarged endothelial cell that demonstrates characteristics of CMV cytopathic effects—a large oval intranuclear inclusion and many smaller, round intracytoplasmic inclusions (hematoxylin and eosin stain; original magnification, ×250).

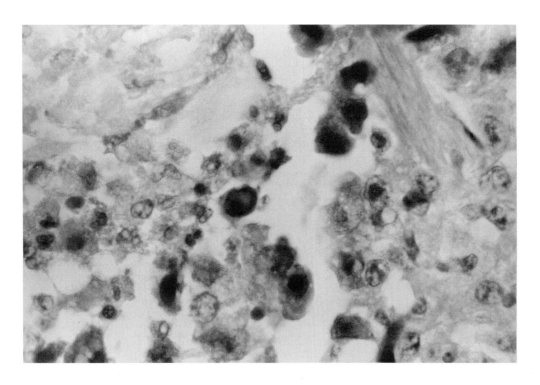

FIGURE A-4. Section of lung shows the cytopathic effects typical of infection with adenovirus. The infected alveolar epithelial cells are only moderately enlarged or of normal size, and they have either large, discrete intranuclear inclusions (early infection) or diffuse, smudgy inclusions (late infection) and a thin rim of cytoplasm (hematoxylin and eosin stain; original magnification, ×250).

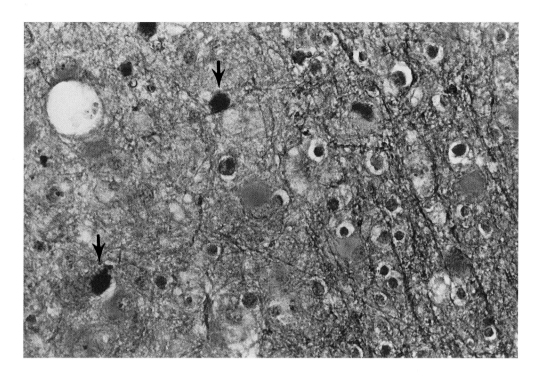

FIGURE A-5. Section of brain from a patient with progressive multifocal leukoencephalopathy shows the typical cytopathic effects induced by infection with JC virus. Infected oligodendrogliocytes are enlarged and have prominent, homogeneous intranuclear inclusions (*arrows*). Other findings include extensive demyelination; enlarged, reactive astrocytes; and phagocytosis of myelin by macrophages (Luxol Fast Blue stain; original magnification, ×100).

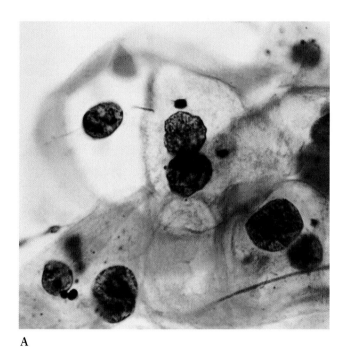

A

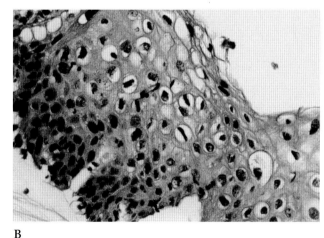

B

FIGURE A-6. (**A**) Cervical Papanicolaou smear shows the typical cytopathic effects induced by infection with human papillomavirus (HPV). A few binucleate cells are present, and the nuclei are slightly enlarged, hyperchromatic, and surrounded by a well-demarcated perinuclear clear space (Papanicolaou stain; original magnification, ×250). (**B**) Section of a cervical biopsy specimen illustrates the cytopathic effects characteristic of HPV infection: koilocytotic atypia of the squamous epithelial cells characterized by enlarged, hyperchromatic nuclei with smudged nuclear chromatin and the presence of large, well-demarcated perinuclear clear spaces (hematoxylin and eosin stain; original magnification, ×100).

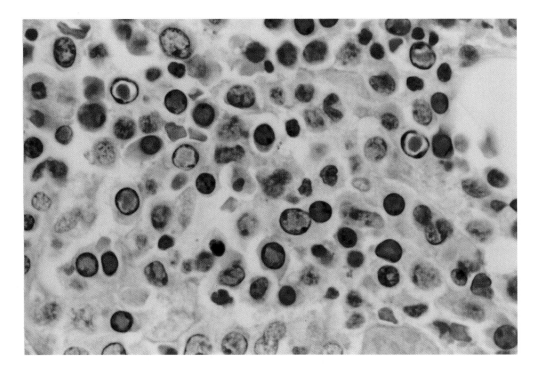

FIGURE A-7. Section of bone marrow illustrates the cytopathic effects characteristic of infection of erythroid precursors with parvovirus B19. Infected erythroid cells are enlarged and have prominent intranuclear inclusions and peripheral margination of the chromatin (hematoxylin and eosin stain; original magnification, ×250).

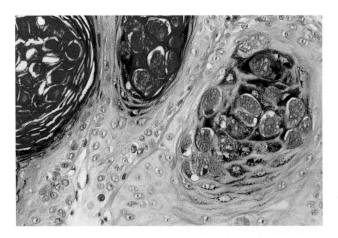

FIGURE A-8. Section of lip shows the cytopathic effects typical of infection with molluscum contagiosum virus. The squamous epithelial cells are enlarged and contain an acidophilic intracytoplasmic granular mass (the molluscum body) that almost fills the entire cell (hematoxylin and eosin stain; original magnification, ×50).

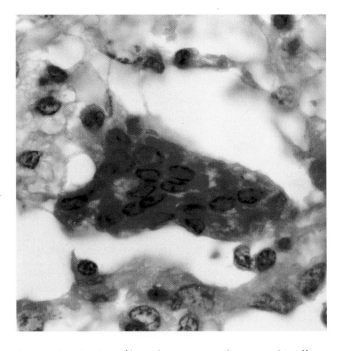

FIGURE A-9. Section of lung demonstrates the cytopathic effects typical of infection with measles virus: multinucleate giant cells with prominent intranuclear and intracytoplasmic inclusions (hematoxylin and eosin stain; original magnification, ×250).

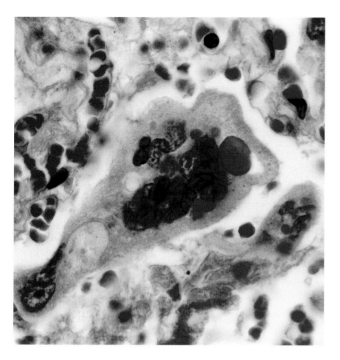

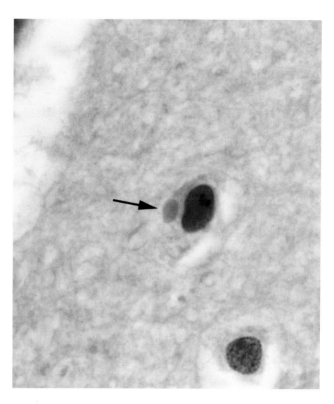

FIGURE A-10. Section of lung from an immunocompromised patient shows the cytopathic effects induced by prolonged infection with respiratory syncytial virus (i.e., multinucleate giant cells with prominent pink intracytoplasmic inclusions; hematoxylin and eosin stain; original magnification, ×250). These findings, however, are not usual. In immunocompetent patients, inclusions are rare; when they are present, they are found in the cytoplasm of epithelial cells, often in a paranuclear location, and are smaller and less prominent than those illustrated here.

FIGURE A-11. Section of brain illustrates the cytopathic effect typical of infection with rabies virus. The infected neuron has a well-defined eosinophilic, round to oblong intracytoplasmic inclusion (Negri body) 2–10 μm with internal basophilic stippling (*arrow*; hematoxylin and eosin stain; original magnification, ×250).

APPENDIX
B

Appearance of Bacteria in Smears and Tissue

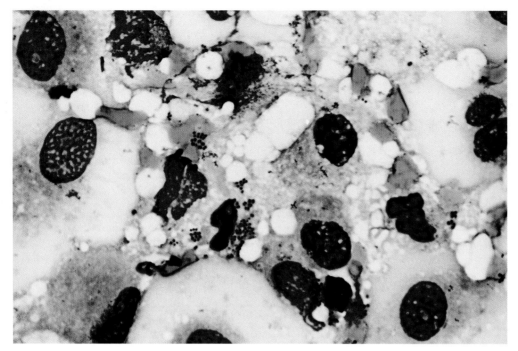

A

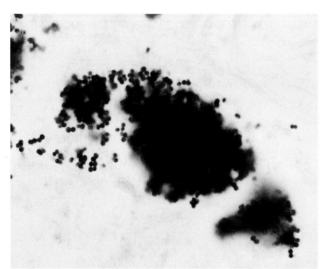

B

FIGURE B-1. (**A**) Cytocentrifuge preparation of cells collected by bronchoalveolar lavage shows macrophages, neutrophils, and clusters of bacterial cocci. Culture grew *Staphylococcus aureus*. (Giemsa stain; original magnification, ×250). (**B**) Section of kidney stained with a tissue Gram stain illustrates gram-positive cocci in pairs and clusters. Blood culture grew *S. aureus*. (Brown-Brenn modification of the tissue Gram stain; original magnification, ×250).

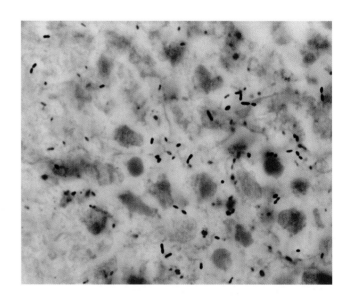

FIGURE B-2. Section of lung stained with a tissue Gram stain shows many gram-positive diplococci, some of which appear more elongated or lancet-shaped than coccoid (Gram-Weigert method; original magnification, ×250). The appearance of these bacteria is very suggestive of *Streptococcus pneumoniae*, which was recovered from blood cultures in this case; however, definitive differentiation from diphtheroid bacilli and *Rhodococcus* (shown in Figure B-3) may be difficult.

FIGURE B-3. (**A**) Cytocentrifuge preparation of cells collected by bronchoalveolar lavage shows histiocytes that have gram-positive coccobacillary organisms within their cytoplasm (Gram-Weigert method; original magnification, ×250). Culture grew *Rhodococcus equi*. (**B**) Section of lung from the same patient shows numerous gram-positive cocci and coccobacilli of *R. equi* within the cytoplasm of histiocytes (Gram-Weigert method; original magnification, ×250).

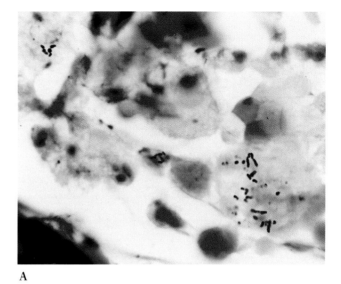

A

B

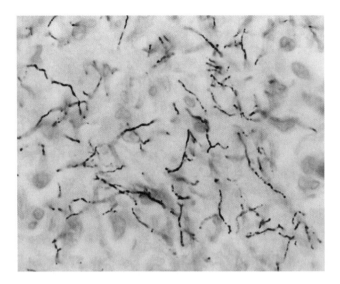

FIGURE B-4. Section of lung stained with a tissue Gram stain shows many narrow, branching, beaded filamentous gram-positive bacilli (Gram-Weigert method; original magnification, ×250). This feature is characteristic of *Nocardia* species; *Nocardia asteroides*, which is the most common human nocardial pathogen, was cultured from lung tissue.

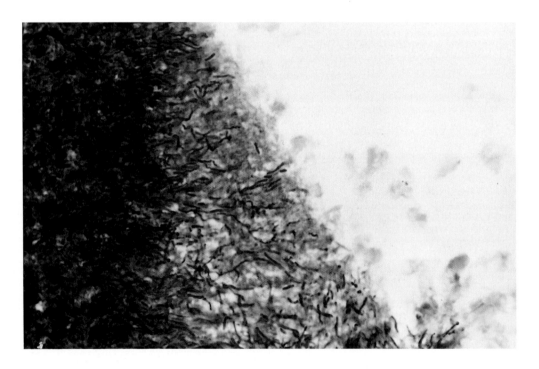

FIGURE B-5. Section of lung stained with a tissue Gram stain shows a typical bacterial sulfur granule. *Actinomyces* species was recovered in the bacterial culture (Gram-Weigert method; original magnification, ×250). Slender, branching, beaded gram-positive bacilli radiate toward the periphery of the granule.

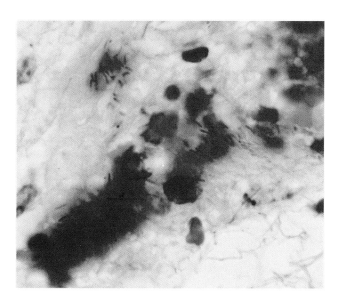

FIGURE B-6. Section of lung stained with a tissue Gram stain shows many long, gram-negative bacilli. *Pseudomonas aeruginosa* was recovered by bacterial culture (Brown-Hopps stain; original magnification, ×250).

FIGURE B-7. Section of a cutaneous ulcer from a patient with granuloma inguinale shows a mixed inflammatory infiltrate composed of neutrophils, plasma cells, and histiocytes with numerous short bacilli (*Calymmatobacterium granulomatis*; Donovan bodies) in their cytoplasm (hematoxylin and eosin stain; original magnification, ×250).

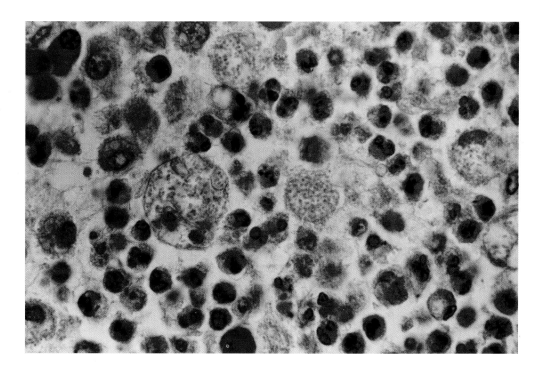

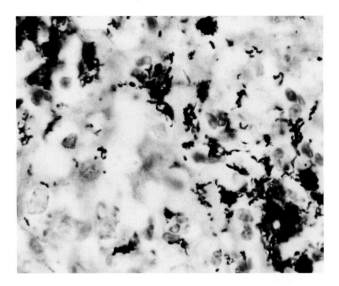

FIGURE B-8. Section of a lymph node stained by the Warthin-Starry method shows many small, pleomorphic coccobacilli within an area of necrosis, characteristic of *Bartonella henselae*, the principal agent of cat-scratch disease (Warthin-Starry stain; original magnification, ×250). In this patient, the diagnosis of cat-scratch disease was based on clinical manifestations, characteristic histologic findings, and results of serologic tests for *B. henselae*; culture was not performed and is not required for diagnosis.

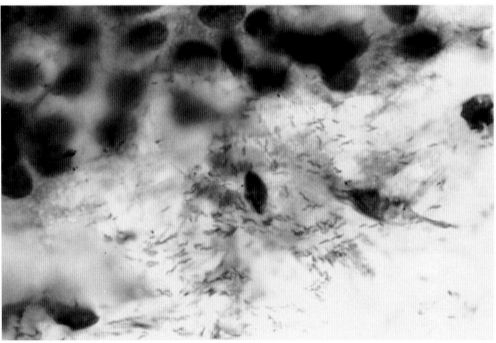

A

FIGURE B-9. (**A**) A smear of cells from a gastric brushing demonstrates numerous, spiral bacilli within the mucous layer covering the gastric epithelial cells (Papanicolaou smear; original magnification, ×250). These features are characteristic of *Helicobacter pylori* infection.

FIGURE B-9. *Continued.* (**B**) Section of a gastric biopsy specimen shows many curved and S-shaped bacilli, characteristic of *H. pylori*, within the mucous layer on the surface of and between the gastric epithelial cells (hematoxylin and eosin stain; original magnification, ×250). (**C**) Although bacilli of *H. pylori* can be seen in sections stained with hematoxylin and eosin, they often are more easily identified in sections stained with a silver impregnation stain, such as the Steiner stain (Steiner stain; original magnification, ×250).

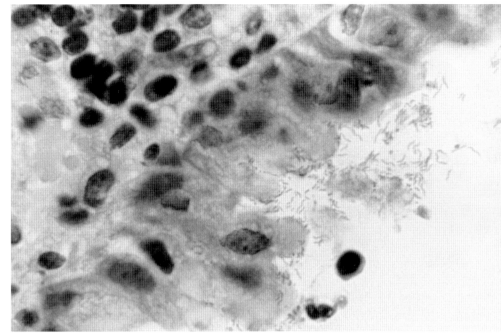

B

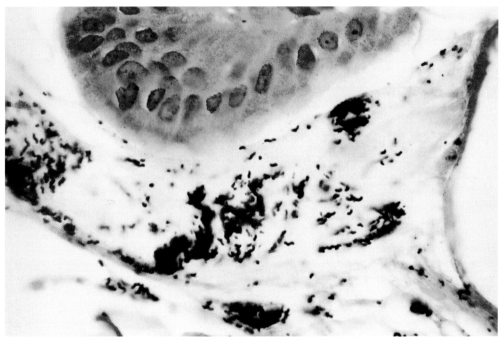

C

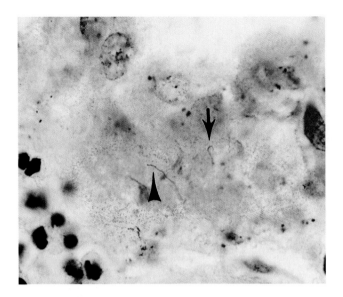

FIGURE B-10. Section of kidney from a patient with leptospirosis (diagnosed based on results of serologic tests)
demonstrates spirochetes of *Leptospira*, which characteristically have curved or hooked ends (*arrow*), are more tightly
coiled (*arrowhead*) than spirochetes of *Treponema pallidum*,
and appear granular rather than wavy (Warthin-Starry stain;
original magnification, ×250).

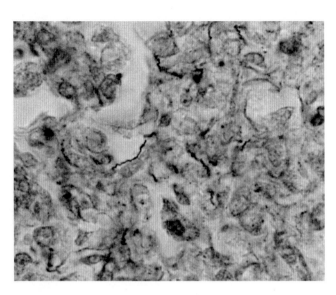

FIGURE B-11. Section of lung from a neonate with congenital
syphilis demonstrates the thin, coiled spirochetes of *Treponema
pallidum* (Steiner stain; original magnification, ×250).

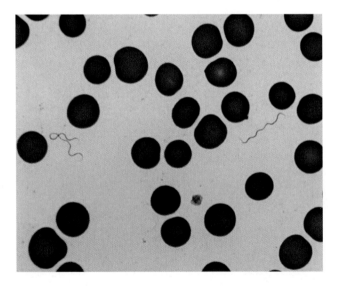

FIGURE B-12. Smear of peripheral blood from a patient with
relapsing fever shows spirochetes of *Borrelia* species
(Romanovsky stain; original magnification, ×250). Borreliae
are motile, helical bacteria that are 5–25 μm long and 0.2–0.5
μm wide.

FIGURE B-13. A smear of sputum stained with a modified acid-fast method shows many delicate, finely beaded, branching filamentous bacilli (modified Kinyoun carbol fuchsin stain; original magnification, ×250). These features are characteristic of *Nocardia* species (*Nocardia asteroides* was recovered from the sputum culture). It is important to remember, however, that mycobacteria also stain acid-fast with a modified acid-fast stain and occasionally may appear filamentous, as illustrated in Figure B-14.

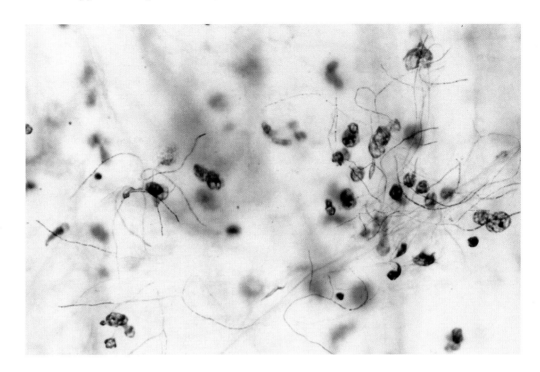

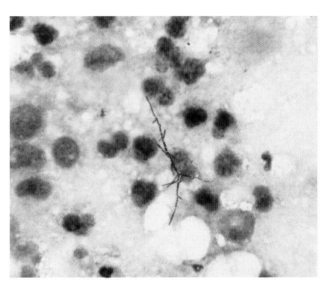

FIGURE B-14. Smear of cells from a fine-needle aspirate of a cervical lymph node stained with a modified acid-fast stain shows beaded, filamentous acid-fast bacilli. Mycobacterial culture grew *Mycobacterium fortuitum* (modified Kinyoun stain; original magnification, ×250). These bacilli are longer than those of *Mycobacterium tuberculosis*, and they are not as delicate and usually have more rudimentary branching than is typical of *Nocardia* species (see Figure B-13).

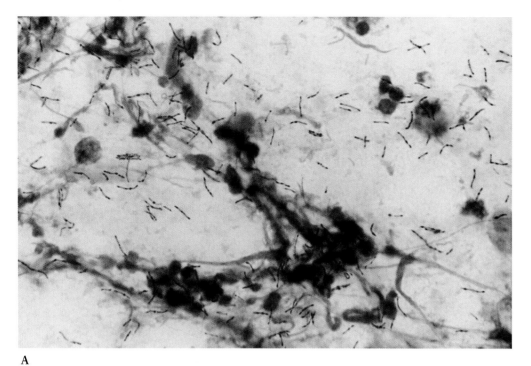

A

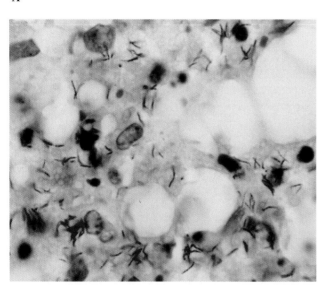

B

FIGURE B-15. (A) Smear of cells from a fine-needle aspirate of a supraclavicular lymph node stained with an acid-fast stain shows many beaded (non-branching), acid-fast bacilli. Culture grew *Mycobacterium tuberculosis* (Kinyoun carbol fuchsin stain; original magnification, ×250). (B) Section of lung from a patient with acquired immunodeficiency syndrome shows numerous slender, finely beaded, acid-fast bacilli (Ziehl-Neelsen stain; original magnification, ×250). Mycobacterial cultures of sputum from this patient grew *M. tuberculosis.*

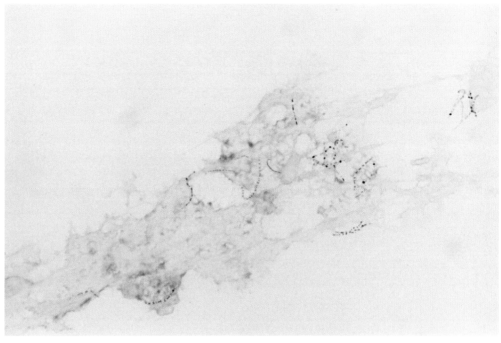

A

FIGURE B-16. (**A**) Smear of cells from a fine-needle aspirate of an osteolytic lesion of the ulna stained with an acid-fast stain shows long (i.e., longer than bacilli of *Mycobacterium tuberculosis*, but not filamentous like *Nocardia* species), prominently beaded, acid-fast bacilli, some of which have the appearance of a shepherd's crook or candy cane (Kinyoun carbol fuchsin stain; original magnification, ×250). The latter feature is typical of *Mycobacterium kansasii*, which was recovered by mycobacterial culture. (**B**) Section of an area of caseous necrosis in the lung from a patient with acquired immunodeficiency syndrome demonstrates acid-fast bacilli with the features of *M. kansasii* described above (Ziehl-Neelsen stain; original magnification, ×250). Mycobacterial cultures of sputum and lung tissue from this patient grew *M. kansasii*.

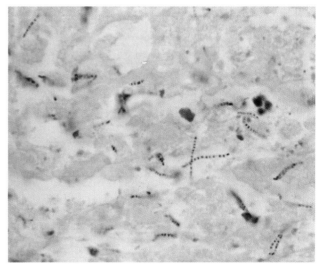

B

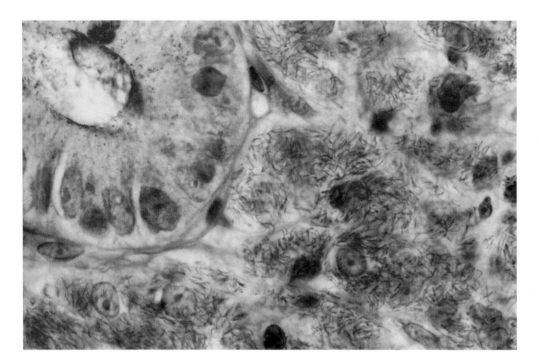

FIGURE B-17. Section of small intestine stained by the periodic acid-Schiff stain shows numerous slender bacilli within histiocyte cytoplasm (periodic acid-Schiff/hematoxylin stain with diastase digestion; original magnification, ×250). This feature is characteristic of infection with *Mycobacterium avium* complex, which was recovered from a mycobacterial blood culture in this case.

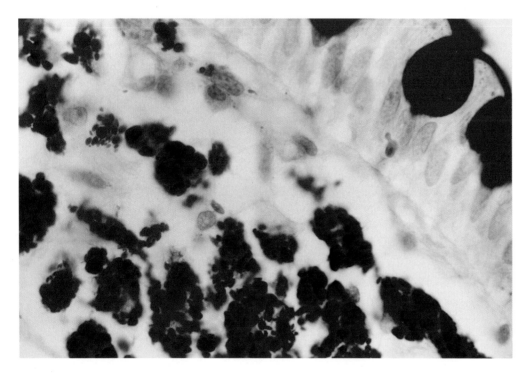

FIGURE B-18. Section of small intestine stained by periodic acid-Schiff stain shows numerous globular, intensely staining bacteria within histiocyte cytoplasm (periodic acid-Schiff/hematoxylin stain with diastase digestion; original magnification, ×250). This feature is characteristic of Whipple's disease.

Appearance of Fungi and Algae in Cytologic Preparations and Tissue Sections

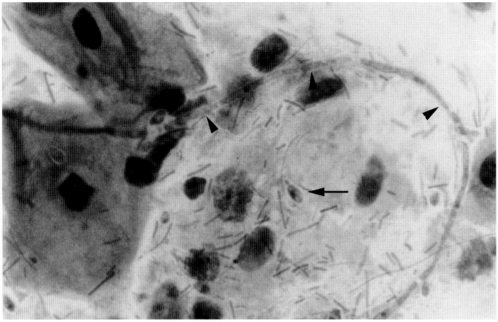

A

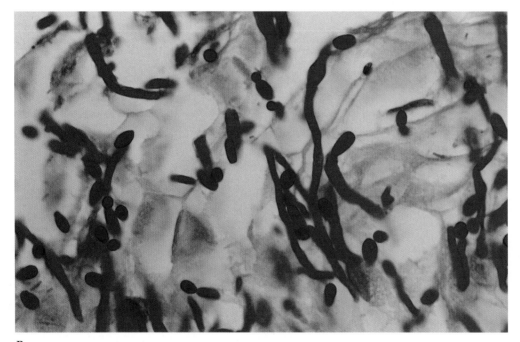

B

FIGURE C-1. (A) Smear of cells collected by esophageal brushing shows pseudohyphae (*arrowheads*) and budding (*arrow*) and nonbudding yeast cells of *Candida* species. Numerous smaller, thinner bacilli are present in the background (Papanicolaou stain; original magnification, ×250). (B) Section of an esophageal ulcer from a patient infected with human immunodeficiency virus who had oral thrush shows budding yeast cells and pseudohyphae admixed with keratin, diagnostic of *Candida* esophagitis (periodic acid-Schiff/hematoxylin stain; original magnification, ×250).

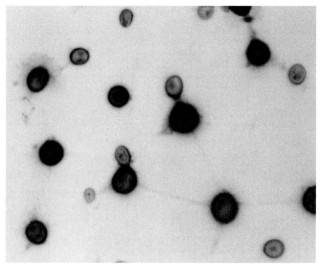

A

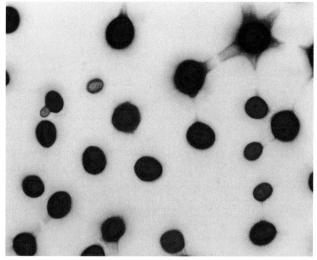

B

FIGURE C-2. (**A**) Cytocentrifuge preparation of cerebrospinal fluid from a patient with acquired immunodeficiency syndrome (AIDS) shows many magenta-colored, budding and nonbudding, variably-sized, round yeast cells with no accompanying inflammatory cells (Papanicolaou stain; original magnification, ×250). The magenta color, variability in size (3–15 μm in diameter), and single buds with narrow necks are characteristic of *Cryptococcus neoformans*. (**B**) To confirm the diagnosis, a mucicarmine stain may be performed directly over a partially destained Papanicolaou-stained preparation. Yeast cells of *C. neoformans* stain positively with mucicarmine, and some cells are surrounded by a "fuzzy" circular or stellate-shaped halo (mucicarmine stain; original magnification, ×250). (**C**) Sputum specimen from this patient shows budding and nonbudding yeast cells and a few pseudohyphae (Papanicolaou stain; original magnification, ×250). The fungal culture of this specimen grew *C. neoformans*, which rarely produces pseudohyphae in tissue.

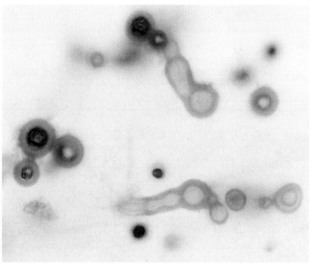

C

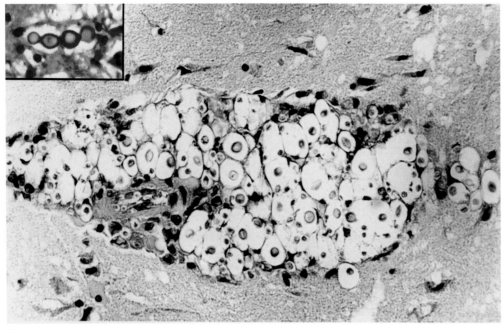

D

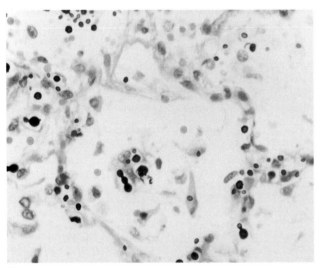

E

FIGURE C-2. *Continued*. (**D**) Section of brain from a patient with AIDS shows many yeast cells, a few of which are budding, surrounded by large clear spaces with no accompanying inflammatory infiltrate (hematoxylin and eosin stain; original magnification, ×100). *Inset*: The capsular material of the yeast cells also stains with the mucicarmine stain (Mayer's mucicarmine stain; original magnification, ×100). These features are typical of cryptococcal meningoencephalitis. *C. neoformans* was recovered from cerebrospinal fluid antemortem. (**E**) Section of lung stained with the Fontana-Masson stain shows black budding yeast cells (Fontana-Masson stain; original magnification, ×100). This stain, which demonstrates the melanin in the yeast cell wall, is especially helpful in cases with capsule-deficient *C. neoformans*.

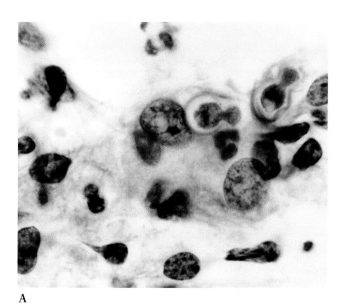
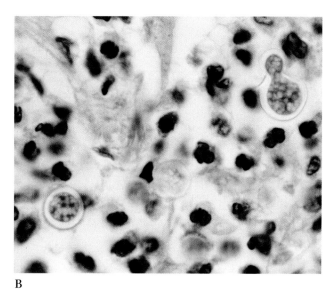

A   B

FIGURE C-3. (**A**) Cytologic preparation of bronchial epithelial cells collected by bronchoscopy and brushing shows histiocytes and yeast cells 10–12 µm in diameter with broad-based buds, thick refractile cell walls, and centrally retracted cytoplasm, leaving a clear space between the endoplasm and cell wall (Papanicolaou stain; original magnification, ×250). These features are characteristic of *Blastomyces dermatitidis*, which was recovered from the fungal culture of the specimen. (**B**) Section of lung from a patient with fatal pulmonary blastomycosis illustrates the typical features of yeast cells of *B. dermatitidis*: uniform size (12–15 µm in diameter), broad-based buds, centrally retracted endoplasm, and a thick hyaline cell wall (hematoxylin and eosin stain; original magnification, ×250).

FIGURE C-4. Section of an ulcerative skin lesion shows oval to cigar–shaped budding yeast cells, 4–6 µm in diameter (methenamine silver stain; original magnification, ×250). These features are typical of *Sporothrix schenckii*, which was recovered from the fungal culture of this specimen.

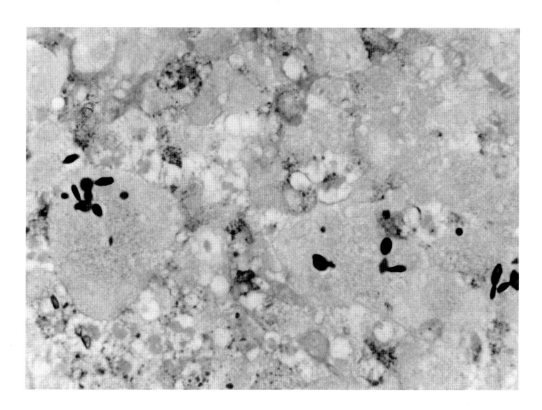

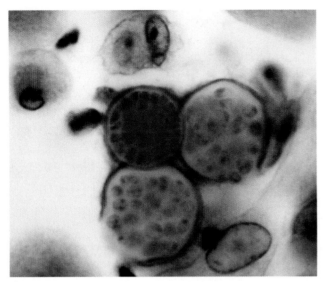

A

FIGURE C-5. (A) Cytologic preparation of bronchoalveolar lavage fluid shows mature spherules containing well-developed endospores (Papanicolaou stain; original magnification, ×250). The presence of spherules measuring up to 200 μm in diameter with clearly visualized endospores is diagnostic of *Coccidioides immitis*, which was recovered from the fungal culture of this specimen. (B) Section of a core bone marrow biopsy shows a mature spherule of *C. immitis* that contains many endospores (*arrow*) and several immature spherules, some of which are similar in size to *Blastomyces dermatitidis* (hematoxylin and eosin stain; original magnification, ×250).

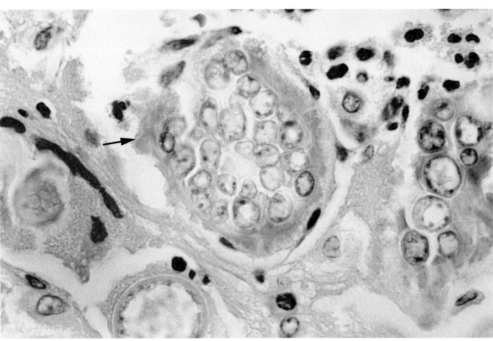

B

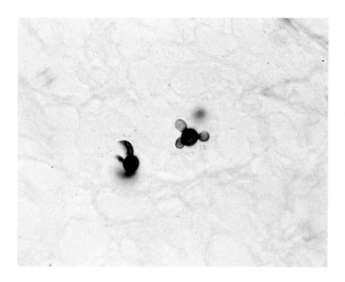

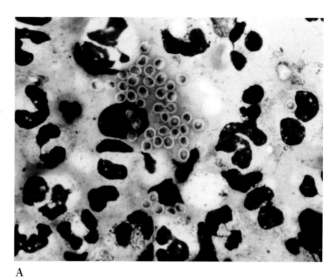

A

FIGURE C-6. Section of a laryngeal biopsy shows a spherical yeast cell with multiple buds (methenamine silver stain; original magnification, ×250). The presence of multiple buds that give the appearance of a "ship's wheel" is typical of *Paracoccidioides brasiliensis*, which was recovered from the fungal culture of this specimen.

FIGURE C-7. (**A**) Cytologic preparation of cells scraped from a vulvar ulcer shows many small (2–3 μm in diameter), single yeast cells that appear to be surrounded by a narrow clear space or halo within the cytoplasm of a histiocyte (Giemsa stain; original magnification, ×250). These features are characteristic of yeast cells of *Histoplasma capsulatum* in cytologic preparations; this fungus was recovered from the fungal culture of this specimen. (**B**) Section of lung stained by the methenamine silver method shows small (3–5 μm in diameter) budding yeast cells within macrophages (methenamine silver stain; original magnification, ×250). These features are characteristic of *H. capsulatum* in tissue, which grew from the fungal culture of the specimen.

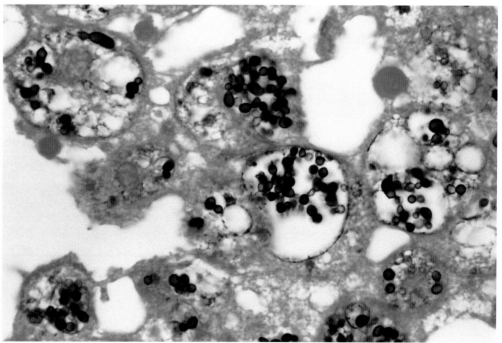

B

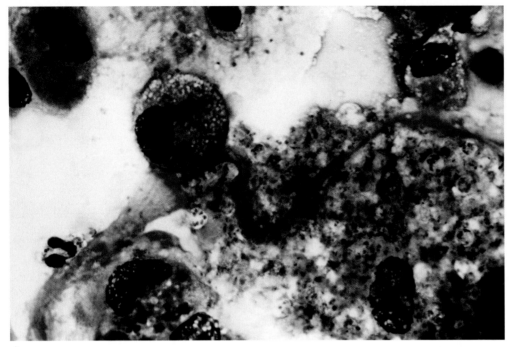

A

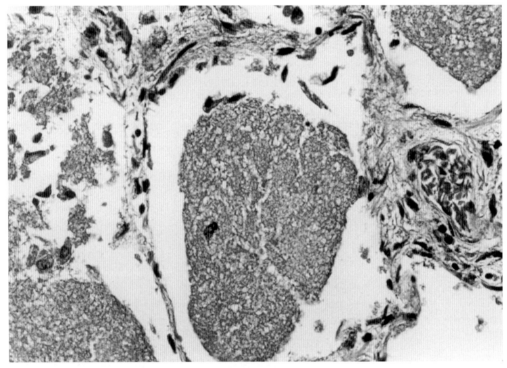

B

FIGURE C-8. (A) Cytologic preparation of bronchoalveolar lavage fluid stained with the Giemsa stain reveals classic features of *Pneumocystis carinii* (Giemsa stain; original magnification, ×250). The foamy material contains cysts of the organism, which appear as clear spheres containing up to eight intracystic bodies, and free trophozoites. (B) Section of lung from a patient with acquired immunodeficiency syndrome shows an accumulation of foamy-appearing material within the alveolar spaces (hematoxylin and eosin stain; original magnification, ×100). This feature is typical of *P. carinii*. To confirm the diagnosis, a silver stain may be performed.

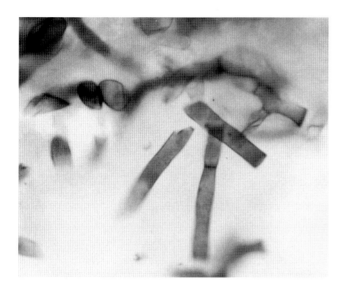

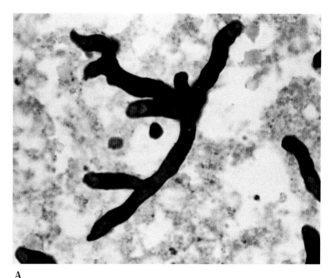

A

FIGURE C-9. Smear of material collected from the sclera of a patient with keratitis shows branching, septate hyphae (methenamine silver stain; original magnification, ×250). Based only on the appearance of these hyphae, a specific diagnosis is not possible. Identification of the responsible organism requires fungal culture of the material, which in this case grew *Fusarium* species.

FIGURE C-10. (**A**) Section of lung tissue shows branching, septate hyphae (methenamine silver stain; original magnification, ×250). The most likely diagnosis is aspergillosis, but hyphae of other fungi (particularly *Fusarium* species and *Pseudallescheria boydii*) have a similar appearance. Identification of *Aspergillus* species in tissue requires the presence of fruiting heads, which were not observed in this case; therefore, fungal culture, which in this case grew *Aspergillus* species, is necessary for diagnosis. (**B**) Section of nasal septum shows fruiting heads (i.e., a vesicle surrounded by conidia) of *Aspergillus flavus* (*arrows*; hematoxylin and eosin stain; original magnification, ×100). *A. flavus* also was recovered from the fungal culture of the tissue.

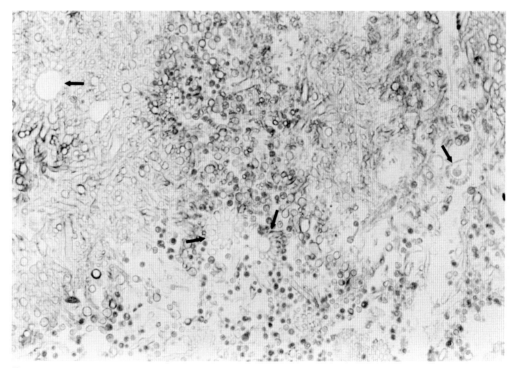

B

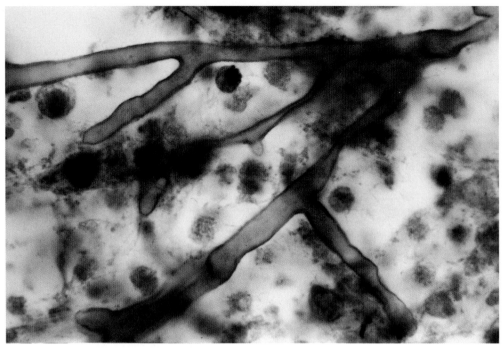

A

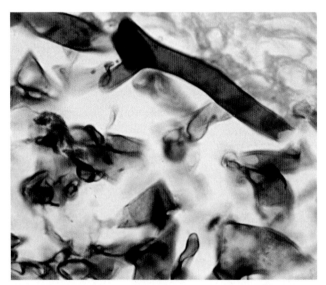

B

FIGURE C-11. (A) Sputum smear shows broad, nonseptate hyphae, one of which is branching at 90 degrees (Papanicolaou stain; original magnification, ×250). This appearance is consistent with zygomycetes; however, species identification requires fungal culture, which in this case grew *Rhizopus* species. (B) Section of lung from the patient whose sputum cytology is illustrated in **A** shows the broad, nonseptate, ribbonlike hyphae of zygomycetes (methenamine silver stain; original magnification, ×250).

FIGURE C-11. *Continued.*
(**C**) Section of a mass removed from the nasal sinus shows sporangia, the presence of which allows the diagnosis of zygomycosis (hematoxylin and eosin stain; original magnification, ×100).

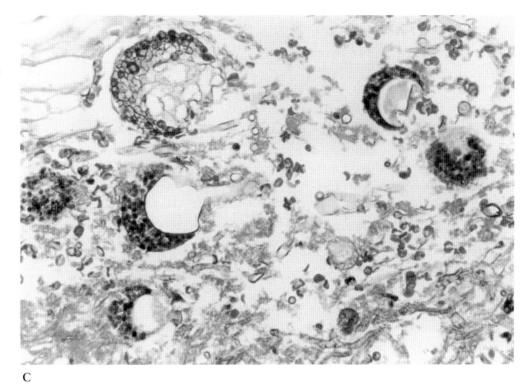

C

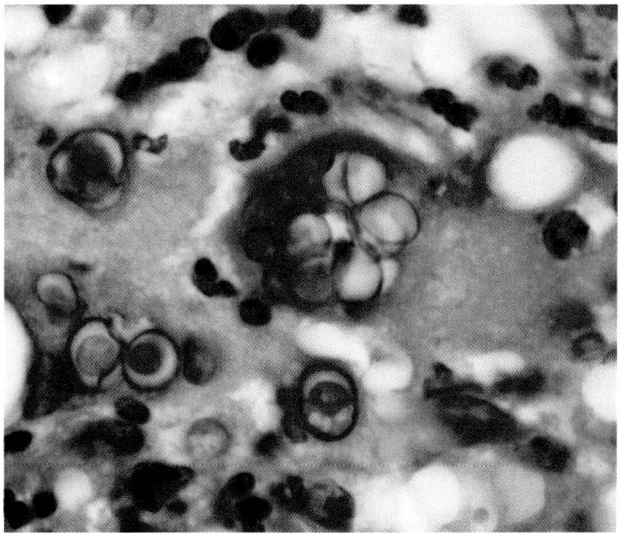

FIGURE C-12. Section of tissue from a verrucous, ulcerated skin lesion shows a mixed granulomatous and suppurative inflammatory cell infiltrate in the dermis and several brown, thick-walled fungal cells with one or more septations, called *sclerotic bodies* (hematoxylin and eosin stain; original magnification, ×250). These features are characteristic of chromoblastomycosis; however, identification of the responsible dematiaceous fungus requires fungal culture, which in this case grew *Fonsecaea pedrosoi*.

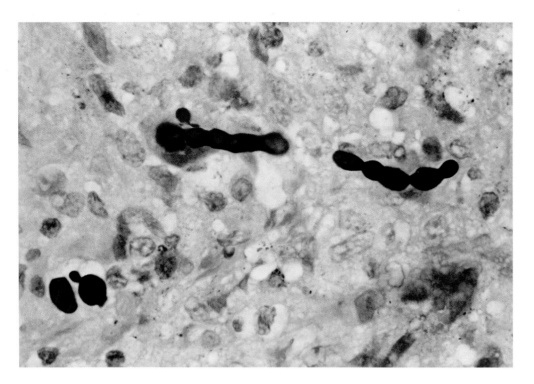

FIGURE C-13. Section of tissue from a subcutaneous mass shows chains of moniliform pseudohyphae (methenamine silver stain; original magnification, ×250). This appearance is characteristic of phaeohyphomycosis; however, identification of the responsible fungus requires fungal culture, which in this case grew *Bipolaris spicifera*.

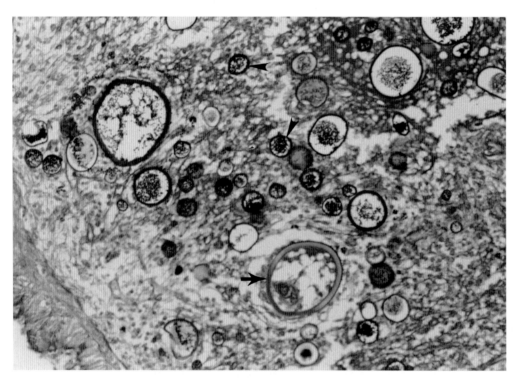

FIGURE C-14. Section of nasal polyp shows a few mature thick-walled sporangia (*arrow*) and several smaller trophocytes (*arrowheads*) of *Rhinosporidium seeberi* (Gridley stain; original magnification, ×250). Sporangia typically measure 100–200 μm in diameter but may be as large as 350 μm. Trophocytes, the immature form of *R. seeberi*, are 10–100 μm in diameter and contain a central nucleus or karyosome and granular-to-flocculent cytoplasm.

FIGURE C-15. Section of a lesion of cutaneous protothecosis shows both nonendosporulating cells and sporangia, a few of which have the typical configuration of a morula form (hematoxylin and eosin stain; high-power magnification). The characteristic morula form is a sporangium with a central endospore that is surrounded by a single layer of polygonal or wedge-shaped, molded endospores.

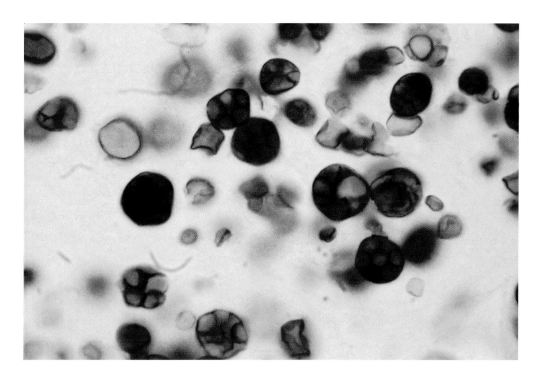

APPENDIX

D

Appearance of Parasites in Cytologic Preparations and Tissue Sections

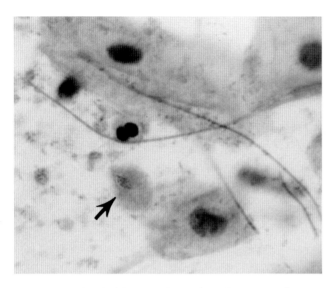

FIGURE D-1. Cervical Papanicolaou smear shows a small, pear-shaped protozoan typical of *Trichomonas vaginalis* (*arrow*; Papanicolaou stain; original magnification, ×250). The tropho-zoite of *T. vaginalis* measures 10–25 µm × 7–8 µm and has a prominent nucleus in the anterior third of the cytoplasm. Also present in the smear are long, filamentous bacilli, typically called *Leptothrix*.

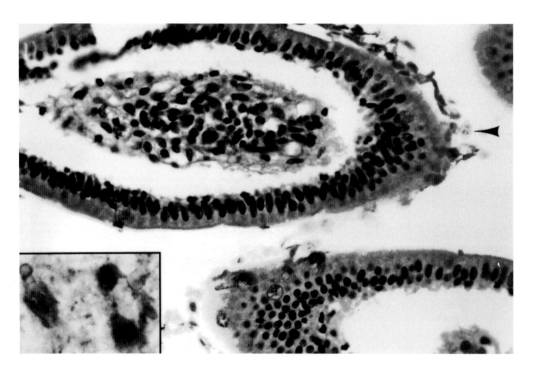

FIGURE D-2. Section of duodenal biopsy shows many organisms, approx-imately 15 µm long, lying along the mucosal sur-face (iron-hematoxylin stain; original magnifica-tion, ×100). A few pear-shaped organisms, with two parallel nuclei, are viewed *en face* (*arrow-head*). *Inset*: These fea-tures, which often are more clearly visualized in cytologic preparations of duodenal brush biopsy specimens (Papanicolaou stain; original magnifica-tion, ×250), are charac-teristic of *Giardia*.

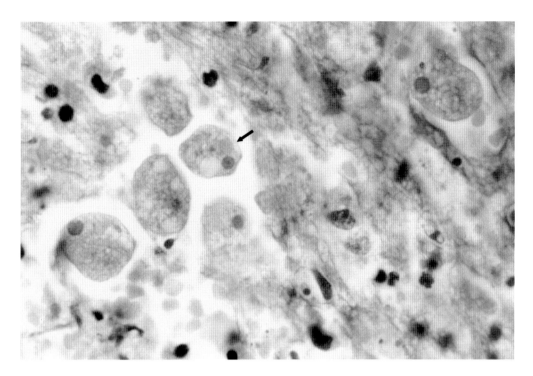

FIGURE D-3. Section of a rectal biopsy illustrates trophozoites of *Entamoeba histolytica* (hematoxylin and eosin stain; original magnification, ×250). In tissue sections, amebic trophozoites are smaller (i.e., 15–25 μm in diameter) than they appear in wet mounts or smears due to shrinkage during fixation and processing. The trophozoite cytoplasm is finely granular and may contain phagocytized erythrocytes (*arrow*). The nucleus of the organism may or may not be present in the section, and when visible, it must be differentiated from that of histiocytes. The histiocyte nucleus is more convoluted and has a variable chromatin pattern; because it is larger than that of a trophozoite nucleus, it generally is present in almost all sections. In contrast, the amebic nuclei are multiple, round, and contain a prominent karyosome.

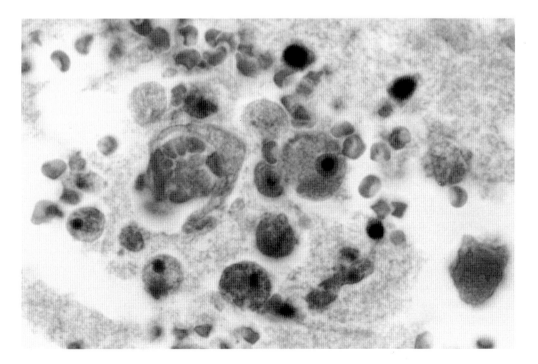

FIGURE D-4. Section of brain demonstrates trophozoites of *Balamuthia mandrillaris* (hematoxylin and eosin stain; original magnification, ×250). In tissue sections, *Balamuthia* trophozoites measure an average of 22 μm in diameter. The nucleus has a large nucleolus, and the cytoplasm is vacuolated. Cysts have a thick, irregular wall containing the endocyst, which often is shrunken and represented by a dark mass with a nucleus that appears similar to that of the trophozoite.

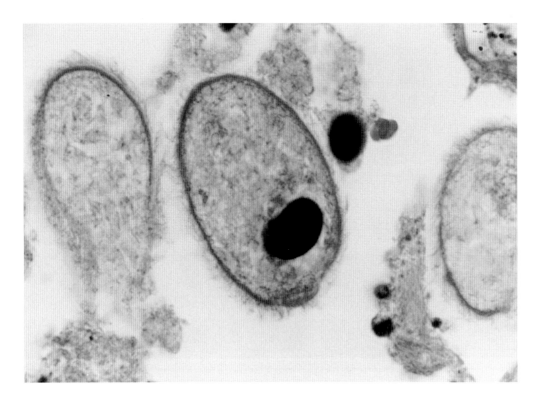

Figure D-5. Section of colon shows oval, ciliated trophozoites of *Balantidium coli* (hematoxylin and eosin stain; original magnification, ×250). These organisms measure up to 200 µm in diameter, have a prominent, reniform macronucleus and a small micronucleus (rarely visible in tissue sections, as is the case in this illustration), and a thin outer cuticle covered by numerous cilia.

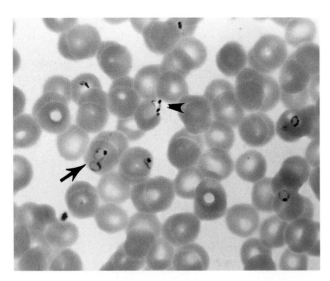

Figure D-6. Smear of peripheral blood from a patient with falciparum malaria shows several red blood cells containing small, ring-stage trophozoites of *Plasmodium falciparum* (Romanovsky stain; original magnification, ×250). Infected erythrocytes are not enlarged, and multiple infections in a single red blood cell (*arrow*) are common. Rings often show two distinct chromatin dots (*arrowhead*). Trophozoites become sequestered in the capillaries of internal organs as they mature. Therefore, maturing parasites generally are not present in the peripheral circulation, although banana-shaped gametocytes occasionally are found.

FIGURE D-7. Section of liver from a patient with falciparum malaria shows enlarged Kupffer cells filled with coarsely granular brown-black pigment (hematoxylin and eosin stain; original magnification, ×250). This malarial pigment (called *hemozoin* or *hematin*) is microscopically indistinguishable from formalin pigment, which may present a problem in countries where malaria is endemic, if unbuffered formalin is used.

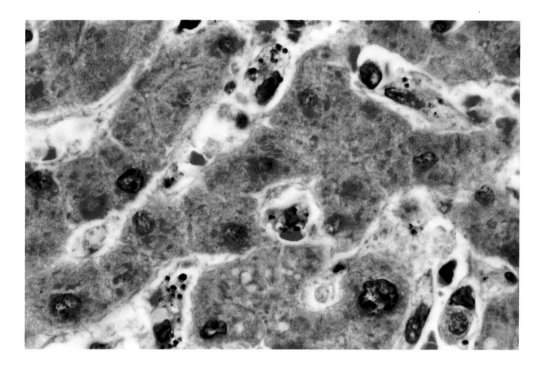

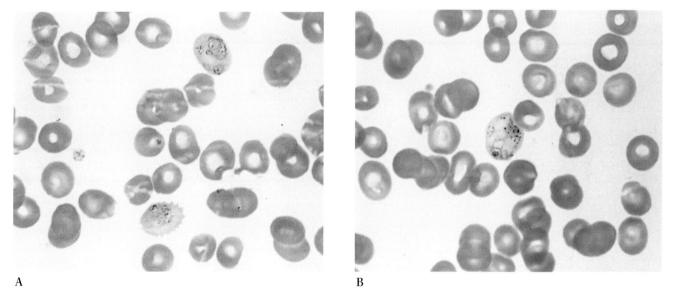

A   B

FIGURE D-8. (**A** and **B**) Two fields from a smear of peripheral blood from a patient with vivax malaria show ameboid trophozoites in enlarged, pale erythrocytes (Romanovsky stain; original magnification, ×250). The main features of *Plasmodium vivax* infection are large, pale red blood cells; irregularly shaped trophozoites that almost fill the entire cell; fine, golden-brown pigment (present in this case); and several phases of growth seen in one smear. Fine Schüffner's dots are not always present (they were not seen in this case) but are helpful for diagnosis when they are.

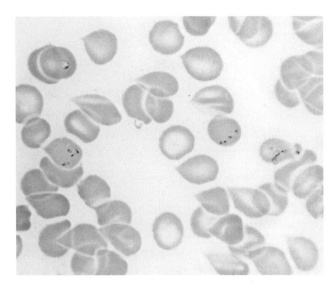

FIGURE D-9. Smear of peripheral blood from a patient with babesiosis shows intracellular parasites of *Babesia microti* (Romanovsky stain; original magnification, ×250). A few of the erythrocytes contain four merozoites. *Babesia* rings can be confused with ring forms of *Plasmodium* species. Features that are helpful in differentiating the two include the occasional presence of tetrads (Maltese crosses, not observed in this case), which are diagnostic of *Babesia*, and the absence of pigment accompanying *Babesia*. Additionally, *B. microti* rings are more variable in size than those of *P. falciparum*, and extracellular parasites are more common in *B. microti* infections.

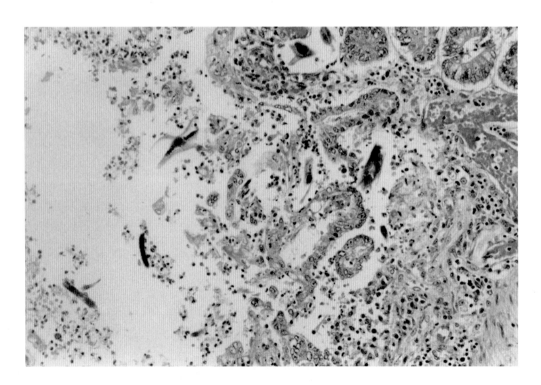

FIGURE D-10. Section of small intestine shows features of intestinal strongyloidiasis (hematoxylin and eosin stain; original magnification, ×50). The villi are ulcerated and flattened, and several adult worms and larvae are present within the bowel lumen and intestinal crypts.

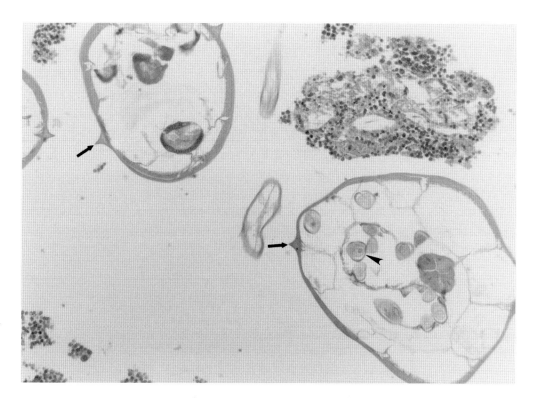

FIGURE D-11. Section of appendix shows cross sections of male (upper left) and female (lower right) *Enterobius vermicularis* (hematoxylin and eosin stain; original magnification, ×50). The diameter of the worm varies, depending on the level of the section, the sex of the worm, and its stage of maturation. At their midbody, females measure up to 350 μm in diameter, and males measure up to 150 μm. Both worms illustrated here demonstrate the prominent lateral alae (*arrow*) that are characteristic of *E. vermicularis*. Within the uterus of the female worm, there are several embryonated ova (*arrowhead*).

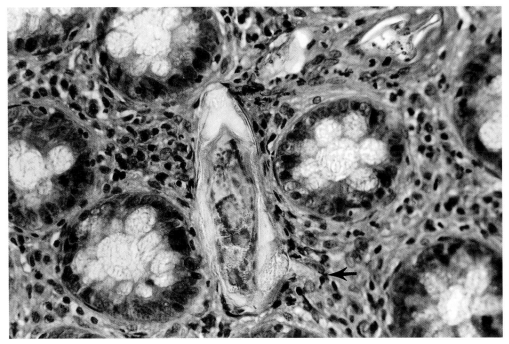

A

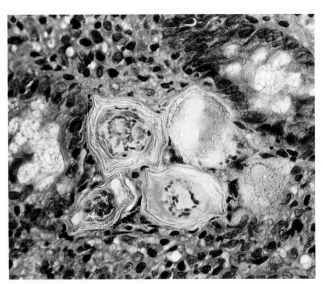

B

FIGURE D-12. Two fields from a section of a rectal biopsy show (A) a full length and (B) cross-sections of eggs of *Schistosoma mansoni* in the lamina propria (hematoxylin and eosin stain; original magnification, ×100). Eggs of *S. mansoni* are 115–180 µm long and 45–70 µm wide. As shown in A, they have a prominent lateral spine (*arrow*) near the more rounded posterior end; the anterior end is slightly pointed and curved. When embryonated, the ovum may contain a mature miracidium, as illustrated in this case. Species identification in tissue requires visualization of the lateral spine; therefore, if only cross sections of the egg are seen, identification may be difficult. Eggs of *S. haematobium*, which have a terminal spine, do not stain by the modified Ziehl-Neelsen stain, whereas eggs of *S. mansoni* and *S. japonicum* do.

FIGURE D-13. Section of liver from a child with visceral larva migrans shows a portion of a nematode larva (*arrow*) in an inflammatory exudate composed of eosinophils and histiocytes. The species of nematodes most frequently causing visceral larva migrans in humans are *Toxocara canis* and *Toxocara cati*. When the larva invades the liver, the earliest lesion is mild disruption of the parenchyma, accompanied by a few inflammatory cells and a larva. As the lesion progresses, hepatocyte necrosis and more marked infiltrate of granulocytes (predominantly eosinophils), histiocytes, and lymphocytes are evident. This is followed by the development of well-formed granulomas in which the larva usually is viable. The larva may leave the granuloma and travel to another part of the liver or to a different tissue, where it becomes encapsulated and dormant. Granulomas without the larva resorb with complete healing. Diagnosis of visceral larva migrans usually is based on the clinical presentation with or without serologic testing. If tissues containing the parasite are available, identification of the species requires visualization of features evident in cross sections through the mid-gut; oblique and longitudinal sections typically do not permit identification to the species level. The diameter of *T. canis* in tissues ranges from 18 to 20 μm and of *T. cati*, from 14 to 16 μm; both are 290–350 μm long. The larva has small lateral alae that are present in most cross sections of the body. The cuticle is best seen on transverse sections at the level of the lateral alae. Muscles lie underneath the cuticle; internally, two excretory columns that appear as large round structures are present.

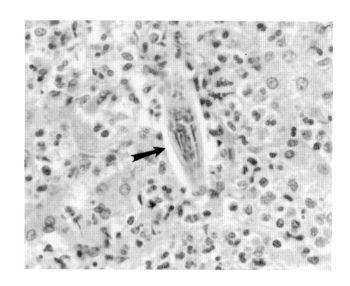

FIGURE D-14. Section of lung shows a pulmonary infarct due to *Dirofilaria* species (hematoxylin and eosin stain; original magnification, ×25). The maximum diameter of *Dirofilaria* in tissue section varies; males measure 140–200 μm in diameter, and females measure up to 300 μm. The worms have a smooth cuticle without longitudinal ridges, except at the ventral posterior end of the male.

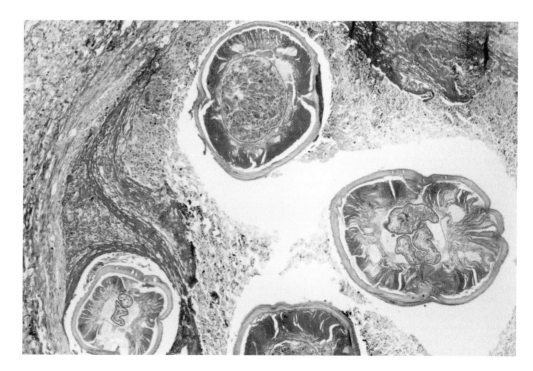

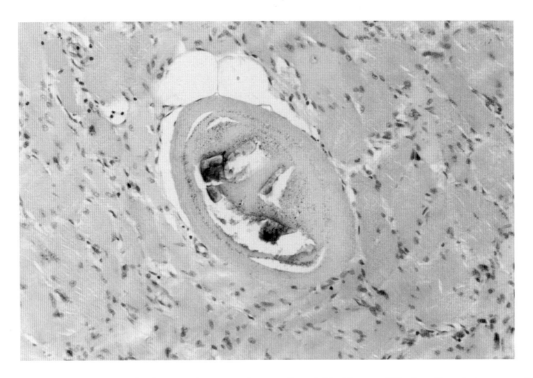

FIGURE D-15. Section of skeletal muscle shows a degenerated, partially calcified larva of *Trichinella spiralis* encased in a hyaline sheath with virtually no accompanying inflammatory reaction (hematoxylin and eosin stain; original magnification, ×50). The findings in skeletal muscle associated with trichinosis vary depending on the time after arrival and penetration of the larvae in the muscle fiber. Initially, basophilic degeneration, edema, a slight increase in the size of the fiber, and enlarged nuclei are present. As the larva matures, the muscle cell shrinks, the nuclei are displaced toward the center, and the cytoplasm is replaced by an eosinophilic network of fibers. The parasite is fully developed and encapsulated by week 5, and after 3 months, it is completely surrounded by a wall. Myositis, characterized by fiber degeneration and an infiltrate of eosinophils, lymphocytes, and a few histiocytes, occurs during encystation and subsides as the larva encapsulates. Eventually, the larva dies and becomes calcified, as illustrated in this case.

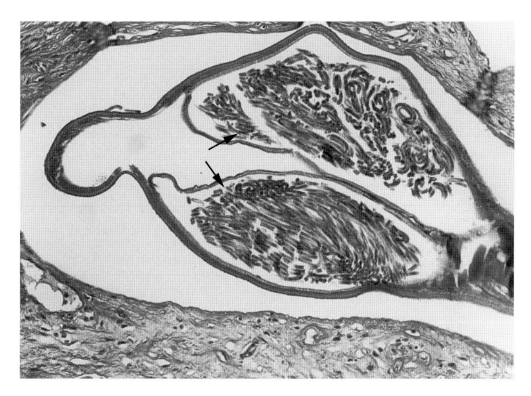

FIGURE D-16. Section of a subcutaneous nodule shows *Onchocerca volvulus* (hematoxylin and eosin stain; original magnification, ×50). In cross section, the maximum diameter of the female worm is 350 μm, and the male measures up to 125 μm. The parasites are covered by a two-layered cuticle. The uterus of the female worm shown here contains numerous microfilariae (*arrows*).

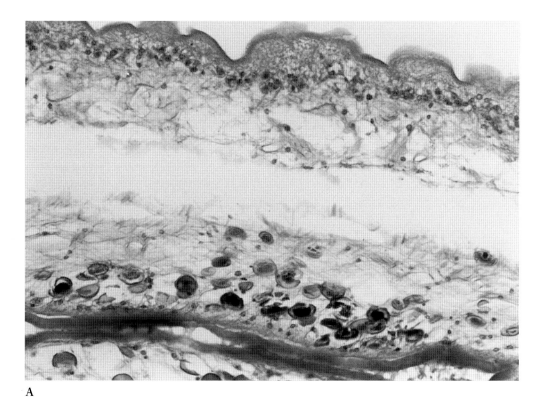

A

FIGURE D-17. (**A**) Section of a cystic lesion of the brain illustrates the characteristic features of cysticercosis (hematoxylin and eosin stain; original magnification, ×100). The outer cuticular wall of the cysticercus consists of a wavy, eosinophilic membrane that overlies a layer of small nuclei. Deeper within the larval wall, oval calcifications are present, which represent calcareous corpuscles found only in cestodes.

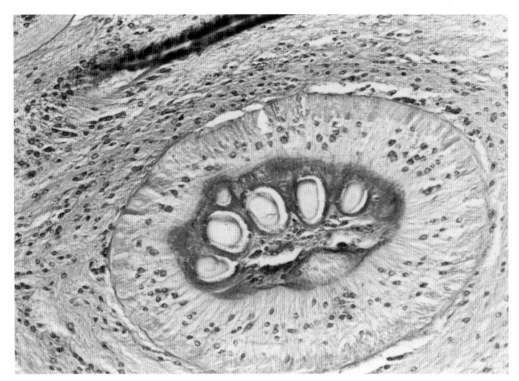

B

FIGURE D-17. *Continued.*
(B) Higher-power magni-
fication of the cysticercus
shows the inverted pro-
toscolex with a portion
of the double row of
hooklets that arm the
rostellum (hematoxylin
and eosin stain; original
magnification, ×100).

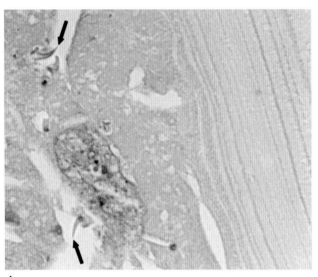

A

FIGURE D-18. (A) Section of the external wall of an echinococcal
cyst illustrates its thick, laminated external cuticle, below which
are degenerated protoscolices and preserved hooklets (*arrows*;
hematoxylin and eosin stain; original magnification, ×50).

FIGURE D-18. *Continued.* (**B**) Section of a degenerated echinococcal cyst of the liver shows disintegrated remains of protoscolices with well-preserved hooklets, shown at higher magnification in the inset (hematoxylin and eosin stain; original magnification, ×50; *inset*: original magnification, ×100).

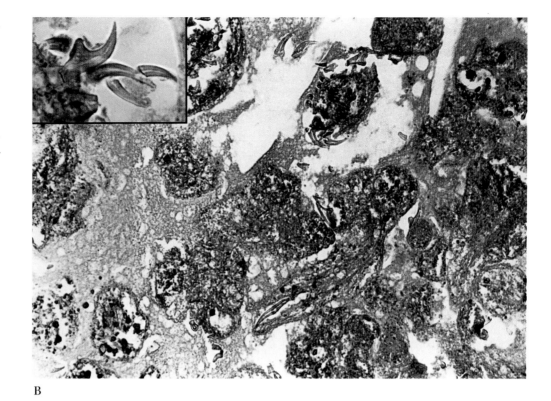

B

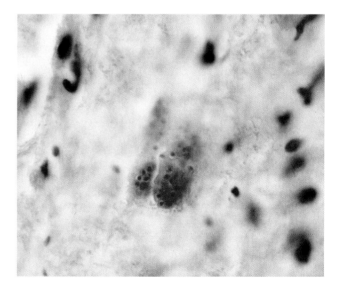

FIGURE D-19. Section of brain shows a pseudocyst of *Toxoplasma gondii* that contains many bradyzoites (hematoxylin and eosin stain; original magnification, ×250). Pseudocysts resemble cysts, except that they do not have a cyst wall.

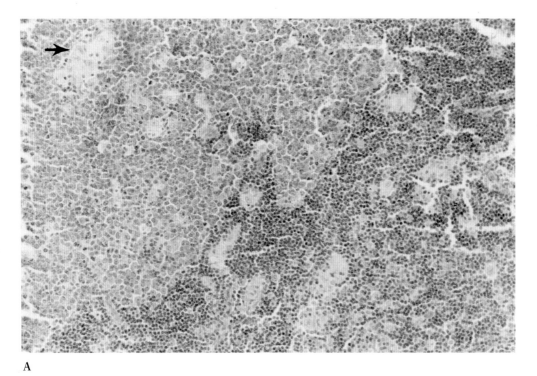

A

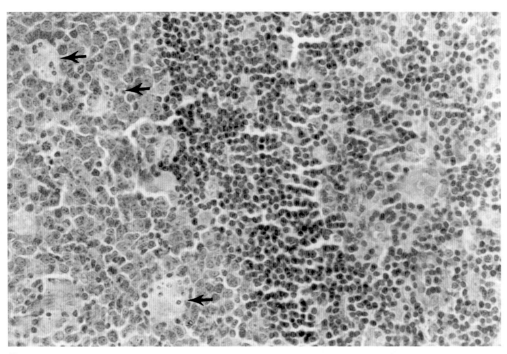

B

FIGURE D-20. (A) Section of lymph node from a patient with acute toxoplasmosis shows prominent follicular hyperplasia, many tingible-body macrophages, and small clusters of epithelioid macrophages (*arrow*; hematoxylin and eosin stain; original magnification, ×50). (B) Higher-power magnification of the section illustrated in **A** demonstrates tingible-body macrophages with a germinal center (*arrows*), and on the right side of the field, epithelioid macrophages are seen in the parafollicular area (hematoxylin and eosin stain; original magnification, ×100).

FIGURE D-21. Cytologic preparation of skin scrapings shows two histiocytes that contain numerous amastigotes of *Leishmania* species within their cytoplasm (Giemsa stain; original magnification, ×250). A few extracellular amastigotes also are present (*arrowhead*). The amastigotes are characterized by their magenta nucleus and darkly-staining rodlike kinetoplast (*arrows*), the latter of which helps distinguish these forms from yeast cells of *Histoplasma capsulatum* (see Figure C-7).

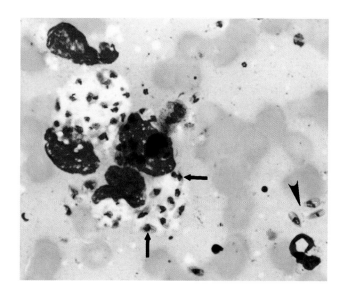

Index